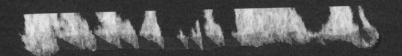

Equine Back Pathology
Diagnosis and Treatment

Equine Back Pathology
Diagnosis and Treatment

Edited by

Dr Frances M.D. Henson, MA, VetMB, PhD, CertES(Orth),
CertEM(Int Med), MRCVS, RCVS Specialist in Equine Surgery
(Orthopaedics)

Department of Veterinary Medicine
University of Cambridge
UK

WILEY-BLACKWELL

A John Wiley & Sons, Ltd., Publication

This edition first published 2009
© 2009 Blackwell Publishing Ltd

Blackwell Publishing was acquired by John Wiley & Sons in February 2007. Blackwell's publishing programme has been merged with Wiley's global Scientific, Technical, and Medical business to form Wiley-Blackwell.

Registered office
John Wiley & Sons Ltd, The Atrium, Southern Gate, Chichester, West Sussex, PO19 8SQ, United Kingdom

Editorial offices
9600 Garsington Road, Oxford, OX4 2DQ, United Kingdom
2121 State Avenue, Ames, Iowa 50014-8300, USA

For details of our global editorial offices, for customer services and for information about how to apply for permission to reuse the copyright material in this book please see our website at www.wiley.com/wiley-blackwell.

Wiley also publishes its books in a variety of electronic formats. Some content that appears in print may not be available in electronic books.

Designations used by companies to distinguish their products are often claimed as trademarks. All brand names and product names used in this book are trade names, service marks, trademarks or registered trademarks of their respective owners. The publisher is not associated with any product or vendor mentioned in this book. This publication is designed to provide accurate and authoritative information in regard to the subject matter covered. It is sold on the understanding that the publisher is not engaged in rendering professional services. If professional advice or other expert assistance is required, the services of a competent professional should be sought.

Library of Congress Cataloging-in-Publication Data
Equine back pathology : diagnosis and treatment / edited by Frances M.D. Henson.
    p. ; cm.
   Includes bibliographical references and index.
   ISBN 978-1-4051-5492-5 (hardback : alk. paper)   1. Horses–Diseases–Diagnosis.   2. Horses–Diseases–Treatment.   3. Back–Diseases–Diagnosis.   4. Back–Diseases–Treatment.   I. Henson, Frances M. D.
   [DNLM: 1. Horse Diseases.   2. Back Pain–veterinary.   3. Spinal Diseases–pathology.   4. Spinal Diseases–veterinary.   5. Spine–anatomy & histology. SF 951 E631 2009]

   SF951.E542 2009
   636.1'089756–dc22

                                                                                                    2008039843

A catalogue record for this book is available from the British Library.

Set in 9.5 on 11.5 pt Palatino by SNP Best-set Typesetter Ltd., Hong Kong
Printed in Singapore by C.O.S. Printers Pte Ltd

2   2009

Contents

Colour plate section follows page 146

Contributors

David Bainbridge, VetMB MA PhD MRCVS
University Clinical Veterinary Anatomist
Department of Physiology, Development and
Neuroscience, University of Cambridge,
Cambridge, UK

Andrew P. Bathe, MA, VetMB, DipECVS, DEO,
MRCVS
RCVS and European Specialist in Equine Surgery
Rossdales Equine Hospital, Cotton End Road,
Exning, Newmarket, Suffolk, UK

Mary Bromiley, FRSP, SRP, RPT(USA)
Downs House Equine, Combeleigh Farm,
Wheddon Cross, Minehead, Somerset, UK

Adam Driver, BVSc, CertVR, MRCVS
Global Equine Group Ltd
9 The Manor, Herringswell, Bury St Edmunds,
UK

Constanze Fintl, BVSc, MSc, PhD,
CertEM(IntMed), DipECEIM, MRCVS
Department of Companion Animal Clinical
Sciences, Norwegian School of Veterinary
Science, Oslo, Norway

Joyce Harman, DVM, MRCVS
Harmany Equine Clinic Ltd, Flint Hill, Virginia,
USA

Marcus J. Head, BVet.Med, MRCVS
Rossdale's Diagnostic Centre, Cotton End Road,
Exning, Newmarket, Suffolk, UK

Frances M.D. Henson, MA, VetMB, PhD,
CertES(Orth), CertEM(Int Med), MRCVS
Queen's Veterinary School Hospital, University
of Cambridge, Cambridge, UK

Leo B. Jeffcott, MA, BVet.Med, PhD, FRCVS,
DVSc, VetMedDr
Dean and Professor of Veterinary Science
Faculty of Veterinary Science, University of
Sydney, JD Stewart Building, New South Wales,
Australia

Jessica A. Kidd, BA, DVM, CertES(Orth),
Diplomate ECVS, MRCVS
The Valley Equine Hospital, Lambourn,
Berkshire, UK

Svend E. Kold, DrMedVet, PhD, CUEW, RFP,
MRCVS
Willesley Equine Clinic Ltd, Byams Farm,
Willesley, Tetbury, Gloucestershire, UK

Luis P. Lamas, DVM CertES(Orth) MRCVS
Queen's Veterinary School Hospital, University
of Cambridge, Cambridge, UK

Graham A. Munroe, BVSc(Hons), PhD, CertEO, DESM, DipECVS, FRCVS
Flanders Veterinary Services, Cowrig Cottage, Greenlaw, Duns, Berwickshire, UK

Alastair Nelson, MA, VetMB, CertVR, MRCVS,
Rainbow Equine Clinic, Old Malton, North Yorkshire, UK

Richard J. Piercy, MA, VetMB, MS, PhD, DipACVIM, MRCVS
Comparative Neuromuscular Diseases Laboratory, Royal Veterinary College, Hawkshead Lane, North Mymms, Hatfield, UK

Rob Pilsworth, BSc(Hons), MA, VetMB, CertVR, MRCVS
Newmarket Equine Hospital, Newmarket, Suffolk, UK

Mimi Porter, MS
Equine Therapy Inc., 4350 Harrodsburg Road, Lexington, Kentucky, USA

Tracy A. Turner, DVM, MS, DiplACVS, DiplABT
Anoka Equine Veterinary Services, Elk River, Minnesota, USA

P. René van Weeren, DVM, PhD, DiplECVS
Professor of Equine Musculoskeletal Biology
Department of Equine Sciences, Faculty of Veterinary Medicine, Utrecht University, The Netherlands

Renate Weller, Drmedvet, PhD, MRVCS
Lecturer in Diagnostic Imaging
Department of Veterinary Clinical Sciences, The Royal Veterinary College, Hawkshead Lane, North Mymms, Hatfield, UK

Mary Beth Whitcomb, DVM
Assistant Professor
Clinical Large Animal Ultrasound, Department of Surgical and Radiological Sciences, School of Veterinary Medicine, University of California, Davis, California, USA

Foreword

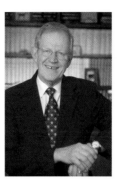

In the fourth Sir Frederick Hobday Memorial Lecture that I delivered 30 years ago to the British Equine Veterinary Association, I ended with a quote from Mohammed. He wrote some 3000 years earlier "Care for your mares – their bellies are your treasure, **their backs your safety**, and God will help their owners". For me this was proof indeed that the horse's back is of considerable importance for their function and athletic ability.

At the time of the Hobday Lecture I highlighted six areas that I considered to be important limiting factors in the evaluation of back problems in the horse:

1. Lack of knowledge of the natural history of disorders
2. Difficulties in establishing a specific diagnosis
3. Insufficient research being performed (particularly in biomechanics)
4. Few controlled studies on therapy and outcome
5. Lack of common ground between veterinary surgeons and paraprofessionals
6. Lack of definitive studies on back pathology.

Much has happened in the intervening years and a great deal more interest has been paid to the horse's back, both clinically and in research. This book serves to identify the considerable progress that has been made in addressing all these factors. So now it is possible to establish definitive diagnoses, to appreciate huge advances in our understanding of the biomechanics of the back, to evaluate the results of controlled studies on therapy and outcome, and to work really closely with our paraprofessional colleagues to better evaluate and treat horses with back problems. Despite these important advances there is still much work to be done. However, it is hoped that this book will help to maintain the interest in the horse's back by informing interested people, teaching students, enthusing "old hands" who have been treating back cases for years and, most importantly, improving the diagnosis and management of all horses with back pathology.

Leo Jeffcott

Acknowledgements

This book would not have been written without the leadership, inspiration and support that Professor Leo Jeffcott has shown me throughout my career. Anything I know about the equine back comes from the foundations that he taught me.

I would also like to thank all of the horses that I have had the pleasure of examining and treating, the clinicians with whom I have worked for teaching me so much, all of the staff in the Equine Hospital, University of Cambridge (particularly Alison Smith and Graham Munroe), for supporting and humouring me, and all of the contributors to this book for putting up with my electronic nagging.

My grateful thanks to my mother and father, Joan and Mike, for giving me a love of horses and a scientific mind, and to my daughters, Claudia and Sofia, for being a delight and joy.

Special thanks, of course, to my wonderful husband, Mike, for simply everything.

Frances Henson

Abbreviations

ACP	aceptomazine	IT	intertransverse
AP	articular process	L	lumbar
AR	axial rotation	LB	lateral bending
AF	articular facet	LMN	lower motor neuron
AMP	angular movement pattern	NSAID	non-steroidal anti-inflammatory
BHV	between-horse variability		drug
C	cervical	OA	osteoarthritis
CNS	central nervous system	ORDSP	overriding dorsal spinous processes
Cy	coccygeal	p.o.	per os
DLVMO	dorsolateral–ventromedial–oblique	PNS	peripheral nervous system
DMVLO	dorsomedial–ventrolateral–oblique	ROI	region of interest
DSIL	dorsal sacroiliac ligament	ROM	range of motion
DSP	dorsal spinous process	S	sacral
EEE	eastern equine encephalitis	SID	sacroiliac dysfunction
EHV	equine herpesvirus	SIJ	sacroiliac joint
EPM	equine protozoal myeloencephalitis	SIL	sacroiliac ligament
FE	flexion–extension	SSL	supraspinous ligament
GP	general proprioceptive	SWL	shock wave therapy
GSA	general somatic afferent	T	thoracic
GVA	general visceral afferent	TB	thoroughbred
GSE	general somatic efferent	TP	transverse process
GVE	general somatic efferent	UMN	upper motor neuron
HNP	head and neck position	VSL	ventral sacroiliac ligament
i.m.	intramuscularly	WEE	western equine encephalitis
ISL	interspinous ligament	WHV	within-horse variability

Section 1

Anatomy and Function

1

The Normal Anatomy of the Osseous Structures of the Back and Pelvis

Leo B. Jeffcott

Introduction

In order to understand the pathological conditions that affect a horse's back it is necessary to have an excellent working knowledge of its structure. The back and pelvis are made up of osseous structures, joints, muscles, ligaments, blood vessels and nerves, all of which can be altered or affected in disease. In this chapter the osseous structures of the back (i.e. the thoracolumbar spine, sacrum and pelvis) are discussed. The soft tissues (i.e. muscles and ligaments) and the innervation of the back are dealt with in Chapters 2, 3 and 4 respectively.

The vertebral column runs from the atlanto-occipital joint to the last coccygeal vertebra (Figure 1.1). As it passes through the body the vertebral column does not form a straight-line structure; rather it descends sharply from the atlanto-occipital joint to reach its lowest point at the cervicothoracic junction. The column then ascends gently to the caudal lumbar region and descends down, via the sacrum, to the coccygeal vertebrae (Figure 1.1). The external appearance of the horse, however, presents a different picture in the cranial thoracic region. Externally the withers (corresponding approximately to T3–7) is the highest point of the back, even though the vertebral bodies are ventral to most other vertebral bodies at this point. This is due to the external elevation provided by the long dorsal spinous processes (DSPs) in the withers region, which creates a contrary impression [1].

Vertebral numbering system

The nomenclature for the classification of different vertebral segments is fairly standardised between different texts and papers, with vertebral segments traditionally counted within spinal regions from a cranial reference point. Within each region the vertebrae are numbered sequentially from cranial to caudal, e.g. T1 (first thoracic vertebra), T2 (second thoracic vertebra). However, occasionally, some authors use modified reference systems, using caudal reference points [2]. It is important to be aware of this alternative numbering system when consulting the literature in this area to avoid confusion. In this book the standard cranial reference system will be used.

Standard vertebral formula

The spine of the horse is made up of cervical, thoracic, lumbar, sacral and coccygeal vertebrae (Figure 1.2). The standard vertebral formula for the horse is 7 cervical vertebrae, 18 thoracic vertebrae, 6 lumbar vertebrae, 5 sacral vertebrae and between 15 and 21 coccygeal vertebrae [3] (Table 1.1).

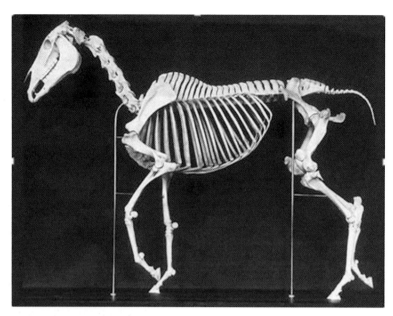

Figure 1.1   A photograph of the skeleton of the horse. The vertebral column runs from the atlanto-occipital joint to the last coccygeal vertebra. The vertebral column descends sharply from the atlanto-occipital joint to reach its lowest point at the cervicothoracic junction. The column then ascends gently to the caudal lumbar region and descends down, via the sacrum, to the coccygeal vertebrae.

Cervical
($n = 7$)

Thoracic
($n = 18$)

Lumbar
($n = 6$)

Sacral
($n = 5$)

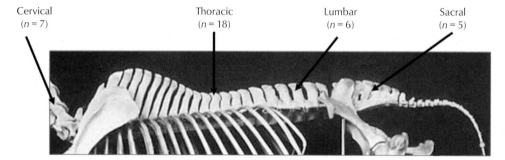

Figure 1.2   The bones of the vertebral column from the seventh cervical vertebra to the penultimate coccygeal vertebra. The vertebral column is divided into cervical, thoracic, lumbar, sacral and coccygeal regions. There are 7 cervical vertebrae, 18 thoracic vertebrae, 6 lumbar vertebrae, 5 sacral vertebrae and 15–21 coccygeal vertebrae in the normal horse.

Table 1.1   Average vertebral formula for the horse

Anatomical site	Number of vertebrae
Cervical	7
Thoracic	18
Lumbar	6
Sacral	5
Coccygeal	15–21

Variations in the vertebral formula

Although there may be some variation in the number of specific vertebrae in the axial skeleton, the total number in the formula is more constant. Anecdotally, so-called "short-backed" horses, such as Arabians, have been reported as having fewer vertebrae than other horses [4]. More objective data on the numbers of vertebrae have come from studies investigating the numbers of vertebrae within a population, with a number of studies designed to investigate the frequency of occurrence of the standard six lumbar vertebrae. Haussler et al. [2], in a study on thoroughbred horses, showed that only 69% of horses had the expected six lumbar vertebrae. However, it has been suggested that variations in the number of vertebrae within one spinal region are compensated for by an alteration in number in an adjacent vertebral region, in many cases to give a constant overall total vertebral number. There has been no proven association between the numbers of vertebrae that a horse has and any pathological condition.

Transitional vertebrae

Before a description of the different anatomical features of vertebrae at different anatomical sites in the vertebral column, "transitional vertebrae" must be considered. Transitional vertebrae are located between two adjacent vertebral regions and have the morphological characteristics of both these regions, i.e. they are "hybrid" vertebrae. They occur, therefore at the cervicothoracic, thoracolumbar or lumbosacral junction. A few studies have documented the incidence of transitional vertebrae. Haussler et al. [2] showed that 22% of their study population had thoracolumbar transitional vertebrae, none had lumbosacral transitional vertebrae and 36% had sacrococcygeal transitional vertebrae. Transitional vertebrae may exhibit their unusual morphology either through left-to-right asymmetry or via altered cranial-to-caudal graduation in the morphology. In large-scale studies of lumbosacral transitional vertebrae in humans and dogs, the morphological characteristics of the transitional vertebrae have been demonstrated to occur at the vertebral arches and transverse processes rather than at the vertebral body.

In clinical practice the most common transitional vertebra is transitional C7, which is often detected on lateromedial radiographs of the base of the spine and is characterised by having a short DSP, when it would normally have none at all.

Developmental aspects and growth plate closure times

The primary ossification centres of the vertebral bodies and neural arches (i.e. those surrounding the embryonic notochord in the centrum and lateral to the neural tube in the vertebral arch) fuse shortly after birth [5], whereas the secondary separate centres of ossification do not fuse until later on in life, if at all.

Secondary centres of ossification occur in the summits of the DSPs of the cranial thoracic vertebrae (the caudal thoracic and lumbar DSPs have fibrocartilaginous caps), the extremities of the transverse processes (TPs) of the lumbar vertebrae, the epiphyses of the vertebral bodies and the ventral crest.

The age at which these secondary centres of ossification fuse to the parent bone depends on the method of estimation of growth plate closure. Postmortem and histological growth plate closure times will always report an older age of closure than radiographic surveys because radiography is a less sensitive method of identifying the presence of an open growth plate.

The secondary centres of ossification present in the summits of the DSPs of the cranial thoracic region from T2 to around T9 are reported to fuse to the parent bone between 9 and 14 years of age [3], but in many cases, in the author's experience, they never fuse to the parent bone, even in aged horses. Thus they can be confused with fractured summits of the DSPs on radiographs if this developmental feature is not appreciated (see Figure 8.6 in Chapter 8).

The secondary centres of ossification at the cranial and caudal epiphyses of the vertebral bodies have reported closure times of between 3 and 3½ years of age using radiographic techniques (see Figure 8.4 in Chapter 8) [5]. However, gross anatomical studies suggest that the plates fully close later and asynchronously. The physes are reported to close between 4.9 and 6.7 years, with the cranial physis closing first, usually 1–2 years before the caudal physis [2].

The secondary centres of ossification of the TPs close in the first few months of life, although specific reports of this are not available.

Structure of the thoracic and lumbar vertebrae

A typical thoracic vertebra is made up of a vertebral body, a vertebral arch and vertebral processes (Figure 1.3). The vertebral body provides the surface against which the intervertebral disc sits, whereas the vertebral arch provides a gap in the osseous structure through which the spinal cord runs. The vertebral processes are the sites of attachment for various ligaments and muscles and are named the dorsal spinous processes, the transverse processes and the articular processes (APs) (Figure 1.3). These processes vary subtly within each anatomical region and this variation reflects the functional and structural demands at that particular anatomical site, e.g. the length of the DSP varies from region to region, being particularly long between T3 and T7. The lumbar vertebrae, in contrast, have long TPs and medium height DSPs.

Vertebral bodies

The vertebral bodies of the equine thoracolumbar spine (see Figure 1.4) provide support for weight-bearing and attachment sites for soft tissues and muscles. They are convex in shape cranially and concave in shape caudally. Ventrally a ridge of bone, the "ventral crest" (see Figure 1.3) is observed on approximately four to eight vertebrae (mean 5.5 ± 0.8 [2]) centred around the thoracolumbar junction.

The shape of the vertebral bodies changes from a rounded shape in the thoracic region to a dorsoventrally flattened shape in the caudal lumbar and sacral regions. It has been hypothesised that this shape change limits movement laterally between these vertebrae, but not dorsoventrally. Other anatomical variations between sites include the observation that prominent ventral body ventral crests are found in the cranial thoracic area and between

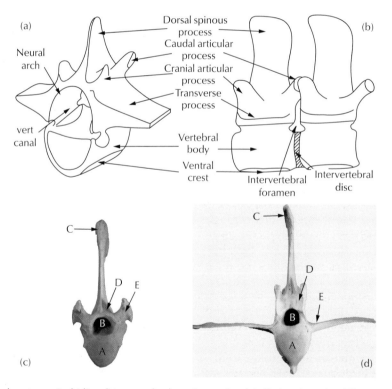

Figure 1.3 Vertebral anatomy: (a, b) line diagrams of a thoracic vertebra labelled to show the different anatomical regions of the vertebra: (a) a craniocaudal oblique diagram, (b) a lateral diagram. (c, d) Photographs of typical vertebrae: (c) thoracic vertebra, (d) lumbar vertebra; A, vertebral body; B, vertebral canal; C, dorsal spinous process; D, articular facet; E, transverse process. Note the much longer transverse processes in the lumbar vertebra compared with the thoracic vertebra.

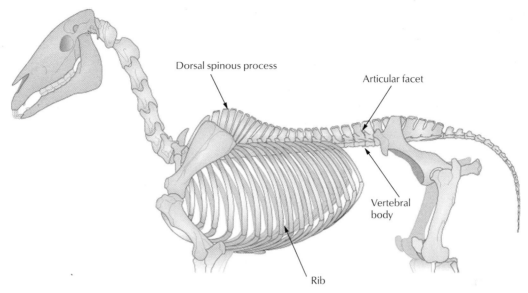

Dorsal spinous process

Articular facet

Vertebral body

Rib

Figure 1.4 A line drawing of the skeleton showing the relative positions of the dorsal spinous processes, articular facets, vertebral bodies and ribs.

T15 and L3. The ventral crest at the latter site, which can vary in the number of vertebrae involved, is believed to be the site of insertion of the crura of the diaphragm.

Intervertebral discs

The intervertebral discs (or fibrocartilages) are positioned between adjacent vertebral bodies and, together, they are correctly described as fibrocartilaginous articulations. They function to aid weight bearing, axial shock absorption and the maintenance of vertebral flexibility; they have both proprioceptive and nociceptive fibres in the outer third of the disc. The discs are made up of a gelatinous central *nucleus pulposus* and an outer fibrous *annulus fibrosus*; this *annulus fibrosus* is designed to provide rotational stability to the intervertebral joint by being formed of concentric layers of fibres angled relative to each other.

The width of the intervertebral discs differs between anatomical sites. In one study it was demonstrated that the intervertebral discs were thicker at T1–2 (average 5.9 mm, [6]) than elsewhere in the thoracic spine, with the average diameter of an intervertebral disc in the mid-

thoracic region being 2.5 mm. It was also shown that the lumbosacral junction has a wider intervertebral disc compared with elsewhere in the spine (average 3.6 mm).

In the horse, relatively few clinical problems arise from intervertebral disc pathology, particularly compared with the high frequency of pathology at this site in dogs and humans. However, discospondylitis and intervertebral disc degeneration are occasionally seen (see Chapter 15). Intervertebral disc herniation is extremely rare in the horse, possibly because of the poorly developed *nucleus pulposus* and thin intervertebral disc.

Vertebral arch

The spinal cord runs through the vertebral arch, which is made up of the dorsal part of the vertebral body ventrally, the vertebral lamina dorsally and the pedicles laterally. Dorsally in the vertebral arch the ventral laminae are connected by the ligamenta flava. The vertebral arches of the spinal vertebrae together form the continuous vertebral canal housing the spinal cord and its associated structures up to the cranial sacral region where the spinal cord terminates in the *cauda equina* (see

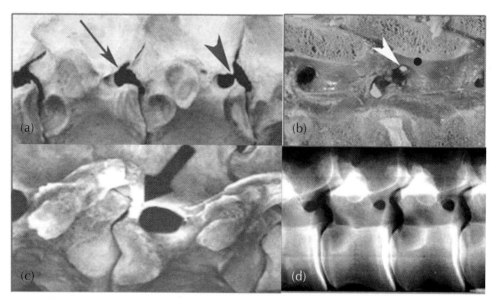

Figure 1.5   Intervertebral and lateral foramina of the thoracic spine: (a, c) photographs of a skeleton; (b) a cross-section from a postmortem specimen; (d) a lateromedial radiograph. In (a) an open intervertebral foramen is seen (black arrow) in the vertebral segment cranial to an intervertebral foramen that has spurs of bone formation protruding into it from dorsal and ventral (arrow head). In (b) this new bone formation is seen on the postmortem specimen. In (c) a strut of new bone is seen bridging the intervertebral foramen to form a lateral foramen. In (d) an open intervertebral foramen is seen cranial to two lateral foramina (circular radiolucencies).

Chapter 4). The vertebral arch is relatively large compared with the diameter of the spinal cord, ensuring no compression of the cord during movements of the spinal segments in the normal spine. However, in pathological conditions narrowing of the vertebral arch can occur (i.e. if there is displaced bone secondary to a fracture or new bone formation in osteoarthritis). In these cases spinal cord compression may result in onset of neurological signs.

Intervertebral foramina

Between the vertebral arches of each vertebra there is a small opening on either side – the intervertebral foramina (Figure 1.5a). These intervertebral foramina are formed by ventral notches in the cranial and caudal margins of the vertebral arch. The intervertebral foramina permit soft tissue structures (nerves, blood vessels and lymphatics) to exit the bony vertebral canal at each segment.

Lateral foramina

In addition to the intervertebral foramina that are observed on either side of the spine at each segmental junction between vertebrae, a second lateralised opening out of the bony canal is also present intermittently in some individuals. These are known as the lateral foramina (Figure 1.5c and d). Thoracic vertebrae T11, T15 and T16 have been reported as showing the highest incidence of fully formed lateral foramina in the thoracolumbar spine [7].

The origin of the lateral foramina is not known; however, it has been proposed that they arise from the intervertebral foramina as a consequence of spur formation in the caudal ventral notch of the vertebral arch (Figure 1.5a). Progressive calcification of the caudal ventral notch can occur, similar to that seen in ventral spondylitis (Figure 1.5c) (see Chapter 15). In addition to a fully enclosed lateral foramen, there are a number of other variations in the anatomy of the caudal notch of the vertebral arch, including one or more spurs protruding into the notch [7]. It has been demonstrated that, where present, the lateral foramen contains spinal nerves and some vessels, and the presence of lateral foramina may possibly be associated with spinal nerve impingement during and subsequent to this calcification.

Sacral foramina

In the sacrum the soft tissue structures exit the fused vertebral arches via either dorsal or ventral (pelvic) sacral foramina. The dorsal branches of the sacral spinal nerves exit via the dorsal sacral foramina. The pelvic sacral foramina communicate with the vertebral canal ventrally and contain the ventral branches of the sacral spinal nerves.

Vertebral canal contents

The vertebral canal contains the spinal cord and the structures surrounding the spinal cord (i.e. the cerebrospinal fluid, meninges, fat and vascular plexus). The spinal cord has segmentally paired dorsal and ventral motor roots that converge within the intervertebral foramen to form the spinal nerves (see Chapter 4).

Dorsal spinous processes

The DSPs project dorsally from the vertebral arch to rise above the vertebra into the epaxial musculature. The function of the DSPs is considered to be as levers for the muscular and ligamentous attachments of the vertebral column; bilateral contraction of the muscles that attach to the DSPs causes spinal extension, and unilateral contraction causes rotation.

The DSPs vary in their length, shape and angulation in different regions and will be considered anatomically from T1 running caudally. T1 has an extremely small DSP, rising approximately to twice the height of the vertebral body dorsally (Figure 1.6). This is the first elongated DSP in the vertebral column in most horses; however, occasionally an elongated DSP is seen on C7 (i.e. C7 has the properties of a transitional vertebra). Care must be taken not to automatically assume that

the first obvious DSP on a lateromedial radiograph is therefore T1.

Although T1 has a small spinous process, the DSPs in the cranial thoracic vertebral region are markedly elongated in the region of T2–8 to form the withers (Figure 1.7). The apex of the withers is formed by the DSPs of T4–7 (Figure 1.7a). As noted above the tips of the DSP of approximately T4–7 have separate centres of ossification. From an apex at T6 or T7 the length of the DSP decreases down to approximately T12; the height of the DSP decreases slightly down to the anticlinal vertebra (the vertebra at which the angulation of the DSPs changes, see below; Figure 1.7b) and then increases gently to the last lumbar vertebra (Figure 1.7c).

The shape of the DSPs also depends on the anatomical site from which they arise. DSPs from vertebrae T1–10 are narrow and tend to be quite straight (Figure 1.7a). At T11–16 they have a marked beak-shaped outline, wider at their base than at their apex and forming a cranial beak with a rounded caudal aspect at their summits. The cranial and caudal borders of the DSPs are often roughened due to new bone formation on these edges, which are the insertions of the interspinous ligaments; the dorsal summits of the DSPs are also often roughened at the sites of attachment of the supraspinous ligament (see Chapter 10).

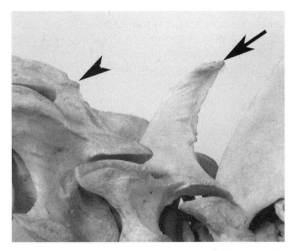

Figure 1.6   A photograph of vertebrae cervical 7 (C7) and thoracic 1 (T1). Note the elongated dorsal spinous process on T1 (arrow) compared with C7 (arrow head).

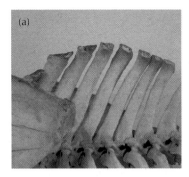
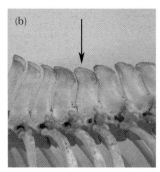
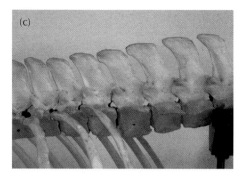

Figure 1.7   Three photographs of the vertebral column of a horse showing the shape and angulation of the dorsal spinous processes (DSPs): (a) cranial thoracic region (withers); the DSPs are markedly elongated and angle caudally. Note the separate centres of ossification in the most cranial vertebrae. In (b) the DSPs of the mid-thoracic region are seen. At this site the DSPs are shorter than in the cranial thoracic region and have a 'beak shape' at their summits. The DSPs of the more cranial vertebrae angle caudally until the 'anticlinal' vertebra (black arrow). From this point caudally the DSPs angle cranially. In (c) the DSPs of the caudal thoracic and first four lumbar vertebrae are seen. The DSPs angle cranially.

The angulation of the thoracolumbar DSPs changes from T1 caudally to the lumbosacral junction. From T1 to T14 the DSPs are angled dorsocaudally (i.e. towards the tail; Figure 1.7a). At T15, the so-called "anticlinal vertebra" (Figure 1.7b), the DSP is upright and then from T17 to L6 the DSPs are angled dorsocranially (towards the head) (Figure 1.7c). The anatomical reason for this alteration in DSP angulation is suggested to be due to attached soft tissue interactions. The position of the anticlinal vertebra suggests an alteration, at this anatomical site, of the soft tissue forces acting on the spine. The cranial thoracic region transmits forces from the head, neck and forelimbs, whereas the caudal thoracic and lumbosacral regions transmit forces associated with the hindlimbs; therefore the pull of the associated soft tissue structures does indeed alter either side of the anticlinal vertebra.

A further change in DSP angulation is observed in the sacrum, which is inclined dorsocaudally (Figure 1.8). The anatomical consequence of this alteration in angulation, without the intermediary of an anticlinal vertebra as occurs in the thoracic spine, is that a wide interspinous space is formed at the lumbosacral junction (Figure 1.8). It has been suggested that this wide interspinous space allows an increased range of motion at this site without the risk of process impingement. The wide space between L6 and S1 is a relatively consistent finding; however, in one study 36% of

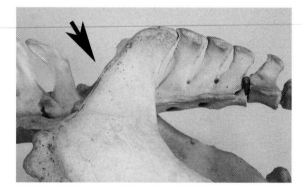

Figure 1.8   A photograph of the lumbosacral region: the wing of the ilium is seen in front of the cranial part of the sacrum. The last lumbar vertebra angles cranially and the sacrum angles caudally. The lumbosacral space is wide compared with any other interspinal space in the vertebral column (black arrow).

horses had an equally wide interspinous space between L5 and L6 [2]. This has, at the current time, little clinical relevance apart from possibly making more difficult the identification of the landmarks for cerebrospinal fluid retrieval from the lumbosacral space.

The distance between the summits of the DSPs varies between anatomical sites and between individuals. In most horses there is a small but clear gap between the DSP in the region T1 to T11; however, after T11 the DSPs become closer together. In some cases, *post mortem* or on lateromedial radiographs, the DSPs are seen to overlap with no evidence of bony contact (i.e. they are not quite in the same sagittal plane). Thus there is no bony contact and no evidence of bony remodelling. However, in many cases the close proximity of the DSPs does lead to bony contact, remodelling and, in some cases, false joint formation. This condition is known variously as "kissing spines" or "overriding dorsal spinous processes" and can cause back pain (see Chapter 14).

Articular processes (facets)

Paired articular processes (facets) arise both cranially and caudally from the vertebral arch and extend dorsally laterally. Between the cranial articular process of one vertebra and the caudal articular process of an adjacent vertebra a synovial joint is formed (i.e. a zygapophyseal joint). At each vertebral junction a pair of these joints is thus formed. The size, shape and orientation of the articular facets and hence joint surface differ within the vertebral column. In the cervical region and T1 the articular surfaces are large and lie at 45° to the horizontal. At T2 there is a transition from a 45° angle to a horizontal positioning of the articular facets. In the remainder of the thoracic region until about T16 (in 11 of 21 horses [6]), the articular surfaces continue to lie approximately horizontal with the cranial articular surfaces facing dorsally and the caudal articular surfaces facing ventrally (Figure 1.9a). The morphology of the articular facets is, however, not always symmetrical; one study reported that 83% of horses had asymmetrical facets [2]. At T16 and then into the lumbar region the articular surface orientation changes from horizontal to vertical (Figure 1.9b). In addition to the change in orientation of the articular facets, changes are also seen in the actual shape of the processes. In the thoracic region the facets are relatively flat; from T16 onwards their articular surfaces change such that the cranial articular surfaces are dorsally concave and the caudal articular surfaces ventrally convex. The alteration in the angulation and shape of the articular processes may reflect the movements of the different parts of the spine; in the thoracic vertebral region vertebral motion is mostly rotation and

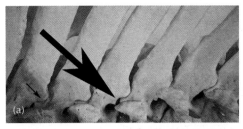

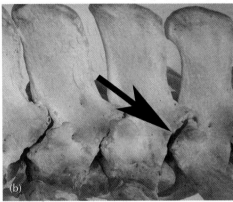

Figure 1.9 Two photographs to show the angulation of the articular facets at different regions of the vertebral column: (a) cranial thoracic vertebrae; articulations are close to horizontal (black arrows). (b) Caudal thoracic vertebrae: articulations are more vertically oriented (black arrow).

lateral flexion. In the lumbosacral region motion is mainly dorsoventral.

It has been proposed, based on the morphology of the articular facets, that the equine thoracolumbar spine can be divided into four regions: the first thoracic intervertebral joint (T1–2), the cranial and mid-thoracic region (T2–16), the caudal thoracic and lumbar region (T16–L6), and the lumbosacral joint (L6–S1) [6]. Studies on the amount and type of movement at each of these sites have indicated that each of these four sites does have a characteristic movement [8] and thus a structure–function relationship at these sites is likely (Table 1.2).

Transverse processes

The TPs exit the vertebrae at right angles to the direction of travel of the spinal cord and protrude out into the soft tissues of the back. Their function seems to be as lever arms to provide support to

Table 1.2 The relative amounts of movement in the joint complexes of the four regions of the equine thoracolumbar spine and the structure of the articular facets at each site

Region	Angle of articular facets	Shape of articular facets	Flexion and extension	Axial rotation	Lateral bending
T1–2	45°	Flat	++	+	+
T2–16	Horizontal	Flat	+	+++	+++
T16–L6	Vertical	Concavity	+	+	+
L6–S1	Vertical	Small, flat	++++	+	+

Adapted from Townsend et al. [8] and Townsend and Leach [6].

the vertebral column, and permit movement of the column via the muscles and ligaments that attach to them. Thus the TPs serve to maintain posture and permit rotation and lateral flexion. TPs alter in length at different sites within the vertebral column. In the cranial thoracic vertebral region the TPs are short and blunt in the thoracic region. In the lumbar region the TPs are markedly elongated and flattened horizontally (see Figs 1.3 and 10.4 in Chapter 10). These TPs provide attachment sites for a number of muscles, including iliopsoas.

The TPs have articulations with a number of different osseous structures, again dependent on site. In the thoracic region the TPs articulate with the ribs at the costotransverse articulations. In the lumbar region the horse is unusual in that there are intertransverse synovial articulations between the TPs of the last two or three lumbar vertebrae and the lumbosacral articulation [6, 9]. The latter articulation has the largest surface area, with more cranial articulations being smaller. These intertransverse articulations usually occur as paired structures at any given anatomical site; however, asymmetrical distributions of these articulations have been reported (9% [9] and 14% [2]). The number is not constant between horses and it has been suggested that the number of lumbar vertebrae dictates the numbers of intertransverse articulations (i.e. horses with six lumbar vertebrae have an extra articulation [10]). The genus *Equus* and the rhinoceroses are the only mammals with this particular anatomical feature.

In addition to intertransverse articulations found in all horses, intertransverse ankylosis has also been a relatively common finding [6, 11], with Smythe [12] reporting its occurrence in 50% of horses. The relationship between intertransverse ankylosis and back pain has not been proved in the horse.

Lumbosacral junction

The lumbosacral junction is the articulation between the last lumbar vertebra and the sacrum (see Figure 1.8). As discussed above, in most individuals, the DSPs of the lumbar vertebrae point cranially, whereas the sacral DSPs point caudally, giving an 'open' lumbosacral space (i.e. a large gap between DSPs dorsal to the bony roof of the vertebral arch). In some cases a large open interspinous space is also noted between L5 and L6.

Sacrum

The sacrum of the horse is a triangular structure with slightly convex dorsal and concave ventral surfaces. In most horses it is made up of five vertebrae that become fused by the age of 5 years (Figure 1.10 and see Figure 1.8). The sacral vertebrae have two secondary centres of ossification, which can be visualised radiographically after birth: the cranial and caudal sacral internal physes. The cranial physis closes at 5.4 ± 1.5 years, the caudal one at 5.0 ± 1.5 years [2].

In the sacrum the spinal cord passes through the vertebral canal, which is formed from the fused vertebral arches. The spinal nerves exit the sacrum via dorsal and ventral sacral foramina – the sacral version of the thoracic and lumbar intervertebral foramina as discussed above. The sacral spinal nerves and the lumbar spinal nerves form the lumbosacral plexus.

Sacroiliac joint

The vertebral column articulates with the pelvis at the bilateral sacroiliac joints (see Chapter 18). It is at this site that the propulsive forces of the hindlimb are transferred to the vertebral column. The sacroiliac joint is actually a highly specialised point of contact, essentially between two flat bony surfaces. The point of contact is a synovial joint with unusual histological characteristics. Most synovial joints in the body are formed between two hyaline cartilage surfaces; in the sacroiliac region the joint is formed between a hyaline cartilage surface (sacral surface) and a fibrocartilage surface (ilial surface) [13].

Unlike other important synovial joints in the body the sacroiliac joint does not have the advantage of osseous contouring to aid the maintenance of joint integrity, as is found, for example, in ball-and-socket joints. Therefore, in order to provide biomechanical stability to the meeting of two flat surfaces, the horse uses three strong sacroiliac ligaments: the dorsal sacroiliac, ventral sacroiliac and interosseous sacral ligaments. These ligaments are discussed in detail in Chapter 3.

Articulations of the vertebral column

Haussler [10] points out that an often overlooked aspect of the vertebral column is the large number of articulations present. He considered that the vertebral column was unique because of the potential for the presence of two types of articulation at each vertebral segment: a synovial articulation between the articular processes and a fibrocartilaginous articulation at the intervertebral disc. The exact number of articulations at each anatomical site varies (Table 1.3).

The pelvis

The bony pelvis of the horse is made up of the os coxae, the sacrum and the first two or three coccygeal vertebrae. The os coxae has three parts – the ilium (*os ilii*), the ischium (*os ischii*) and the pubis (*os pubis*) – which meet at the acetabulum (i.e. the cavity into which the head of the femur fits and articulates) (see Figure 1.11). The three parts of the *os coxae* are present in the developing fetus but

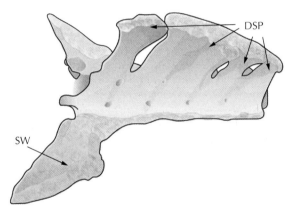

Figure 1.10 Line diagram of the sacrum: DSP, dorsal spinous processes of sacral vertebrae; SW, sacral wing.

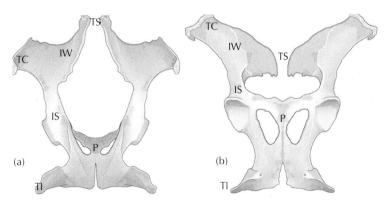

Figure 1.11 Line diagrams of the dorsal and ventral surfaces of the pelvis to demonstrate the anatomy: (a) dorsal pelvis; (b) ventral view. TC, tuber coxae; TS, tuber sacrale; TI, tuber ischii; IS, ilial shaft; IW, ilial wing; P, pubic symphysis.

Table 1.3 The number of articulations at different anatomical regions of the spine

Anatomical site	No. of articulations	Articular surfaces
Thoracic vertebrae	12	2 intervertebral discs 4 synovial intervertebral 4 costovertebral 2 costotransverse
Cranial lumbar vertebrae	6	2 intervertebral discs 4 synovial intervertebral
Caudal lumbar vertebrae	10	2 intervertebral discs 4 synovial intervertebral 4 synovial intertransverse processes
Sacral vertebrae	0	Fused; no articulations

Table 1.4 The growth plate closure times of the equine pelvis

Anatomical site	Growth plate closure time (years)
Tuber sacrale	5.8 ± 1.2
Tuber coxae	5.8 ± 1.5
Ischial tuberosity	5.2 ± 1.4
Pubic symphysis	5.7 ± 1.4

become fused by 1 year of age. The growth plate closure times of the pelvis are detailed in Table 1.4.

The ilium

The ilium, the largest of the three bones. can be subdivided into different structural and functional areas (see Figure 1.11). The largest and widest part of the bone is the ilial wing, the most dorsal part of the ilium is the *tuber sacrale*, the most ventral and lateral part of the ilium is the *tuber coxae*, and the most medial part is the ischiatic spine.

The ilial wing itself has two surfaces: the gluteal (outer) and the pelvic (inner) surfaces. The surface of the ilium has a number of modifications of structural importance. The gluteal line is found running from the *tuber coxae* to the middle of the medial border. The middle and deep gluteal muscles attach here. The ilium is also modified to allow the passage of important vessels and nerves to cross its surface. The iliolumbar artery crosses the lateral border of the ilium, the iliacofemoral artery also crosses the lateral border more ventrally, just above the psoas tubercle (site of attachment of *psoas minor*), and the sciatic nerve runs over the medial surface of the bone at the greater sciatic notch.

The *tuber sacrale* is the highest point of the skeleton in most horses. At this point the ilial wing curves upwards and caudally and, at the summit, the *tuber sacrale* is roughened to provide the attachment for the dorsal sacroiliac ligament.

The *tuber coxae* is the most lateral part of the pelvis and forms the "point of the hip". The *tuber coxae* is the elongated lateral angle of the pelvis, narrow in the middle of the angle and enlarged at either end.

The ischiatic spine is smooth medially and roughened laterally and is attached to the wing of the ilium by the ilial shaft. Medially there are grooves for the obturator vessels and nerve.

The ischium

The ischium forms the caudal part of the ventral floor of the pelvis (see Figure 1.11). When *in situ* it is approximately horizontal in the body and has two surfaces: the pelvic (interior) surface and the ventral (exterior) surface. The paired *tuber ischii* are the most caudal part of the ischium. These are triangular structures that are palpable either side of the tail.

The pubis

The pubis forms the anterior part of the ventral floor of the bony pelvis (see Figure 1.11). Of note are the reported anatomical differences between the sexes in the anatomy of the pubis. In the stallion the pelvic surface (interior) is convex, whereas in the mare the pelvic surface is smooth and concave. Also the medial angle of the pubis (where the two pubic bones meet at the cranial end of the pubic symphysis) is much thinner in mares than it is in stallions.

Obturator foramen

The obturator foramen is an oval hole in the pelvis, situated between the pubis and ischium, with its margin grooved for the obturator nerve and vessels.

Coccygeal vertebrae

The number of coccygeal vertebrae ranges from 15 to 21. The first coccygeal vertebra is separate from the sacrum in most horses but can become fused to the sacrum in older horses.

The coccygeal vertebrae have a number of modifications compared with the thoracic and lumbar vertebrae. Notably both the cranial and caudal surfaces of the vertebral bodies are convex. The articulations between the bodies are therefore mediated via a thick intervertebral disc. The coccygeal vertebrae have TPs but these steadily decrease in size towards the last coccygeal vertebra. Other anatomical features of note are that the DSPs of the first two coccygeal vertebrae are bifid (as is occasionally seen in the sacrum) and that DSPs are essentially absent from the rest of the vertebrae. The coccygeal vertebrae have articular processes; small cranial APs with expanded extremities are usually found down to coccygeal Cy7 but caudal APs are usually absent.

The vertebral canal gradually peters out in the coccygeal region. From a point beyond Cy3–6 the neural processes do not meet and the canal is merely an open groove, which itself stops at approximately Cy8. From Cy8 onwards the vertebrae are cylindrical with no vertebral arches.

References

1. Jeffcott, L.B. and Dalin, G. Natural rigidity of the horse's backbone. *Equine Veterinary Journal* 1980;**12**: 101–108.
2. Haussler, K.K., Stover, S.M. and Willits, N.H. Developmental variation in lumbosacropelvic anatomy of Thoroughbred racehorses. *American Journal of Veterinary Research* 1997;**58**:1083–1087.
3. Getty, R., ed. *Sisson and Grossman's The Anatomy of Domestic Animals*, 5th edn. Philadelphia: W.B. Saunders, 1975.
4. Dyce, K.M., Sack, W.O. and Wensing, C.J.G. *Textbook of Veterinary Anatomy*, 3rd edn. Philadelphia: Saunders, 2002.
5. Jeffcott, L.B. Radiographic examination of the equine vertebral column. *Veterinary Radiology* 1979;**20**:135–139.
6. Townsend, H.G.G. and Leach, D.H. Relationship of intervertebral joint morphology and mobility in the equine thoracolumbar spine. *Equine Veterinary Journal* 1984;**16**:461–466.
7. Gloobe, H. Lateral foramina in the equine thoracolumbar vertebral column: An anatomical study. *Equine Veterinary Journal* 1984;**16**:469–470.
8. Townsend, H.G.G., Leach, D.H. and Fretz, P.B. Kinematics of the equine thoracolumbar spine. *Equine Veterinary Journal* 1983;**15**:117–122.
9. Stecher, R.M. Lateral facets and lateral joints in the lumbar spine of the horse. A descriptive and statistical study. *American Journal of Veterinary Research* 1962;**23**:939–947.
10. Haussler, K.K. Osseous spinal pathology. *Veterinary Clinics of North America: Equine Practice* 1999;**15.1**: 103–111.
11. Townsend, H.G.G., Leach, D.H., Doige, C.E. and Kirkaldy-Willis, W.H. Relationship between spinal biomechanics and pathological changes in the equine thoracolumbar spine. *Equine Veterinary Journal* 1986;**18**:107–112.
12. Smythe, R.H. Ankylosis of the equine spine: pathologic or biologic? *Modern Veterinary Practice* 1962;**43**: 50–51.
13. Dalin, G. and Jeffcott, L.B. Sacroiliac joint of the horse. 1. Gross morphology. *Anatomia, Histologia, Embryologia* 1986;**15**:80–94.

2 The Normal Anatomy of the Soft Tissue Structures of the Thoracolumbar Spine

Jessica A. Kidd

Introduction

The soft tissue structures of the equine back are myriad. Put simply, the soft tissue structures can be grouped into their types, i.e. muscles, ligaments, and other, miscellaneous, soft tissue structures (e.g. fascia). In order to provide a comprehensive reference point for these structures, the names, origins, insertions and functions of these structures are listed alphabetically in Table 2.1. Additional information about selected structures is discussed in the text below.

Musculature

There are numerous muscles in the equine thoracolumbar region, which can be classified according to a number of different schemes. The intrinsic back muscles attach only to the axial skeleton and originate from the vertebrae, ribs or fascia. One of the simplest classification schemes is, therefore, to divide the muscles into two groups, depending on where they are positioned relative to the transverse processes (TPs) of the vertebrae (see Chapter 1), i.e. into epaxial or hypaxial muscle groups. Epaxial muscles are those that are dorsal to the TPs whereas hypaxial muscles are ventral to the TPs (Figure 2.1). The epaxial muscles function to extend the spine but can also create lateral movement when contracted unilaterally. The hypaxial muscles function to flex the spine and can also induce lateral movements (Plates 1–3).

Epaxial musculature

Within the epaxial muscle group, there are nine pairs of muscles in the thoracolumbar area. These pairs of muscles can be divided into three layers [1].

First layer

- *Trapezius thoracalis*
- *Latissimus dorsi*.

These two muscles are extremely superficial. *Trapezius thoracalis* originates from the supraspinous ligament between T3 and T7 and inserts on the scapular spine. Running just under the skin and fascia, *trapezius thoracalis* acts to elevate the shoulder. *Latissimus dorsi*, so called because it is the widest muscle of the back, has a broad origin in the thoracolumbar fascia and from the ribs. Caudally it tapers into the lumbar region. It inserts onto the tendon of *teres major* and other related cervical muscles, and functions to aid neck extension via its cervical attachments.

Table 2.1 Soft tissue structures of the back

Structure	Other names	Latin/Greek origin/derivation	Function	Origin	Insertion
Muscles		Latin *musculus*, diminutive of *mus* = a mouse. A muscle is a little mouse running under the skin			
Iliacus	With psoas collectively called iliopsoas	Pertaining to region of the ilium; Latin *ilium* = flank and iliac bone. Originally, as small intestines are largely supported by this bone, and old term for small intestines was ilia (plural of ilium)	Stabilises vertebral column when hindlimb is fixed	Sacroiliac surface of ilium, wing of sacrum and psoas minor tendon	With psoas major on lesser trochanter of the femur
Iliocostalis thoracis	Iliocostal muscle, thoracic portion; longissimus costarum	From ilium (see iliacus) to ribs (costa/costae); middle English, from Latin *thorax*, breastplate, chest, from Greek	Stabilises thoracic vertebrae; extends spine; lateral flexion	Transverse processes of lumbar vertebrae, and fascial sheet which separates iliocostal muscles from longissimus. (Fascial sheet is also known as "Bogorozky's tendon")	Caudal border of ribs 1–15; deeper tendinous insertions on cranial aspect of ribs 4–18 and to transverse process of C7
Iliocostalis lumborum		Latin *lumbus* = loin	Stabilises lumbar vertebrae and ribs; lateral flexion	Iliac crest	Caudal border of rib 18 and transverse process of middle lumbar vertebrae
Interspinal	Interspinales		Supports ventroflexion	Spinous processes of caudal cervical, thoracic and L1–3	Adjacent spinous processes
Intertransverse	Intertransversarii; intertransversales	Latin *transversus*, from past participle of *transvertere* = to turn across	Assists coordinated movement of vertebral column; stabilises vertebral column; lateral flexion if contracted unilaterally	Mamillary processes of lumbar and thoracic vertebrae	Transverse processes of lumbar and thoracic vertebrae
Latissimus dorsi		Latin *Latissimus* = superlative of *latus* meaning wide; *dorsi* = back	Suspends forelimbs from neck and trunk; retracts leg; draws trunk cranially when leg fixed	Thoracolumbar fascia and supraspinous ligament of thoracic and lumbar vertebrae	Medial aspect of the proximal humerus

Table 2.1 *Continued*

Structure	Other names	Latin/Greek origin/derivation	Function	Origin	Insertion
Longissimus thoracis and lumborum	Longissimus dorsi; erector spinae muscles	Latin *Longissimus* = superlative form of *longus*; "the longest"	Extends and stabilises thoracic and lumbar spine; supports rider and saddle; lateral flexion when not contracted bilaterally; controls stiffness of back at the walk	Spinous processes of the sacral, lumbar and thoracic vertebrae; ventral ilium; thoracolumbar fascia	Articular, mamillary and transverse processes of thoracic vertebrae and proximal ribs
Multifidus	Part of transversospinalis group; multifidus is transversospinalis group in thoracolumbar region; multifidus dorsi; juxtavertebral muscle; multifidous	Latin = many	Extends spine; stabilises and rotates vertebral column; proprioception of spine; coordination of long muscles	Numerous overlapping segments; lateral sacrum, lumbar articular processes and thoracic transverse processes	Spinous process of preceding vertebrae from C7 to S2
Omotransversarius		Greek *omo* = shoulder	Suspends forelimbs from neck and thorax	Shoulder fascia	Transverse processes of C2–4
Psoas major	With iliacus collectively called iliopsoas	Greek *psoas* = muscle of loin; *major*, comparative of *magnus* = great	Flexes hip joint; if hindlimb is fixed, flexes lower back at sacroiliac articulations	Ventral vertebrae of T16–18, transverse processes of L1–6	With iliacus on lesser trochanter of femur
Psoas minor	With iliacus collectively called iliopsoas	Late Latin *minor* = lesser	Flexes hip joint; if hindlimb is fixed, flexes lower back at sacroiliac articulations	Ventral vertebrae of T16–L6	Pelvic inlet on psoas minor tubercle of ilium
Quadratus lumborum		Latin *quadratus* = a square in shape. Latin *lumbus* = the loin	Weak stabiliser of lumbar vertebrae	Proximoventral surface of ribs 17 and 18 and lumbar transverse processes	Ventral sacrum and sacroiliac ligaments
Rectus abdominis		Latin *rectus* = straight	Flexes thoracolumbar spine	Lateral costal cartilages T4–9	Prepubic tendon and head of femur via accessory ligament

Structure	Alternative name	Derivation	Action	Attachment	Attachment
Rhomboideus		Greek *rhombus* = lozenge, *eidos* = resemblance	Draws scapula dorsally and cranially, elevates neck; suspends forelimbs from neck and thorax	Spinous processes of T2–7 via dorsoscapular ligament	Medial surface of scapular cartilage
Serratus dorsalis cranialis	Serratus dorsalis anterior		Used in inspiration; encases iliocostalis	Thoracolumbar fascia and dorsoscapular ligament	Lateral surface of rib 5 or 6 to rib 11 or 12
Serratus dorsalis caudalis	Serratus dorsalis posterior		Used in expiration; encases iliocostalis	Thoracolumbar fascia	Lateral surface of ribs 11 or 12–18
Serratus ventralis	Serrate muscle; serrate face is another name for medial scapula	Latin *serratus* = notched from *serra* = saw	Suspends neck and thorax from forelimbs	First seven ribs	Medial scapula
Spinal	Spinalis thoracis		Extends and fixes spine	Spinous processes of lumbar and last six thoracic vertebrae	Spinous process of T1–6/7 and C3–7
Transverse spinal muscles	Transversospinales			Spinous process	Transverse process of adjacent vertebra
Trapezius		Latin, from Greek *trapeza* = table because of shape formed by muscles	Suspends forelimbs from neck and thorax; elevates scapula	Supraspinous ligament of T3–10	Dorsal portion of spine of scapula
Ligaments		Latin *ligamentum* = ligament; from *ligare* = to bind			
Costotransverse ligament			Stabilises thoracic vertebrae and ribs	Ribs	Transverse processes
Costovertebral ligament			Stabilises thoracic vertebrae and ribs	Ribs	Vertebral body
Dorsal longitudinal ligament	Ligamentum longitudinale dorsales		Supports intervertebral discs; vertebral stability	Spans length of vertebral column along floor of vertebral canal	
Interspinous ligament	Ligamenta interspinalis		Stabilises spinous processes; prevents vertebrae sliding dorsally	Spinous process	Adjacent spinous process
Intertransverse ligament	Ligamenta intertransversaria		Limits lateral flexibility and rotation	Lumbar transverse processes	Transverse process of adjacent vertebrae

Table 2.1 *Continued*

Structure	Other names	Latin/Greek origin/derivation	Function	Origin	Insertion
Ligamentum flavum	Interarcuate ligaments	Latin = yellow ligament	Supports weight of trunk	Fills interarcuate spaces	
Nuchal ligament (laminar portion)	Lamina nuchae	Latin *nucha* = the back of the neck	Supports weight of trunk	Dorsal portion of nuchal ligament and spinous processes of T2 and T3	C2–7
Short spinal ligament			Runs between individual vertebrae to protect the spinal cord	Vertebra	Adjacent vertebra
Supraspinous ligament			Stability of thoracolumbar vertebrae	Caudal continuation of nuchal ligament; in caudal thoracic region it fuses with lumbodorsal fascia and tendinous insertions of latissimus dorsi	With lumbodorsal fascia and tendinous insertions of latissimus dorsi, attaches to periosteum of caudal thoracic and lumbar vertebrae and interspinous ligament
Ventral longitudinal ligament	Ligamentum longitudinale ventralis		Vertebral stability	Spans length of vertebral column on ventral aspect of vertebrae	
Fascia and other soft tissue structures					
Supraspinous bursa	Supraspinal subligamentous bursa		Cushions nuchal ligament as it passes over tallest thoracic spinous process		
Thoracolumbar fascia	Lumbar dorsal fascia		Attachment site for multiple muscles	Attaches to thoracolumbar spinous processes	Also attaches to cranial ilial wing
Dorsoscapular ligament			Limits dorsal movement of scapula; shock absorber for shoulder region	Part of the thoracolumbar fascia; supraspinous ligament over the highest spines of the withers	Deep surface of rhomboideus muscle. Many branches that insert on deep scapula alternating with branches of serratus ventralis

Second layer

- *Rhomboideus thoracalis*
- *Serratus dorsalis anterior*
- *Serratus dorsalis posterior.*

These three muscles form the next layer of the back. *Rhomboideus thoracalis* originates from the dorsal spinous processes (DSPs) between T2 and T7 and inserts on the medial aspect of the cartilage of the scapula. Similar to *trapezius thoracalis*, *rhomboideus thoracalis* acts on the scapula; in this instance it draws the scapula upwards and forwards. *Serratus dorsalis anterior* and *posterior* are thin muscles that lie under *rhomboideus*, *serratus ventralis* and *latissimus dorsi*. The *serratus dorsalis* muscles originate from the lumbodorsal fascia and dorsoscapular ligament and insert on the ribs. *Serratus dorsalis* anterior inserts from ribs 5–6 to 11–12, functioning to draw the ribs forwards and outwards as an aid to the inspiratory phase of respiration. In contrast *serratus dorsalis posterior* inserts on the last seven or eight ribs and functions to draw these ribs backwards, assisting expiration.

Third layer

- *Longissimus costarum (iliocostalis)*
- *Longissimus dorsi*
- *Multifidus dorsi*
- *Intertransversales lumborum.*

The *longissimus costarum* muscle (or *iliocostalis* as it is commonly known) is a long thin muscle consisting of a series of overlapping segments or fascicles. This muscle is the most lateral of the large group of epaxial muscles made up of the *longissimus costarum* and dorsi muscles and the *spinalis* muscles. *Longissimus costarum* is the flattest muscle in the back and originates from the deep layer of the lumbodorsal fascia back to L3–4 and the anterior borders of the last 15 ribs. Each segment spans several vertebrae with the muscle fibres oriented cranioventrally. The muscle lies next to *longissimus dorsi*, dorsal to the angle of the ribs. The short lumbar portion of *longissimus costarum* is not distinct but instead fuses with the lumbar portion of *longissimus dorsi*. *Longissimus costarum* inserts on the posterior border of the ribs and the TPs of the last cervical vertebrae. Its action, when contracting bilaterally, is to assist in expiration by depressing and retracting the ribs. However, when *longissimus costarum* contracts unilaterally, it has been proposed that it may participate in lateral movement of the spine.

Longissimus dorsi is the largest and longest muscle in the body, running from the sacrum and ilium in the pelvis to C7. It is the major muscle of the back, arranged segmentally with multiple individual attachments. *Longissimus dorsi* fills the space between the TPs and DSPs of the vertebrae. It is thickest in the lumbar region where it is

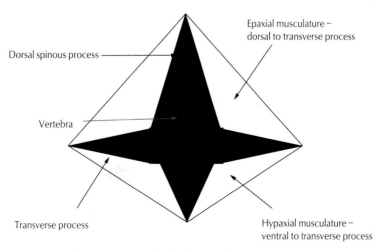

Figure 2.1 Schematic cross-section through spine at level of T12 to show relative positions of epaxial and hypaxial musculature.

covered in thoracolumbar fascia, and narrows in the thoracic region. It originates from the ilium, DSPs of S1–3, DSPs of the lumbar and thoracic vertebrae, and the supraspinous ligament. It inserts on the TPs and articular processes of the lumbar vertebrae, TPs of the thoracic vertebrae, TPs and DSPs of C4–7, and lateral surfaces of the ribs (except the first rib). The *spinalis* muscles sit dorsomedially on the *longissimus dorsi* muscles and are adjacent to the dorsal aspect of the spinous processes. In most diagrammatic representations and text, they are considered to be part of *longissimus dorsi* and they certainly function as such.

Longissimus dorsi is the main extensor of the back and loins of the horse. In addition, via its costal attachments, it helps in expiration. As with *longissimus costarum*, unilateral contraction may assist in lateral movement of the spine. *Longissimus dorsi* also raises the hindlimbs for bucking and the forelimbs for rearing. It has its greatest extension during the swing phase of the hindlimb stride and is used to transmit energy from the hindlimbs to the back during this phase. In well-muscled horses, this muscle can extend above the tops of the dorsal spinous processes; this results in a groove running down the midline of the back.

Multifidus dorsi is the most medial epaxial muscle and is located adjacent to the DSPs. *Multifidus dorsi* is part of the transversospinalis group; in the thoracolumbar region it is the entirety of this group. It is made up of numerous overlapping segments that extend from the lumbar to the cervical regions. *Multifidus dorsi* originates from the lateral part of the sacrum, articular processes of the lumbar vertebrae and TPs of the thoracic vertebrae, and inserts on the DSPs of S1 and S2, lumbar and thoracic vertebrae and C7. The action of *multifidus dorsi* is to extend the back – acting unilaterally it flexes the spine laterally.

The *intertransversales lumborum* muscles are thin, muscular and tendinous structures that occupy the TPs of L1–5. They therefore originate and insert on the TPs and function to assist the flexion of the loins laterally or, conversely, to hold the region in a fixed posture.

The muscles described above complement the long muscles of the back. There are numerous short muscles that are responsible for fine movement of segments of the back, as well as proprio-

ception and proprioceptive correction. It is worth noting that opinion is divided over the presence of the intertransverse muscles in the thoracic and lumbar spine: some anatomists state that the intertransverse muscles are present in the thoracic and lumbar spine, whereas other texts state that the intertransverse muscles occur only in the cervical and tail regions. They are included in Table 2.1 for completeness and not as any definitive statement of their existence.

Hypaxial musculature

- *Psoas major*
- *Psoas minor*
- *Iliacus*
- *Quadratus lumborum.*

Psoas major originates from the ventral surface of the TPs of the lumbar vertebrae and the last two ribs. It inserts on the trochanter minor of the femur and functions to flex the hip joint and rotate the proximal hindlimb outwards. *Psoas minor* originates from the bodies of T15–18, L1 to L4–5 and the vertebral ends of ribs 16–17. It inserts on the *psoas* tubercle of the ilium in the pelvis, and acts to flex the pelvis relative to the loins and move it laterally if contracted unilaterally. *Iliacus* originates from the ventral surface of the ilium lateral to the iliopectineal line, the ventral sacroiliac ligament, the wing of the sacrum and the tendon of psoas minor. It inserts, with *psoas major*, on the trochanter minor of the femur and acts similarly to flex the hip joint and rotate the proximal hindlimb outwards. Finally, in this group, *quadratus lumborum* originates from the last two ribs and the TPs of the lumbar vertebrae, and inserts on the ventral surface of the sacrum and the ventral sacroiliac ligament. The action of *quadratus lumborum* is to hold the last two ribs fixed and, acting unilaterally, to produce lateral flexion of the loins.

Ligaments

The ligamentous structures of the thoracolumbar region of the equine back can be divided into long and short ligaments (see also Chapter 3).

Long ligaments

* Supraspinous ligament
* Dorsal longitudinal ligament
* Ventral longitudinal ligament.

The supraspinous ligament (SSL) is the thoracolumbar continuation of the nuchal ligament of the neck. Compared with the nuchal ligament, the SSL is much narrower. The reason for this decrease in thickness and hence strength has been hypothesised to be because, unlike the nuchal ligament, the SSL does not function to support the head and, therefore, does not need to be as strong as the nuchal ligament. The laminar ligament, or sheetlike portion of the nuchal ligament, runs from the cervical region and attaches to the dorsal processes of C2 to T2–3.

The function of the SSL is to stabilise the thoracolumbar vertebrae and their associated spinous processes. Its dimensions alter as they pass through the body: the SSL is wider and has more elastic properties in the cranial and mid-thoracic spine than in the rest of the thoracolumbar spine; it is also stronger in the cranial thoracic portion. In the caudal thoracic region, the SSL fuses with the lumbodorsal fascia (see below) and the tendinous insertions of *latissimus dorsi*. Collectively these insert on the periosteum of the proximal spinous processes of the caudal thoracic and lumbar vertebrae and the interspinous ligament. The lumbar portion of the SSL is thicker and denser than the thoracic portion, and is absent between the last lumbar and the first sacral vertebrae.

The dorsal longitudinal ligament runs along the floor of the vertebral canal from C2 to the sacrum, and attaches to each intervertebral disc, whereas the ventral longitudinal ligament runs along the ventral aspect of the vertebrae to the sacrum and also attaches to each intervertebral disc.

Short ligaments

* *Interspinous ligament*
* *Ligamentum flavum*
* *Costovertebral ligament*
* *Costotransverse ligament.*

Multiple short ligaments make up a complex mechanism for stabilisation of the thoracolumbar vertebrae. The interspinous ligament (ISL) runs between adjacent DSPs and dorsally fuses with the SSL whereas its ventral fibres attach to the ligamentum flavum. The ISL, similar to the SSL, also stabilises the thoracolumbar vertebrae and their DSPs, and is elastic in the thoracic spine. The *ligamentum flavum* sits in the spaces between the vertebral laminae. It is primarily elastic, which ensures that, when the spine is completely extended, it does not impinge on the dorsal aspect of the vertebral canal. Finally, the costovertebral ligaments attach vertebral bodies to ribs whereas the costotransverse ligaments attach TPs to ribs; both function to stabilise the thoracic vertebrae and ribs. The intertransverse ligaments are only in the lumbar region and link adjacent TPs to limit lateral flexibility.

Miscellaneous soft tissue structures

* Supraspinous bursa
* Thoracolumbar fascia
* Dorsoscapular ligament.

The supraspinous bursa is always present in horses and is situated between the SSL and the highest DSP of the withers, usually T6. Other bursae are sporadically recorded in this region on the summits of the DSPs.

The thoracolumbar fascia (TLF) is a part of the deep fascia of the trunk and it has a number of components. It is the attachment site for many muscles and courses between the thoracolumbar DSPs and the cranial aspect of the ilial wing. Part of the TLF forms an aponeurosis with *latissimus dorsi* and the caudal portion of *serratus dorsalis caudalis*. Caudally it becomes the gluteal fascia and cranioventrally it merges with the axillary fascia. Cranially it also becomes the *spinocostotransversal fascia* in the shoulder region, where it forms three layers. The superficial layer attaches to *serratus ventralis*. The middle layer surrounds and separates *longissimus dorsi* and *longissimus costarum*.

The dorsoscapular ligament, part of the TLF, originates in the SSL over the highest DSP of the withers, at which point it is mostly fibrous. It courses ventrally deep to *rhomboideus thoracalis*, attaching to the deep surface of this muscle, at which point it is mainly elastic. It has multiple branches that interdigitate with portions of *serratus ventralis* and insert on the medial aspect of the scapula. It functions as a shock absorber for the shoulder as well as restricting the range of dorsal movement of the scapula. Finally, the superficial fascia of the trunk includes the cutaneous trunci muscle and fans into the TLF and attaches to the DSPs.

Reference

1. Getty, R., ed. *Sisson and Grossman's The Anatomy of Domestic Animals*, 5th edn. Philadelphia: W.B. Saunders, 1975.

3 The Normal Anatomy of the Soft Tissue Structures of the Pelvis

David Bainbridge

Introduction

Over hundreds of millions of years, the pelvis of land vertebrates has evolved in concert with nearby structures to perform a variety of functions. The pelvis/sacrum/cranial tail complex is the musculoskeletal unit which:

- transfers supportive and propulsive forces from the hindlimb to the trunk
- is itself a portion of the spinal column
- serves as the point of attachment of many spinal, abdominal and hindlimb muscles
- contains within it major components of the alimentary, urinary, reproductive, vascular, lymphatic and nervous systems.

While conforming to the basic mammalian plan, the equine pelvis shows specialisations for the natural way of life of the species. The horse is thought to have evolved to survive on pasture of an unpredictable and frequently extremely low quality, leading to a large abdominal mass, which has in turn meant that the soft tissues of the pelvis have become extremely strong and fibrous to support the weight. Some other adaptations are often termed "cursorial specialisations", although they probably reflect a need to walk and graze efficiently for long periods, interspersed with only occasional bursts of speed to evade predators, for example, hindlimb movement is more restricted to the sagittal plane in horses than in any other major domestic species. Also, the hindlimb muscle mass is unusually concentrated at the proximal end in horses to reduce the moment of inertia of the swinging limb – by loss of distal muscle mass and the proximal "creep" of muscle origins [1]. Presumably also related to the need to escape predators is the fact that the equine birth process is relatively rapid; to allow this the birth canal is wide and straight compared with that of some other large ungulates.

In this chapter the non-osseous locomotor structures of the pelvis are reviewed [2–5]. The author has divided them into three groups:

1. The sacroiliac joint: the main route of transfer of compressive forces from hindlimb to trunk is considered, along with other structures that support its function.
2. The diverse structures that form the dorsolateral and caudal walls of the pelvic cavity – limb muscles, ligaments, the pelvic diaphragm, and the structures of the anal and perineal regions.
3. The complex network of thick connective tissue that strengthens the ventral aspect of the pelvis.

Sacroiliac joint

The sacroiliac joint is essentially a synovial joint, although the synovial component is considerably augmented by additional connective tissue. The nomenclature of some structures can vary confusingly between written sources [6].

The synovial joint is formed between the roughened articular surfaces of the medial ilium and the modified transverse processes, or wing, of the sacrum (see Chapter 18). The equine iliac wing runs obliquely between its two distinct prominences, the ventrolateral *tuber coxae* and the dorsomedial *tuber sacrale*. The joint is formed closer to the latter prominence and the joint space is angled at approximately 30° to the horizontal. The irregularities of the bony facets on the sacrum and ilium are complementary and both surfaces are lined with a thin layer of articular cartilage. In life the articular surfaces are separated by a narrow cleft filled with fluid secreted by the encircling synovial membrane. The joint is surrounded by a tight fibrous capsule, but much of the strength of the joint itself is conferred by strong bands of connecting tissue that span the joint space [7].

The synovial joint is surrounded by the strong ventral sacroiliac ligament (Figure 3.1), a series of fibres radiating from around the articular circumference of the sacrum to insert on the ventromedial aspects of the *tuber sacrale* and iliac wing. The ligament is strongest dorsally and serves to reduce rotational and sliding movements of the joint.

Even more substantial is the dorsal sacroiliac ligament, which consists of two dissimilar parts (Figure 3.2). The first is the cord-like "funicular" portion, which passes in a caudocranial direction from the neural spines of the sacral vertebrae to the tuber sacrale. The relationship of this portion to the adjacent lumbodorsal fascia (or thoracolumbar fascia) can differ between individual horses – being lateral in some and ventral in others. The second part of the ligament is the "membranous part", a triangular sheet fanning out ventrocaudally from the lateral sacrum (and medial tuber sacrale) to blend with the lateral surface of the sacrosciatic ligament (discussed later). This second portion is also occasionally called the "lateral sacroiliac ligament".

The movements of the joint are dramatically restricted by this ligament support and it is assumed that it undergoes only small sliding (planar), pivoting (trochoid) and impact-absorbing movements. These movements are so small as to be almost impossible to measure *in vivo*, although in vivo a tiny pivoting movement of 0.8 ± 0.5° has been reported, which occurs alongside a much larger movement at the lumbosacral joint [8, 9].

An additional degree of stabilisation is conferred by the iliolumbar ligament (see Figure 3.1). This sheet of thick connective tissue is a lateral extension of the intertransverse ligament, which lies between all the lumbar vertebrae. These broad triangular ligaments widen caudally until they insert on the wing of the ilium, ventral to the origin of the *longissimus* musculature. Thus, they indirectly bridge the junction between the pelvis and vertebral column and resist extreme tension on either side of that junction – possibly as an adaptation to rearing.

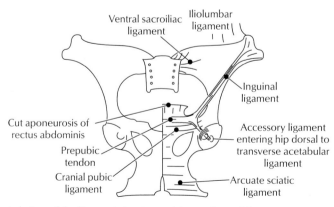

Figure 3.1 Schematic ventral view of the ligament structures of the equine pelvis.

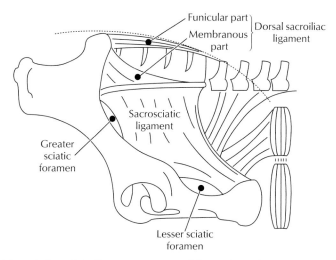

Figure 3.2   Schematic left lateral view of the ligament structures of the equine pelvis.

The dorsolateral and caudal walls

With the exception of the necks and wings of the *ilia*, and the cranial tail, the pelvic cavity is not bounded dorsolaterally or caudally by bone. Instead, a variety of soft tissue structures perform this role, including the pelvic diaphragm and perineal structures. There are considerable differences between their configuration in the horse and that in other domestic species. To complicate matters further, human anatomical terminology is often unhelpful here – horses do not have a muscular "pelvic floor"; they have a "coccygeus" muscle but no coccyx and their "*levator ani*" muscle does not "lift the anus". The relevant structures are described in order from superficial to deep [10].

This area is covered by thick fasciae. The *gluteal fasciae* are the caudal continuation of the lumbodorsal fascia and cover the prominent buttock region of the horse. The main points of attachment of the fasciae are the *tubera sacrale* and *coxae*, the neural spines of the sacral vertebrae and the sacrosciatic ligaments. Their function is thought to be to provide general mechanical support to the region and to constrain the movements of underlying muscles within "fascial tunnels". Thus, the gluteal fasciae send off a series of intermuscular septa between the *middle gluteal, biceps femoris, semitendinosus* and *semimembranosus* muscles. Although in the most part separated from the true

"pelvic diaphragm" by the muscles of the hip region, these fasciae are important in allowing those muscles to maintain tone that supports the soft tissue boundaries of the pelvic cavity. From the *gluteal fasciae* and dorsal sacroiliac ligament arise the tail fasciae, which, although simply surrounding the cranial tail musculature, are tightly adherent caudal to the anus [11].

Several skeletal muscles (Figure 3.3) are important in indirectly maintaining the integrity of the walls of the pelvis, by exerting pressure on the ligamentar sheets deep to them. However, they can also confound veterinary attempts to image the structures beneath. The important muscles include the following:

- The middle gluteal muscle is extensive in the horse and supports much of the cranial part of the underlying sacrosciatic ligament. Its origin on the concavity of the lateral iliac wing is supplemented by attachments on the gluteal fasciae, the lateral surfaces of the sacrosciatic and sacroiliac ligaments, and via an aponeurosis as far cranially as the first lumbar vertebra. The relative enlargement of this muscle has also been proposed to be an adaptation for rearing.
- The equine superficial gluteal muscle originates more proximally that that of other domestic species, from the gluteal fasciae and the *tuber coxae*. It effectively fills a shallow

depression between the middle gluteal and *biceps femoris* muscles.

- *Biceps femoris* has additional proximal origins, or 'long heads', which lie caudal to the middle gluteal muscle. As well as its origin on the sciatic tuberosity, it has attachments on the gluteal and tail fasciae and the sacrosciatic and sacroiliac ligaments. Thus, it covers the lateral aspect of the middle region of the sacrosciatic ligament in this species.
- The equine *semitendinosus* muscle also supplements its attachments with more proximal origins on the transverse processes of the first two caudal vertebrae and the tail fasciae. Thus, this muscle, readily delineated in the standing animal, completes the triad that confers additional lateral support on the dorsolateral pelvic wall.
- The *semimembranosus* muscle is more on the caudal aspect of the limb, but it too has extensive proximal origins, in this case on the caudal sacrosciatic ligament. Its origins, and its bulk in horses, mean that the left and right *semimembranosus* muscles bulge towards each other on either side of the anus, covering the sciatic tuberosities and ischiorectal fossae in a way that is quite unlike the arrangement in carnivores and ruminants.
- A final muscle that deserves brief mention is *sacrocaudalis ventralis*, the most ventral muscle of the tail which, covered by the tail fasciae, forms the dorsal boundary of the caudal pelvic cavity.

Deep to the rump and thigh muscles lies the sacrosciatic ligament (see Figure 3.2), also known as the sacrotuberous ligament. The development of this ligament appears to be related to absolute species body size – small species lack it; in dogs it is a taut cord passing from the sacrum to the sciatic tuberosity; in horses and cattle it is very extensive. The dorsal attachment of the equine sacrosciatic ligament runs along the lateral aspect of the sacrum and the transverse processes of the first two caudal vertebrae, where it blends with the fibres of the membranous part of the dorsal sacroiliac ligament. From here the sheet-like ligament courses caudoventrolaterally to attach along the dorsal edge of the iliac neck and ischium. The free caudal edge of the ligament is strengthened by a strong "funicular" component which inserts on the dorsal aspect of the sciatic tuberosity, and is further supported by the long head of semimembranosus. Thus, the left and right sacrosciatic ligaments may be compared with a tent over the pelvic cavity, suspended from the "ridge pole" of the sacral and caudal vertebrae, and "tethered down" ventrally to the pelvis. Each ligament is fenestrated at two points: the greater sciatic foramen lies in the dorsocaudal concavity of the iliac neck and allows passage of the sciatic nerve; the lesser sciatic foramen lies caudal to the sciatic spine and permits passage of the internal obturator muscle. The tautness of the sacrosciatic ligaments (and indeed the sacroiliac ligaments) is under hormonal control – they become laxer before birth, although this is less clinically evident

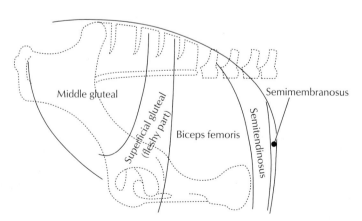

Figure 3.3 Schematic left lateral view of the outlines of the rump muscles covering the equine pelvic region.

in horses than cattle due to the presence of thick overlying muscles.

The caudal part of the sacrosciatic ligament overlies the pelvic diaphragm (the internal surface of the cranial part is lined only by peritoneum). Important features of this region include the following:

- Interposed between the ligament and the diaphragm, and bounded ventrally by the ischium, is a fat-filled space called the ischiorectal fossa, although in this species this cannot be palpated lateral to the anus because it is overlain by *semimembranosus*.
- The coccygeus muscle is the only convincing "diaphragm" muscle in the horse, resembling another "ridge tent" nestling inside the caudal part of the larger, fibrous sacrosciatic ligaments. It originates on the caudoventral part of the internal surface of that ligament, and its fibres course caudodorsomedially to insert via two leaves of tendon on the first four tail vertebrae and the tail fasciae. Thus, the muscle serves to enclose the caudal parts of the pelvic viscera, and to flex the tail.
- Whereas *levator ani* of the carnivores inserts primarily on the tail and supplements the action of coccygeus, the same muscle in the horse inserts mainly on the circumference of the external anal sphincter in a complex manner. It originates on the sciatic spine and nearby regions of the sacrosciatic ligament. Thus, it does not provide such complete enclosure for the pelvic contents and acts mainly to resist eversion and prolapse of the anus.

The caudal wall of the pelvis (Figure 3.4) is bounded by a series of structures related to the termination of the gastrointestinal and reproductive tracts. The anus and the vulva or bulb of the penis are suspended from the tail in the pelvic outlet. They are bounded dorsolaterally by the free edges of the sacrosciatic ligament and the pelvic diaphragm. In horses, considerable lateral support is also given by *semimembranosus*. In mares, the *rima vulvae* often hangs ventrally so that much of it is ventral to the sciatic arch of the pelvis; indeed, it is considered good conformation for it to do so, because it may reduce the incidence of ascending genital infections. The following are the structures that make up the caudal wall of the pelvis:

- The anal sphincters are suspended from the caudal fascia dorsally and themselves suspend the perineal fascia ventrally. The striated external sphincter blends with the fibres of *levator ani*, retractor muscles (see below) and especially the *constrictor vulvae* of the female. The smaller, smooth muscle, internal sphincter lies cranial to the external sphincter, and represents a terminal thickening of the wall of the rectum. Further cranially lies *rectococcygeus*, a band of rectal smooth muscle that extends to the ventral surfaces of the fourth and fifth caudal vertebrae, thus suspending the rectum from the vertebral column.
- The *constrictores vulvae et vestibuli* are well-developed oval rings of muscle that act to constrict the respective portions of the female urogenital opening. The more caudal of the two, the *constrictor vulvae*, blends its fibres extensively with those of the external anal sphincter. The *constrictor vestibuli* is intermixed with the fibres of the retractor muscle.
- The *retractor penis/clitoridis muscles* course ventrally from the caudal vertebrae, run deep to *levator ani* and fuse in the midline ventral to the anus. Further fibres continue ventrally to insert on the penis or to blend with the fibres of the constrictor muscles of the female.
- The perineal body is a fibrous and muscular node between the anus and vulva or bulb of the penis. It contains a complex arrangement of connective tissue and intermixed strands of all the striated muscles mentioned above. It is of clinical relevance due to its importance in the conformation of mares and its propensity for laceration during dystocia.

The innermost layer of the pelvic wall is the thick pelvic fascia, which lines the inner surface of the above structures. Cranially, in the pelvic cavity, this is supplemented by the peritoneal reflections, which protrude into the pelvis from the abdominal cavity.

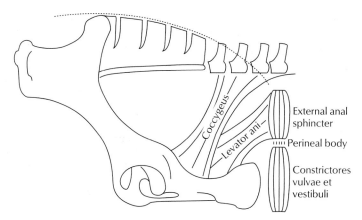

Figure 3.4 Schematic left lateral view of the equine pelvic diaphragm and caudal pelvic wall.

The ventral fibrous structures

The major components of the ventral boundary of the pelvis are, of course, the *pubes* and *ischia*. In foals these bones are fused in the midline by a symphysis, although this ossifies relatively rapidly in horses, with the cranial part mineralising first. Once a synostosis has formed, what little movement existed at the joint is lost. The bony floor of the pelvis is augmented by a series of interconnected fibrous structures both dorsally and ventrally, although it is the ventral structures that predominate. Some of these have other functions unrelated to the integrity of the pelvis, but all are now considered, in a cranial-to-caudal order (see Figure 3.1).

The inguinal ligament is the free caudal margin of the external abdominal oblique muscle, which is largely tendinous in this region. It runs caudoventromedially from the *tuber coxae* to the iliopubic eminence where it blends with the prepubic tendon. The ligament spans the cranioventral concavity of the neck of the ilium and thus bounds a D-shaped opening, the femoral canal, which conveys the femoral artery, vein and nerve, iliopsoas and the deep inguinal lymph nodes.

The prepubic tendon is a complex structure, especially in the large ungulates [11]. Although often described rather like a ligament running between the right and left iliopubic eminences, it actually represents the blended tendons of *rectus abdominis, pectinei, graciles,* and even the *external* and *internal abdominal oblique* muscles, via its connection with the inguinal ligament. Cranially, it is also continuous with *tunica flava* and *linea alba* of the abdomen. Its caudal relations are also complex; it blends into the pelvic symphysis, gives rise to the accessory ligaments of the hip, and is really the most cranial part of the extensive sheet of fibrous material that covers the ventral aspect of the pelvis. Thus, the prepubic tendon of the horse is one of the most important nexuses of connective tissue in the entire body.

Among the major domestic species, the accessory ligament of the hip is unique to equids. Arising from the caudal aspect of the prepubic tendon, this ligament runs caudolaterally to enter the hip joint via the ventral notch in the acetabulum. To do this, it passes dorsal ("deep") to the transverse acetabular ligament to insert on the fovea of the head of the femur. The accessory ligaments reduce the ability of horses to abduct their hips, presumably to minimise inefficient mediolateral movements of the hindlimb. Some abduction is still allowed, however, partly because the ligaments insert close to the point of rotation of the hip joints, rendering them less effective than might be expected. There is some evidence that the accessory ligament may represent a bizarre additional head of the contralateral pectineus muscle.

Caudal to the prepubic tendon, the ventral connective tissue is profuse and strong and occasionally denoted by specific terms:

- The taut transverse band ventral to the pubes is the cranial pubic ligament.

- The curved fibres running along the sciatic arch at the caudal-most part of the bony pelvic floor are the arcuate sciatic ligament.
- These ventral structures are continuous with, and support, the mammary fascia.
- The obturator foramen is almost entirely closed by the obturator membrane although in life this is covered by the laterally directed fibres of the internal obturator (dorsally) and external obturator (ventrally) muscles. A small hole in the cranial membrane permits passage of the obturator nerve. Unlike some ungulates, horses do not have an obvious bony notch through which this nerve passes.

Conclusion

As can be seen, the soft tissues of the equine pelvis are a heterogeneous collection of structures with a variety of functions. Some are dedicated to supporting the structure of the pelvis or sacroiliac joints, whereas others have more varied functions to enclose the pelvic viscera, move the tail, hindlimb or abdomen, or constrain the movement of those parts of the body. Also, the equine pelvis can be seen to exhibit specialisations related to the equine way of life – high body mass, continual walking and grazing, and a speedy birth process.

References

1. Barone, R. *Anatomie Comparée des Mammifères Domestiques*. Lyon: Ecole Nationale Vétérinaire, 1968.
2. Stashak, E. *Adams' Lameness in Horses*, 4th edn. Philadelphia: Lea & Febiger, 1976.
3. Getty, R. *Sisson and Grossman's Anatomy of The Domestic Animals*, 5th edn. Philadelphia: W.B. Saunders, 1975.
4. Pasquini, C., Spurgeon, T. and Pasquini, S. *Anatomy of the Domestic Animals*, 9th edn. Sudz: Pilot Point, 1995.
5. Share-Jones, J.T. *The Surgical Anatomy of the Horse*. London: Baillière, Tindall & Cox, 1908.
6. Tomlinson, J.E., Sage, A.M. and Turner, T.A. Ultrasonographic abnormalities detected in the sacroiliac area in twenty cases of upper hindlimb lameness. *Equine Veterinary Journal* 2003;**35**:48–54.
7. Erichsen, C., Berger, M. and Eksell, P. The scintigraphic anatomy of the equine sacroiliac joint. *Veterinary Radiology and Ultrasound* 2002;**43**:287–292.
8. Degueurce, C., Chateau, H. and Denoix, J-M. In vitro assessment of movements of the sacroiliac joint in the horse. *Equine Veterinary Journal* 2004;**36**:694–698.
9. Engeli, E., Yeager, A.E., Erb, H.N. and Haussler, K.K. Ultrasonographic technique and normal anatomic features of the sacroiliac region in horses. *Veterinary Radiology and Ultrasound* 2006;**47**:391–403.
10. Tomlinson, J.E., Sage, A.M., Turner, T.A. and Feeney, D.A. Detailed ultrasonographic mapping of the pelvis in clinically normal horses and ponies. *American Journal of Veterinary Research* 2001;**62**:1768–1775.
11. Haussler, K.K., Stover, S.M. and Willits, N.H. Developmental variation in lumbosacropelvic anatomy of thoroughbred racehorses. *American Journal of Veterinary Research* 1997;**58**:1083–1091.
12. Habel, R.E and Budras, K.D. Anatomy of the prepubic tendon in the horse, cow, sheep, goat, and dog. *American Journal of Veterinary Research* 1992;**53**:2183–2195.

4 The Normal Anatomy of the Nervous System

Constanze Fintl

Introduction

A working knowledge of the neuroanatomy of the equine back and pelvis is important to the understanding of the diagnosis and treatment of equine back pathology. This chapter describes the neuroanatomical features of the central and peripheral nerves of the equine back and pelvis. As there are currently few studies published on this subject, some extrapolation from other species is necessary.

The vertebral column and spinal cord segments

The horse normally has 7 cervical (C), 18 thoracic (T), 6 lumbar (L), 5 sacral (S) and 20–25 coccygeal (Cy) vertebrae (see Chapter 1), although some individual variation may be present. Typically, this variation involves the numbers of the lumbar and sacral vertebrae, where compensation for reduction or increase in one of these regions will occur in the other. The most common variation appears to be five lumbar and six sacral vertebrae [1, 2], although the number of coccygeal vertebrae is also quite varied but less clinically important.

The equine spinal cord consists of 8 cervical, 18 thoracic, 6 lumbar, 5 sacral and 5 or 6 caudal segments [3]. However, the positioning of the spinal cord segments and the positioning of the corresponding vertebrae are not perfectly matched. During embryonic development, the vertebral and neural components develop closely and, during the initial stages, the spinal cord fills the entire vertebral canal [4]. However, at the latter stages of fetal development, the vertebral column begins to grow in length relatively faster than the spinal cord [3, 4]. The consequence of this is that, in the adult horse, the first three sacral segments are over the body of L6 and the last two sacral and the first few caudal segments are over the body of S1 and cranial part of S2 [3, 5]. Thus the spinal cord containing the last three to four caudal segments ends at S2 [5].

The spinal cord segments also vary in their relative size with the larger segments supplying the peripheral nerves to the appendages. For the forelimb these include parts of segments C6–T1 whereas for the pelvic limbs parts of L4–S1 are involved [6, 7]. These enlarged regions form the cervicothoracic and lumbosacral intumescences respectively.

The caudal extremity of the spinal cord is made up of the *cauda equina*. Caudal to the lumbosacral intumescence, the spinal cord tapers gradually into an elongated cone, the *conus medullaris*, which is finally reduced to a uniform strand of glial and ependymal cells, the terminal filament (*filum terminale*). The terminal filament continues caudally where it soon becomes enveloped by *dura mater* to form the spinal *dura mater* filament (caudal ligament) [8]. The caudal ligament is joined by sacral and caudal spinal nerves that stream caudally through the vertebral canal to exit at their respective intervertebral foramina. The *conus medullaris*, the caudal ligament, as well as the long spinal nerves that run caudally through this distal part of the vertebral canal, together constitute the *cauda equina*.

The spinal nerves

From the dorsal and ventral surfaces of each spinal cord segment emerging nerve rootlets ultimately fuse to form paired spinal nerves containing afferent (sensory) and efferent (motor) nerve fibres. These rootlets contain thousands of nerve fibres that become enveloped within the meninges, join together, and are known as the dorsal and ventral nerve fibres (or 'roots') (Figs 4.1 and 4.2). At each segmental level, a ganglion is present; this is found in the dorsal root at the level of the intervertebral foramen. Just beyond this the dorsal and ventral roots join and intermix to form the segmental spinal nerve (Figure 4.3). The sacral vertebrae have a slightly different arrangement to that described above because of the fusion of these vertebrae. Rather than having intervertebral foramina the sacrum has dorsal and pelvic foramina. This means that, after the spinal nerves have formed within the sacral vertebral canal, they divide into dorsal and ventral branches before exiting through the dorsal and pelvic foramina respectively [5].

The dorsal and ventral nerve roots each have a different function. The dorsal roots carry sensory (afferent) input to the spinal cord through general somatic and visceral afferent neurons, as well as through the general proprioceptive system [6]. The ventral roots carry motor (efferent) innervation from general somatic and visceral efferent neurons respectively.

The position from which spinal nerves innervating a particular spinal cord segment emerge differs at different anatomical sites. Most cervical spinal nerves arising from a particular spinal cord segment emerge through the vertebral foramen cranial to the corresponding vertebra. The exceptions to this are the first and last cervical spinal

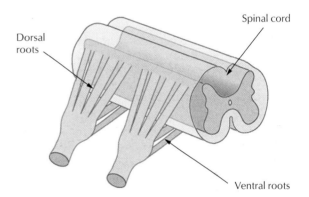

Figure 4.1   A schematic diagram to show the dorsal and ventral rootlets of a typical spinal nerve. (Reproduced from Dellman and McClure [3] with permission from Elsevier.)

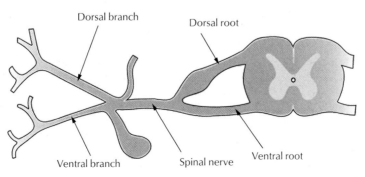

Figure 4.2   A schematic diagram of the divisions of a typical spinal nerve. (Reproduced from Dellman and McClure [3] with permission from Elsevier.)

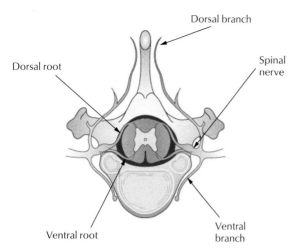

Figure 4.3 A schematic diagram of a cross-section through a vertebra to show the anatomy of the spinal nerve outflow. (Reproduced from Dellman and McClure [3] with permission from Elsevier.)

nerves, which emerge through the lateral vertebral foramina of the atlas and caudal to the seventh cervical vertebrae (and thereby cranial to the first thoracic vertebra), respectively. The spinal nerves from the remaining thoracic and lumbar segments exit through the intervertebral foramen caudal to the corresponding vertebrae.

One consequence of the spinal cord segment is vertebrae mismatch: because the spinal nerves always travel to the intervertebral foramina formed by the corresponding vertebrae, spinal root length reflects the location of the spinal cord segment relative to its numerical vertebra [8], and the spinal nerve length increases as the spinal cord is descended. This is particularly evident in the caudal part of the spinal cord where the spinal nerves from the last segments travel a considerable distance to exit at their respective foramina.

Before describing the distribution of the spinal nerves of the back and pelvis, a brief review of the sensory and motor systems is given.

The sensory system

Sensory information arising from the back and pelvis is mediated through the general somatic afferent (GSA), the general visceral afferent (GVA) and the general proprioceptive (GP) functional systems.

General somatic afferent

GSA activity arises through input from peripheral receptor organs that are specialised to mediate the sensations of pain, pressure, touch and temperature. The cell body of these unipolar neurons is located in the dorsal spinal ganglion whereas the axon continues proximally through the dorsal root [6]. The axon subsequently divides into branches coursing cranially and caudally through the adjacent two or three spinal segments, forming a pathway referred to as the *dorsolateral fasciculus* [6]. Connections from these branches enter the dorsal grey column at several points over the segments, covered by a particular neuron.

General visceral afferent

GVA neurons have their receptor structures located within the internal viscera of the body. Their cell bodies are also located in the spinal ganglion but, unlike the GSA system, the axons of the GVA neurons of the abdominal cavity travel to the spinal cord in nerves that contain neurons from the sympathetic and parasympathetic general visceral efferent (GVE) systems [6]. Once in the spinal cord, the axons terminate on neuronal cell bodies located in the dorsal grey column [6].

It is likely that the pathway for conscious projection of both GSA and GVA neurons follows a similar course through a multisynaptic system involving the thalamus, with further projections to the cerebral cortex [6].

The general proprioceptive pathway

The GP pathway provides important information to the animal regarding the position of the body in relation to the world around it. This information, when analysed with information from the eyes and vestibular system, provides the basis of maintaining posture and a base from which movements can be made – either a simple segmental reflex action, or more complex reflex and conscious responses. The receptor organs (muscle spindles, Golgi tendon organs, etc.) for this system relay information through afferent neurons that join the particular spinal nerves. As for the GSA and GVA systems, the cell body of the GP neuron is located in the spinal ganglion. From the spinal ganglion, the axon continues in the dorsal root to enter the dorsal grey column of the spinal cord where it may synapse directly on α motor neurons (GSE neurons) to complete a reflex arc, whereas others indirectly complete a reflex arc by synapsing on one or more interneurons [6].

Other pathways relay both conscious and unconscious proprioceptive information from the trunk, pelvis and pelvic limbs to the brain. Conscious proprioception is relayed to the cerebral cortex via the dorsal funiculus of the spinal cord in the *fasciculus gracilis* whereas unconscious proprioception is relayed to the cerebellum through the spinocerebellar tracts of the lateral funiculus of the spinal cord [6].

The motor system

The efferent motor neurons of the back, pelvis and pelvic limbs include the general somatic efferent (GSE) and general visceral efferent (GVE) systems. As their names imply, the GSE system innervates voluntary striated muscles whereas the GVE innervates involuntary smooth muscles of the visceral structures, blood vessels and glands. However, both systems consist of lower motor neurons (LMNs) that connect the central nervous system (CNS) with the muscle to be innervated [6]. The cell bodies of the LMNs are topographically organised in the ventral grey horn of the spinal cord. The GSE neurons innervating the axial musculature populate the medial portion of the column, whereas the GSE neurons innervating the appendicular musculature are located laterally and cause the lateral bulge of the ventral grey column that is evident at the cervicothoracic and lumbosacral intumescences [6]. From the neuronal cell body located in the ventral grey column, the axon of GSE neurons courses through the white matter via the ventral root, and joins the spinal nerve on course to its final destination on a skeletal muscle as part of a specific peripheral nerve. A motor neuron and all of the muscle fibres that it innervates constitute a motor unit.

In contrast to the GSE system, GVE lower motor neurons represent involuntary effector responses as part of the autonomic nervous system. The GVE

is composed of two neurons interposed between the CNS and the organ innervated, where the first cell body is located in the grey matter of the CNS and its axon courses through a spinal nerve to a peripheral ganglion [6]. This neuron synapses with a second (postganglionic), peripheral motor neuron, which subsequently terminates in the structure to be innervated.

Distribution of the spinal nerves of the back and pelvis

Spinal nerves of the thoracolumbar region carrying motor and sensory information emerge through the intervertebral foramen, where they soon divide into four major branches: a dorsal branch, a ventral branch, a *ramus communicans* and a meningeal ramus (Figure 4.4) [5].

Dorsal branches

The dorsal branch (ramus) of the spinal nerves divides into lateral and medial branches.

Dorsolateral branch

In the thoracic and lumbar areas the dorsolateral branches (DLBs) pass laterally under the *longissimus thoracicus* and *longissimus lumborum* muscles to surface among *longissimus dorsi, iliocostalis thoracis* and *iliocostalis lumborum*. These DLBs provide cutaneous sensory innervation of

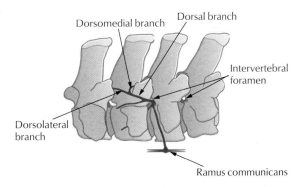

Figure 4.4 A schematic diagram to show lumbar vertebrae 1–4 and the distribution of the branches of the nerves. (Reproduced from Dellman and McClure [3] with permission from Elsevier.)

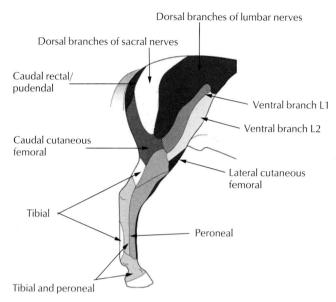

Figure 4.5   A schematic drawing to show cutaneous innervations of the lateral surface of the hindlimb. (Reproduced from Dellman and McClure [3] with permission from Elsevier.)

the thoracic dorsolateral spinous areas. In the lumbar and cranial pelvic areas they provide cutaneous sensory innervation of the dorsum, as well as the areas overlying the superficial gluteal muscles, and are collectively called the cranial clunial nerves. The medial clunial nerves are formed from the DLBs of the sacral nerves and supply the skin from the dorsum, laterally and ventrally, to include the areas overlying the *biceps femoris* muscle mass. The caudal clunial nerves, which are branches of the caudal femoral cutaneous nerve, supply the skin surrounding the ischial tuberosity and caudal thigh areas [9]. A branch of the pudendal nerve provides cutaneous sensory innervation of the perineal area as well as the areas overlying *semitendinosus* whereas dorsal and ventral branches of the caudal spinal nerves innervate the dorsal and ventral aspect of the tail, respectively. Branches of the *iliohypogastric* and *ilioinguinalis* nerves innervate the cranial and caudal areas, respectively, overlying and ventral to the *tuber coxae*.

Cutaneous sensory areas for the equine thoracic limb have been electrophysiologically mapped and areas of single nerve supply (autonomous zones) have been determined [10]. Similar assessment of the equine back and pelvis has not been published and hence assessment of cutaneous

sensory innervation relies on dissection and description of the topographical distribution of the spinal nerve branches discussed above (Figure 4.5) [11]. Currently, areas that display hypalgesia, or even localised sweating indicating change in the autonomic supply to a particular region, can only be approximately localised to particular spinal cord segments and spinal nerves, hence further diagnostic investigations are usually necessary in order to more precisely locate the anatomical site(s) of a lesion.

Dorsomedial branch

The dorsomedial branches (DMBs) of the spinal nerve are directed caudodorsally deep to the multifidus muscles, to which they send branches [5]. They then continue caudodorsally to innervate the vertebral rotator muscles (in the thoracic region) and proceed to provide sensory innervation from the laminae and periosteum of the vertebral arch [5]. The terminal DMBs also supply the caudal aspect of the articular processes of its corresponding segment [5]. In addition, branches of the same nerve terminate on the cranial aspect of the articular processes caudal to its adjacent vertebrae [5]. This means that, for example, the DMB that innervates the caudal aspect of the articular process of

L1 also innervates the cranial aspect of the articular process of L3.

Ventral branches

The ventral rami provide motor innervation to the muscles ventral to the transverse vertebral processes, including the hypaxial musculature as well as the intercostal and abdominal muscles [9]. The ventral branches (VBs) usually divide into two primary branches, the first in the middle of the abdomen and the second close to the linea alba [9]. The VBs of the last three lumbar and first two sacral nerves also give rise to the lumbosacral plexus.

At the current time innervation of the intervertebral disc in the horse has not been determined, although in the dog it was established that the *annulus fibrosus* was innervated but not the *nucleus pulposus* [12]. In addition, each *annulus* was found to be innervated by nerves from the cell bodies in the dorsal root ganglia of two spinal nerve segments cranial and caudal to the disc in question [5, 12]. Clearly, similar studies will need to be performed in the horse to establish the innervation of the intervertebral discs but this study will at the very least give an indication of the arrangement that may also be present in the horse.

Sympathetic innervation

The *ramus communicans* carries both preganglionic and postganglionic sympathetic fibres as well as visceral sensory fibres, from the body cavities via the splanchnic nerves [5]. This branch soon joins the sympathetic trunk, which lies between the *psoas* musculature and the vertebral bodies, either to synapse directly with a local ganglion or possibly to run caudally or cranially to synapse on other vertebral or visceral ganglia.

The meningeal rami are motor to smooth muscles in the vessels of the meninges and sensory to the *dura mater*, and therefore contain postganglionic sympathetic nerve fibres and visceral sensory fibres [5]. However, the meningeal rami described in humans and primates [5, 13, 14] are not well characterised in the horse and were not observed during dissection by Blythe and Engel [5, 13, 14].

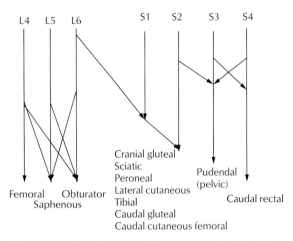

Femoral   Obturator
Saphenous

Cranial gluteal
Sciatic
Peroneal
Lateral cutaneous   Pudendal
Tibial   (pelvic)
Caudal gluteal   Caudal rectal
Caudal cutaneous femoral

Figure 4.6   A line diagram to show an approximation of the origin of the nerves that innervate the pelvis and hindlegs from the lumbosacral plexus.

Lumbosacral plexus

The lumbosacral plexus provides the innervation for the muscles of the pelvis and hindleg; in the horse, it is usually found between L4 and S4, although this may vary between individuals [15]. The lumbosacral plexus gives rise to many important peripheral nerves, each of which usually contains nerve fibres derived from more than one spinal segment (Figure 4.6).

Conclusion

In summary, it is reasonable to assume that the equine central and peripheral neuronal topography and functional distribution to the thoracolumbar region is similar to that in other mammalian species. However, there is still a need to perform detailed anatomical studies to accurately map and determine these important structures of the horse's back.

References

1. Haussler, K.K., Stover, S.M. and Willits, N.H. Developmental variation in lumbosacropelvic anatomy of Thoroughbred racehorses. *American Journal of Veterinary Research* 1997;**58**:1083–1087.

2. Stecher, R.M. Lateral facets and lateral joints in the lumbar spine of the horse. A descriptive and statistical study. *American Journal of Veterinary Research* 1962;**23**:939–947.

3. Dellmann, H.D. and McClure, R.C. Equine nervous system. In: Getty, R. (ed.), *Sisson and Grossman's The Anatomy of the Domestic Animals*, 5th edn. Philadelphia: W.B. Saunders Co., 1975:634–635.

4. Sinowatz, F. Nervensystem. In: Rüsse, I. and Sinowatz, F. (eds), *Lehrbuch der Embryologie der Haustiere*. Berlin: Verlag Paul Parey, 1991:247–286.

5. Blythe, L.L. and Engel, H.N. Neuroanatomy and neurological examination. *Veterinary Clinics of North America* 1999;**15.1**:71–85.

6. De Lahunta, A. *Veterinary Neuroanatomy and Clinical Neurology*. Philadelphia: W.B. Saunders Co., 1983: 318.

7. Fletcher, T.F. Lumbosacral plexus and pelvic myotomes of the dog. *American Journal of Veterinary Research* 1970;**31**:34–41.

8. Fletcher, T.F. Spinal cord and meninges. In: Evans, H.E. (ed.), *Miller's Anatomy of the Dog*. Philadelphia: W.B. Saunders Co. 1996:800–828.

9. König, H.E., Liebich, H-G. and Červeny, C. Nervous system (systema nervosum). In: König, H.E. and Liebich, H-G. (eds), *Veterinary Anatomy of Domestic Mammals*. Stuttgart: Schattauer GmbH, 2004:465–536.

10. Blythe, L.L. and Kitchell, R.L. Electrophysiologic studies of the thoracic limb of the horse. *American Journal of Veterinary Research* 1982;**43**:1511–1524.

11. Sack, W.O. and Habel, R.E. *Rooney's Guide to the Dissection of the Horse*. Ithaca: Veterinary Textbooks, 1982.

12. Forsythe, W.B. and Ghosal, N.G. Innervation of the canine thoracolumbar vertebral column. *Anatomical Record* 1984;**208**:57–63.

13. Kumar, S. and Davies, P.R. Lumbar vertebral innervation and intraabdominal pressure. *Journal of Anatomy* 1973;**114**:47–53.

14. Stillwell, D.L.J. The nerve supply of the vertebral column and its associated structures in the monkey. *Anatomical Record* 1956;**125**:139–169.

15. Getty, R., ed. *Sisson and Grossman's The Anatomy of the Domestic Animals*. Philadelphia: W.B. Saunders Co., 1975.

5 Kinematics of the Equine Back

P. René van Weeren

Introduction

Kinematics is a subdiscipline of mechanics that studies the motions of objects without taking into account the forces that generate this motion. When considering the equine back, one should realise that the back is a segmental, complex structure made up of a large number of separate, but intricately linked, rigid bodies, which are the vertebrae. The motion of the thoracolumbar vertebral column is the sum of motions of the individual vertebrae, which are, however, severely restricted in their movement through numerous anatomical constraints such as muscles, ligaments, intervertebral joints and the presence of ribs. In the same way that kinematics of individual vertebrae contribute to back kinematics, back motion can be considered to be one of the constituting elements of the kinematics of the entire body, hence of the way of moving of the individual. The question of how the back, which bridges the gap between the limbs, functions in quadrupedal locomotion has intrigued scientists for millennia and is an active area of research and discussion today.

In this chapter an overview is first given of the various biomechanical concepts that have been presented as good models for the quadrupedal back. Then, kinematics of the equine back is discussed based on *ex vivo* and *in vivo* research. After that, studies are discussed that have applied newly acquired knowledge on equine back kinematics to answer clinical or equestrian questions. The chapter concludes with a brief evaluation of the importance of equine back kinematics in a general sense, and some ideas on the possible use of data on back kinematics for the management of equine health and performance in the future.

Historical perspective

A scientific interest in the equine gait has existed since horses became an integral part of society and good orthopaedic health was vital for the satisfactory fulfilment of the roles that the animal had in agriculture, transport and, most important of all, the military. Technical advances allowed research in equine gait analysis to flourish from the 1870s until the outbreak of World War II, but the rapid loss of all traditional roles of the horse in society caused interest in this kind of research to wane after World War II. However, the comeback of the species as a sports and leisure animal from the mid-1960s led to what has been called the "second golden age" of equine locomotion research [1]. This second golden age was facilitated by the vast advances in motion capture technology and computational power that simultaneously occurred during this time.

During the second golden age attention focused, during the first decades, principally on limb kinematics and kinetics, with studies on the back being limited to work on cadaver specimens. Only in relatively recent years has more work on the back been done in the living animal. At present, studies are emerging that use the recently acquired fundamental knowledge of equine back kinematics and newly developed, validated analysis techniques for a variety of more applied studies. These studies try to answer questions with respect to the use and mobility of the back that have importance to both veterinary surgeons and a wider equestrian audience.

Biomechanical models of how the equine back works

From Roman times – the "architectural" analogy

Humankind has been thinking about how the mammalian back could best be understood from very earliest times. The famous Roman physician Galen (AD 129–200) described the first known concept [2]. He refers to the prevailing architecture of his days and describes the quadrupedal back as "a vaulted roof sustained by four pillars", the limbs. The spinous processes, pointing in a caudodorsal direction on the ascending part of the arch (or the anterior thoracic part of the trunk) and in a craniodorsal direction on the descending part (posterior thoracic and lumbar part), with the anticlinal (see Chapter 1) vertebrae in top, would prevent the roof from collapsing. Although well thought out, this very first concept cannot be correct because it implies a constant contact between the spinous processes, which is not the case under physiological conditions and in fact may, if present, be a cause of pathology (see Chapter 14).

The nineteenth century – the "bridge" analogy

The next concept was proposed in the middle of the nineteenth century and was again inspired by the technical advances in engineering of those days. This was a time when the railways started

to span continents, crossing rivers and ravines with the help of steel bridges that were masterpieces of daring new construction technology. In the bridge concept of the equine back the limbs are the land abutments of the bridge with the gap between these being spanned by the bridge itself [3–5]. This consists of an upper ledger, (the supraspinous ligament), a lower ledger (the vertebral bodies) and a number of smaller girders, pointing in either a craniodorsal or a caudodorsal direction (the spinous processes and the interspinous ligaments) (Figure 5.1). The bridge concept dominated the veterinary and zoological literature for a long period and has been further elaborated in order to include the biomechanical influences of the head and the tail by using a wide variety of bridge types (Figure 5.2).

Even today the model has its protagonists and is used in the discussions on how the equine back works. The model, however, contains an important conceptual error. The representation of the supraspinous ligament by the upper ledger, and of the string of vertebral bodies by the lower ledger, presumes tensional loading of the former and compressive loading of the latter, because ligamentous structures are not able to withstand compressive loads. In reality, the gravitational forces that act on bridges (and on the mammalian trunk) will cause compression in the upper ledger and tension on the lower one.

The twenty-first century – the "bow-and-string" analogy

The current biomechanical concept of the equine back is that of the bow and string, in which the

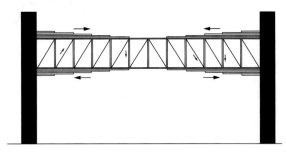

Figure 5.1   A diagram to show the bridge concept of the vertebral column as depicted by Krüger [4]. Open arrows represent tensile forces, closed arrows compressive forces. (Redrawn from Krüger [4].)

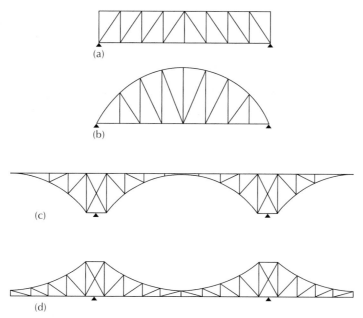

Figure 5.2 A diagram to show various forms of bridges that have been used as a model for the mammalian back. (a) Bridge with parallel girders; (b) parabolic bow-string bridge; (c) parabolic cantilever bridge; (d) inverted parabolic cantilever bridge. (Redrawn from Slijper [2].)

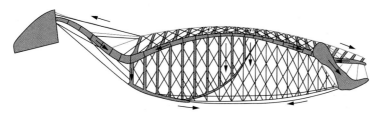

Figure 5.3 A diagram to demonstrate the "bow-and-string" concept of the back according to Slijper [2]. The vertebral column is the bow and the ventral musculature and sternum are the string. The ribs, lateral abdominal musculature, spinous processes and ligamentous connections are additional elements. (Redrawn from Nickel, R., Schummer, A. and Seiferle, E. *Lehrbuch der Anatomie der Haustiere. Band I. Bewegungsapparat*. Berlin: Paul Parey, 1968.)

bow is the thoracolumbar vertebral column and the string the "underline" of the trunk, consisting of the *linea alba*, *rectus abdominis* and related structures. The model was first proposed by Barthez [6], but largely ignored until it was rediscovered by Slijper [2], based on his study of the positions of the spinous processes in a large number of species (Figure 5.3). It is the first concept that takes into account the entire trunk and not just the thoracolumbar vertebral column with adnexa, and presumes that there is a dynamic balance between the tension in the bow and the tension in the string.

Factors that influence the "bow and string"

There are many factors that influence the dynamic balance between tension in the bow and the tension in the string, and the ensuing intrinsic tension of the system (Figure 5.4).

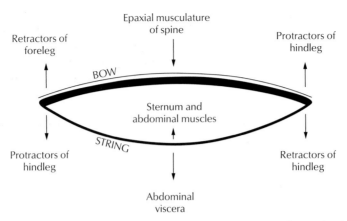

Epaxial musculature
of spine

Retractors of
foreleg

Protractors of
hindleg

BOW

Sternum and
abdominal muscles

STRING

Protractors of
hindleg

Retractors of
hindleg

Abdominal
viscera

Figure 5.4 A diagram to show the factors that determine the motion of the back according to the "bow-and-string" concept. Upward pointing arrows mean a flexing effect on the back; downward pointing arrows represent an extending effect.

Gravitational forces

These will always act in a downward direction and hence tend to straighten the bow, i.e. extend the back or make it more hollow. Gravitational forces act on the back itself, but the gravitational pull on the large intestinal mass of the horse is a more important factor in extending the back. Pregnancy will aggravate this effect and old broodmares typically have a very hollow-backed conformation (acquired lordosis, see Chapter 15). Of course, every load on the back of the horse, including a rider, will have a similar effect.

Active muscular action

This will influence the dynamic equilibrium between the bow and string as well. Contraction of the ventral musculature will tense the bow, i.e. flex the back or make it more arched. In contrast to the belief of many laypeople, contraction of the massive epaxial musculature will have the opposite effect, because the work line of these muscles runs dorsal to the axis through the centres of the vertebral bodies. The only dorsally located muscles that have a flexing effect on the back are the *psoas* muscles. However, these are located between the pelvis and the ventral aspect of the lumbar and last three thoracic vertebrae [7], and will principally affect lumbosacral flexion. There is no musculature ventral to the more cranial thoracic vertebrae that might flex this part of the spine.

Limb movements

Pro- and retraction of the limbs will also affect the balance in the bow-and-string system. Protraction of the hind limbs will, through the forward position of the point of support and the anatomical connection between *gluteus medius* and the lumbar and sacral spinous processes through the gluteal and lumbodorsal fasciae [7], flex the back or tense the bow. In a similar way, retraction of the forelimb will have the same effect. Protraction of the forelimbs and retraction of the hindlimbs will have an opposite effect, i.e. produce a hollow (extended) back.

The head and neck

A last, but not unimportant, factor that should be mentioned is the effect of the head and neck. Lowering the neck will tense the nuchal ligament and exert a forward rotating moment on the spinous processes of thoracic vertebrae T2–6. These long spinous processes forming the basis of the withers provide a long lever arm, and traction on them in a forward direction will provoke tensing of the bow or flexion of the back. Elevation of the head will have an opposite effect.

Kinematics of the equine back – *ex vivo* research

To begin to understand the kinematics of the equine back, it is important to understand that the kinematics of any structure can be described as a product of six basic motions: three rotations and three translations.

Terminology

For the equine spine the three *rotational* movements are the most important. Rotation around the dorsoventral or Z axis represents in most cases lateroflexion or lateral bending (LB), a rotation around the craniocaudal or Y axis represents axial rotation (AR), and a rotation around the axis perpendicular to the sagittal plane or X axis represents ventrodorsal flexion–extension movements (FE) (Figure 5.5a,b). In some studies, X and Y axes are interchanged, which is of course only a matter of definition and does not affect outcome.

In contrast to rotational movements, *translational* movements of vertebrae with respect to each

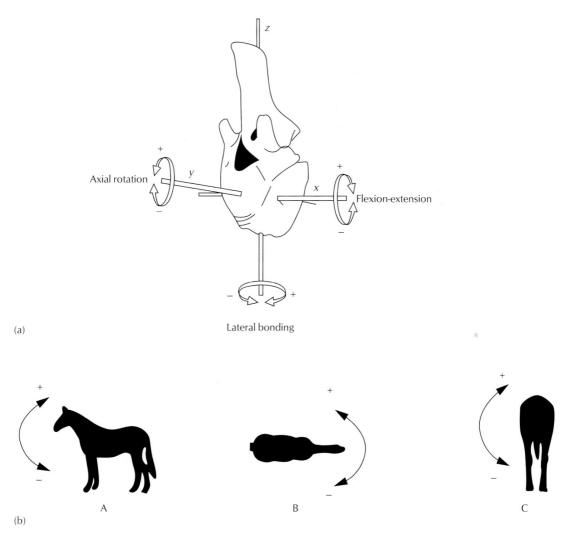

(a)

Axial rotation

Flexion-extension

Lateral bonding

(b)
   A   B   C

Figure 5.5   (a) A diagram to show the basic movements of the back depicted as rotations of an individual vertebra around the three axes of an orthogonal coordinate system. (b) A diagram to show the three basic movements of the equine back: flexion–extension (FE) (A), lateroflexion or lateral bending (LB) (B) and axial rotation (AR) (C).

other are very limited and therefore the translations along the three axes represent in fact the motion of the entire body, which will not be discussed in the context of this chapter. We can, therefore, concentrate solely on the rotational movements of the spine.

Historical in vivo work

Research into equine spinal kinematics has long been mainly limited to work on post mortem specimens due to the large technical problems associated with work in vivo. However, even in the pre-World War II era some *in vivo* work was done. Krüger [4] used two horse cadavers to examine the kinetics of the thoracolumbar column and its movements. This was achieved by manipulating long metal rods that had been inserted in holes drilled in a number of vertebrae, while the pelvis remained fixed. He determined maximal motion in dorsoventral and lateral directions, and compared the outcome with results from *in vivo* work in three horses. The horses were filmed from the side (lateral view) and from above (the camera had been fixed in the branches of a tree!), after marking the midline and two lines perpendicular to it, at the withers and at the pelvis, with white paint. From these experiments Krüger [4] noticed that motion in vivo was considerably less than the maximal ranges of motion found in the cadaver specimens. This observation was confirmed some 40 years later when Jeffcott and Dalin [8] concluded that, in comparison to other species, the natural flexibility of the horse's backbone was very limited.

A number of further studies on back flexibility have taken place. In a large study conducted at the Western College of Veterinary Medicine in Saskatoon, Townsend and coworkers [9] dissected 18 equine spines and marked them with Steinmann pins placed in the geometric centre of the ventral surface of each vertebral body, perpendicular to a plane through the long axis of the thoracolumbar spine and the transverse processes. The sacrum of each spine was fixed in a clamp and manual pressure was used to provoke FE, LB and AR, which were recorded photographically. Conditions before and after removal of the ribcage were compared.

In this study, dorsoventral movement (FE) was found to be maximal in the lumbosacral joint (which may be the transition between either L6 and S1 or L5 and L6). This study demonstrated that the range of motion (ROM) at this site could attain approximately 25°, which was considerably more than in other parts of the spine where FE ROM did not exceed 4° in the area between T2 and L5–6, and was 6–8° at the junction of T1 and T2. LB was largest at T11–12 with 10–11° and decreased in both cranial and caudal directions to about 4° in the cranial thoracic area, and not more than 1° at the last lumbar vertebrae. AR was most prominent in the region T9–14 (up to 5°) and decreased in a cranial (2–3°) and more so in a caudal direction (1°), with the notable exception of the lumbosacral joint (2–3°). Removal of the ribs did not affect FE or LB, but significantly increased AR in the cranial thoracic region. The regional differences in the mobility of the segments of the thoracolumbar spine could be related to anatomical peculiarities of the intervertebral joints and other anatomical or acquired structures, such as the frequent fusion of the transverse processes of the last lumbar vertebrae, explaining the extreme rigidity of this part of the equine spine [10].

Denoix [11] performed a comparable, but more comprehensive *in vitro*, study on cadaver specimens. He included the influence of the position of the head and neck and paid more attention to the effect of the position of a given region of the thoracolumbar spine on the mobility of another region. In this study, FE was found to be larger in the caudal thoracic part (T14–18) than in the rest of the spine, with the obvious exception of the lumbosacral joint. Cervical flexion provoked flexion in the thoracic spine, but also a decrease in FE range of motion in the lumbar area, which was compensated for by an increased mobility at the lumbosacral joint. In the same study, the instantaneous centres of rotation of the intervertebral joints were determined, which appeared to be situated within or near the next adjacent vertebral body. In a study focusing more on the lumbosacral and iliosacral regions, the same author applied forces on isolated pelvises in transverse, axial and dorsoventral directions to assess possible deformations of the structure generated by the forces of locomotion. In the study on the iliosacral region it was shown that the pelvis resisted high loads in the longitudinal direction (i.e. in the direction of impulse in the moving horse), but was more susceptible to forces in the other two directions, which may be substantial under conditions such as taking turns at high speed on insufficiently banked tracks, rearing, and might provoke damage to the pelvic and sacroiliac ligaments. The lumbosacral region was, as in preceding studies, very rigid with respect to FE, with both AR and LB being very limited as well, the latter movement being virtually impossible in the caudal lumbar area (caudal to L4) because of the formation of joints between the transverse processes. It was hypothesised that this high degree of rigidity could lie at the base of the region's tendency to develop intervertebral ankylosis [12].

The relatively frequent diagnosis, or at least suspicion, of iliosacral pathology as a cause of poor performance or subtle and obscure hindlimb lameness (see Chapter 18) has boosted the interest in the kinematics of this very inaccessible area. In an elaborate study using a number of dissected pelvises with pins placed at strategic sites and a state-of-the-art kinematic analysis system, Degueurce et al. [13] showed that the amount of nutation and counternutation (rotation of the sacrum with respect to the pelvic bones in the sagittal plane) did not pass 1°, which is too small to be detected in the living horse. Goff et al. [14] confirmed this observation, but showed a larger range of motion in the transverse plane, when lateral and oblique forces were applied to the pelvis, which may give more insight into the physiological role of iliosacral mobility and might explain the relatively large importance attributed to the area in clinics (see Chapter 18).

Kinematics of the equine back – in vivo research

Whereas studies on the kinematic analysis of limb movement appeared in large numbers from the early 1970s onwards [15], *in vivo* work on back kinematics remained virtually absent for almost another three decades. This was a result of the early days, but partly also of the technical difficulties involved in measuring the small movements of the equine thoracolumbar spine.

Skin marker-based measurement techniques

The first attempts at measuring equine back kinematics in vivo all focused on FE, which is easiest to measure and is influenced least by skin displacement when using skin markers. Audigié et al. [16] used a method developed by Pourcelot et al. [17] and placed five skin markers in the midline over the top of the withers, T12 and T18, the *tuber sacrale* and the sacrocaudal junction. The markers were used to measure what were called the thoracic, thoracolumbar and lumbosacral angles in sound trotting horses. The ROM for all three angles was shown to be less than 4° and variability, both intraindividual and interindividual, was low. Horses extended the back during the first part of each diagonal stance phase and flexed in the last half of the stance phase. Comparison of the kinematic data with electromyographic (EMG) data obtained earlier [18] showed that activity of the epaxial musculature tended to limit FE motion, rather than cause it. A similar conclusion was reached by Licka et al. [19], who presumed, based on an EMG study, that the main action of the *longissimus dorsi* muscle was the stabilisation of the vertebral column against dynamic forces. Licka and Peham [20] used a kinematic analysis system and skin markers on T5, T10, T16, L3, and the sacrum in an attempt to objectify the induction of maximal flexion using manual diagnostic tests. Flexion–extension and LB were investigated and expressed as mean transversal movement (LB) and mean vertical flexion (FE) relative to the height of the withers. Although perhaps not illogical, this measure makes comparison with most of the other literature, where back motion is expressed in degrees, difficult. In a follow-up study, in which LB and FE were induced in the standing horse under simultaneous registration of the positions of markers on the spinous processes of T5, T12, T16 and L3, and S3 and EMG activity of *longissimus dorsi* using surface electrodes, it was concluded that T12 was the best place to take EMG recordings. The EMG data on both sides of the spinous process of T12 showed the highest, and the EMG at the height of L3 the lowest, amplitude [21].

The same research group investigated back kinematics in walking horses on a treadmill. They found maximal LB at L3, which is further caudal than in most other studies. Flexion–extension was maximal at the sacrum. This motion in fact reflects the upward–downward motion of the pelvis as induced by the hind limbs; it cannot be compared with the results of the in vitro studies because in those the pelvis was fixed and thoracolumbar motion was assessed relative to this fixed point.

Kinematic analysis methods using skin markers always suffer to a certain extent from the so-called "skin displacement artefact" that is caused by the fact that the skin will not always exactly follow the motion of the underlying bone, a phenomenon that was actually noted almost 100 years ago [22]. Skin displacement will be of relatively minor importance for FE where the marker will directly follow the movement of the underlying spinous process; however, the coupling of LB and AR during any movement of the spine out of the sagittal plane [23] means that the composed movements of markers under that circumstance cannot be unambiguously broken down into the LB and AR components. Therefore, equine spinal kinematics could never be described fully using skin marker-based techniques.

Invasive marker measurement techniques

The only way to overcome the problems associated with measurements using skin markers was to resort to invasive techniques in which a rigid connection is made between the vertebra and an external marker or measuring device. Haussler et al. [24] used such an approach. They implanted Steinmann pins into a number of spinous processes and connected the pins by liquid metal strain gauges, positioned according to the three axes of rotation. The technique is accurate (resolution of 0.07° in FE and about 0.5° in AR and LB), but laborious, and simultaneous measuring of the motion of a substantial number of vertebrae is difficult. In their first paper, Haussler et al. [24] reported a ROM of FE at the lumbosacral junction at walk of 4°. AR and LB were of the order of 1° at that site. In a follow-up paper [25], the same technique was used to investigate segmental motion at T14–16, L1–3 and L6–S2 at walk, trot and canter. The largest ROM for all three rotations was found at the lumbosacral junction, with the largest ROM for the canter and the smallest for the

trot. ROMs for FE, LB and AR at canter were approximately 5°, 3.5° and 4.5° [25].

The approach chosen by Faber et al. [26] used a technique that was also based on the implantation of Steinmann pins into the spinous processes. Pins were placed under fluoroscopic guidance in the spinous processes of T6, T10, T13, T17, L1, L3, L5 and S3, and in the tips of the *tubera coxae*. To these pins custom-made devices were attached carrying reflective markers that could be detected by the ProReflex kinematic analysis system (Figure 5.6). In this way, a rigid connection was realised between the optical markers and the vertebral body, and the three-dimensional motion of the markers therefore represented the movements of the underlying vertebrae. For data analysis, a newly developed method was used that allowed for the determination of three-dimensional spinal kinematics without defining a local vertebral coordinate system [27]. Measurements were performed on a treadmill at walk, trot and canter (Figure 5.7), and kinematic motion patterns of the vertebrae studied were established [26, 28, 29]. Motion patterns of all three basic rotations had a sinusoidal shape related to the stride cycle. Flexion–extension is induced by pro- and retraction of each hindlimb and therefore shows two peaks for each entire stride cycle, whereas LB and AR have a left and a right component, which is reflected by the positive and negative parts of a single sinus that is generated during a stride cycle (Figure 5.8).

FE at walk was approximately 4° at T6, and remained fairly constant at 8° for all more caudally located vertebrae. LB was maximal for the area round T10 and for the pelvic region (approximately 5°), and less in the more central region of the spine (approx. 3°). AR increased gradually from 4° at T6 to 13° for the tuber coxae. Spinal motion is considerably less at trot than at walk. FE ranged from 2.8° to 4.9°, LB from 1.9° to 3.6° and AR from 3.1° to 5.8° at trot [28]. At canter, maximal ranges of motion for FE, LB and AR were 15.8 ± 1.3°, 5.2 ± 0.7° and 7.8 ± 1.2° respectively [30]. The largest relative FE was, not surprisingly, found between L5 and S3 with 8.6°, which is, however, considerably less than the maximal values found during the *in vitro* experiments alluded to earlier, but a little more than reported by Haussler et al. [25]. Variability of spinal motion appeared to be gait dependent and to vary for the type of motion

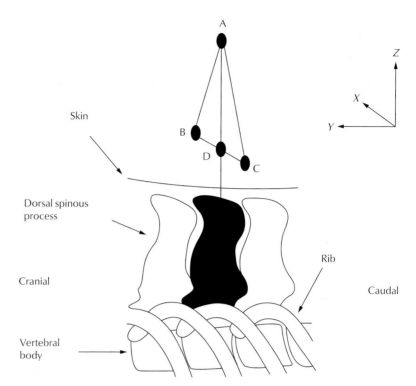

Figure 5.6   A diagram to show a marker device with four markers (A–D) attached via a Steinmann pin to the spinous process of a vertebra and oriented in the laboratory coordinate system (X, Y, Z). (From Faber et al. [26] with permission from the American Veterinary Medical Association.)

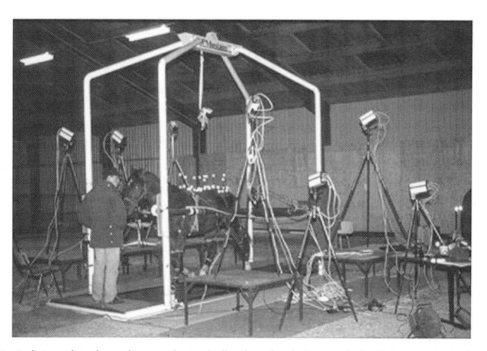

Figure 5.7   A photograph to show a horse on the treadmill with marker devices attached to Steinmann pins implanted into the spinous processes of T6, T10, T13, T17, L1, L3, L5 and S3, and both tubera coxae.

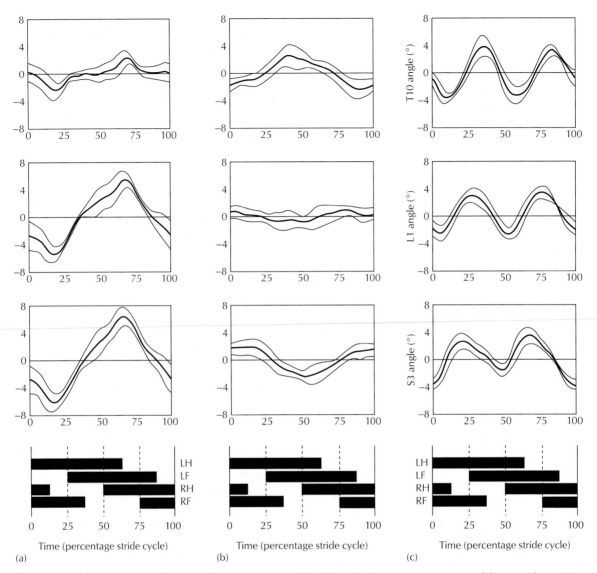

Figure 5.8   A diagram to show the mean (thick line) ± standard deviation (thin lines) motion patterns of three vertebrae (T10, L1 and S3) of five horses walking on a treadmill at a speed of 1.6 m/s. The stride cycle is represented by the bars below (LH: left hind; RH: right hind; LF: left fore; RF: right fore). The bar is closed when the limb is in contact with the ground (stance phase). (a) Axial rotation; (b) lateral bending; (c) flexion–extension. (From Faber et al. [26] with permission from the American Veterinary Medical Association.)

(FE, LB, AR). At walk, within-horse variability (WHV) was lowest at approximately 6% for AR, slightly more for FE (6–8%, but for T6 13.2%) and most for LB (7.8–18.2%). Between-horse variability (BHV) was two to three times higher than WHV for most rotations and vertebrae, and was again higher for LB [26]. At trot LB was the most constant motion (WHV 5.7–8.2%); for FE and AR values ranged from 5.9% to 12.9%, with BHV four to five times higher than WHV [28]. At canter, WHV was lowest for FE (3.1–9.0%), followed by AR (6.3–11.6%) and LB (8.4–12.5%). Here again, BHV values were much higher (Figure 5.9) [30].

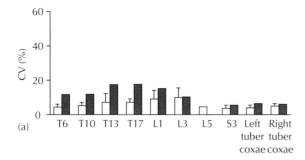

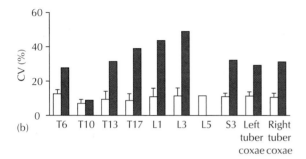

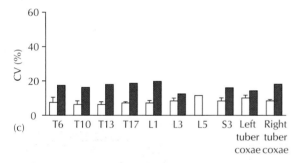

Figure 5.9 A diagram to show the within-horse (open bars) and between-horse (shaded bars) variability at canter in (a) flexion–extension, (b) lateral bending and (c) axial rotation, expressed as a coefficient of variability (CV, as percentage of the range of motion [ROM]). (Redrawn from a thesis by M. Faber – Kinematics of the equine back during locomotion – at Utrecht University, 2001.)

Further modification of the skin marker measurement technique

Based on the invasively acquired data, Faber et al. [29] developed and validated a skin marker-based method of assessing kinematics, which could be used in clinical practice, that is obviously not possible for invasive methods. The method allows for the calculation of ROMs of specific vertebrae,

which gives an indication of overall spinal mobility, but also for the calculation of so-called angular movement patterns (AMPs). The AMP describes the position of a given vertebra in space with respect to two other vertebrae, one on either side, e.g. to calculate the flexion–extension AMP of T10, the three-dimensional coordinates of T6 and T13 are projected onto the Y–Z plane and a line (line 1) is drawn between these points. Assuming that the vertebral column is curved according to the bow-and-string concept [2] and that T10 is located midway between T6 and T13, a second line (line 2) is drawn through the projection of T10 and parallel to the first line. The degree of FE for T10 can then be calculated from the orientation of line 2, relative to the horizontal axis.

For LB, a similar approach is possible with projection on the X–Y plane. AR can be calculated only for the sacrum and is determined from the position of the projection of the *tuber coxae* markers on the X–Z plane, assuming negligible motion in the iliosacral connection [29]. Another parameter that can be used to assess thoracolumbar kinematics is the intravertebral pattern symmetry. For walk and trot, which are symmetrical gaits, the pattern of the AMP during the first half of the stride should be identical to the second half. The amount of similarity, calculated as the correlation coefficient between the patterns during these first and second halves, is called the intravertebral pattern symmetry. The non-invasive, skin marker-based analysis method was tested for repeatability with respect to day-to-day variation by measuring the same horses on five consecutive days, and in two lab settings with different breeds of horses (warmbloods and standardbreds). There was a high degree of between-stride and between-day repeatability in the spatiotemporal variables and in the time–angle diagrams of the vertebrae studied. Variability between horses was considerably larger for all parameters. Between the two labs and breeds small differences were found in range of motion values. It was concluded that this method for the non-invasive analysis of equine back kinematics provided reliable and repeatable data and hence could be used in a more clinical setting [31]. This validated method has further been optimised and is now available as a user-friendly customised program (BacKin), which has been used successfully in several applications of equine back kinematics for the study of clinical and equestrian questions.

Applied kinematics of the equine back

A number of different parameters have been studied using the marker-based analysis system that was developed after the invasive experiments described above. These include physiological factors that may influence back motion, the effects of therapeutic or diagnostic interventions on back movement, the effect of a saddle, the effect of various head and neck positions on back mobility, the influence of induced fore- and hindlimb lameness, the influence of naturally and induced occurring back pain, and the effects of chiropractic treatment.

Physiological factors

Johnston et al. [32, 33] focused on physiological factors. In a study on the effect of conformation on back movement they noticed that horses with longer strides have more FE ROM in the caudal saddle region, which was evident only at walk. A long thoracic back resulted in more LB in the lumbar area and there was a negative relationship between the curvature of the mid-thoracic back and LB at L1–3 and axial rotation of the pelvis [32]. In another study that attempted to create a database for normal kinematics of the equine back as a reference source, they measured 33 normally functioning riding horses and evaluated the effect of physiological variables. Significant differences were found with respect to use and gender with larger LB at T10 and T13 for dressage horses compared with show jumpers. Range of motion for LB was greater at T10 in mares compared with geldings, but less at L5. There was a decrease of FE ROM with increasing age [33].

Therapeutic or diagnostic interventions

Manual manipulation

Faber et al. [34] used the newly developed technique to assess the effect of manual manipulation on back motion and symmetry of movement. Manual treatment of alleged back problems, according to either chiropractic, osteopathic or other principles, has become very popular in recent years, but is not uncontested. Many professionals still take a very sceptical stance and doubt whether the equine thoracolumbar spine can be manipulated at all by human muscular power. Whether or not manipulation may have some effect, it is certain that the popular belief of "realigning a vertebra" after an alleged "subluxation" is not compatible with the anatomical reality and should be discarded as a possible mechanism [35]. In the report on a single case, it was demonstrated that manual treatment could indeed affect vertebral motion patterns and their symmetry, and that the effect lasted (partly) for at least 7 months [34]. The caveat that comes from this study is that the positive clinical effect did not seem to be directly related to the improved symmetry of movement, but was brought about by a change in trainer.

More studies on the effect of chiropractic manipulations on equine spinal kinematics using much larger numbers of horses have recently been performed and have confirmed that chiropractic interventions can alter back kinematics. Haussler et al. [36] showed that spinal manipulative therapy had a beneficial effect on thoracolumbar kinematics in horses in which back pain had been induced by the implantation of fixation pins. Sullivan et al. [37] used chiropractic techniques in various groups of asymptomatic horses and could show that manipulation had a more profound effect on back kinematics than massage or treatment with phenylbutazone. Gómez Álvarez et al. [38] used chiropractic treatment in horses with signs of back pain and showed that the main overall effect of manipulation was a less extended thoracic back, a reduced inclination of the pelvis and improvement of the symmetry of the pelvic motion pattern. However, in this study changes in back kinematics were subtle and not all of them were still measurable at a second measurement session 3 weeks after treatment.

Effect of clinical pathology

The diagnosis of back pain is a controversial item in itself. Recently, Haussler and Erb have introduced the algometer, a device that basically measures the pain threshold when applying pressure to certain areas of the back, as an interesting device that may help in quantifying back pain [39, 40]. However, in many studies back pain is diagnosed by (repeated) palpation, which is a largely subjective procedure. Wennerstrand et al. [41] compared sound horses with horses with back pain, and found a reduction in FE and AR ROM in the symptomatic horses, with a concomitant significant decrease in stride length, which is in accordance with earlier reports [34, 42]. Lateral bending was increased at T13, possibly as a kind of compensatory motion. Most of these horses suffered from kissing spines or muscle soreness.

Diagnoses were made by palpation, radiography and scintigraphy, but no local blocking was performed. The same group assessed the effect of the application of local anaesthetic blocks in the interspinous spaces (T6–L2) of asymptomatic, clinically sound horses. Local blocks resulted at walk in an increase of ROM of FE in virtually all segments of the back and of LB at T10, L3 and L5. Also lateral excursion (defined as the lateral displacement of the markers T10, T13, T17, L1, L3 and L5 in relation to the line connecting T6 and S3) increased for all segments. At trot, the effect was much less. Also the injection of sodium chloride resulted in increased mobility, though to a lesser degree. The mechanism was thought to act via an influence on proprioception of the *multifidus* muscle [43]. This muscle is known to play a very important role in the stabilisation of the back in humans and dysfunction of the muscle is a frequent cause of back pain [44]. Recent research suggests a similar role for this muscle in the horse [45].

The influence of lameness on back kinematics and vice versa has been a controversial item for a long time. In a field study Landman et al. [46] found indications of both lameness and back pain in 26% of the animals belonging to a relatively large ($n = 805$) population of patients presented for orthopaedic problems. In a presumably asymptomatic control population that consisted of horses presented for pre-purchase exams ($n = 399$), concurrence of back problems and lameness was found in 5% only. Dyson [47] diagnosed concurrent forelimb and hindlimb lameness in 46% of horses with thoracolumbar or sacroiliac pain.

Though interesting, the figures, however, give no evidence about a possible causal relationship. In an attempt to learn more about cause and effect, Jeffcott et al. [48] induced transient back pain in trotters by injecting lactic acid into the epaxial musculature. They did not see an effect on linear and temporal stride parameters (stride length, stride frequency, pro- and retraction angles); a stiffer back was noted, but thoracolumbar kinematics were not quantified.

In a very recent study, the same procedure was used in Dutch warmbloods. There were also no effects on the spatial and temporal gait characteristics, but back kinematics were clearly affected, showing a two-stage response that was attributed to an acute reaction to the painful injection and ensuing muscle stiffness in the following days (J. Wennerstrand, unpublished data). From the other side, it has been shown that fore- or hindlimb lameness may alter biomechanics of the back [17, 49]. Horses showed a moderate but evident lameness in these studies. Recently, the effect of very subtle forelimb lameness on back kinematics was studied. It appeared that a very light lameness (maximally two-fifths [50]) increased the vertebral range of motion and changed the pattern of thoracolumbar back movement in the sagittal and horizontal planes, presumably in an attempt to move the centre of gravity away from the lame side and reduce the force in the affected limb [51]. A comparable study in which a subtle lameness was induced in the hindlimbs reported hyperextension and increased ROM of the thoracolumbar back, a decreased ROM of the lumbosacral segment and rotational motion changes of the pelvis [52]. It was concluded that already a slight lameness affects back motion and might hence play a role in the pathogenesis of back problems. It should be stated that these studies have investigated the acute effect of lameness on back motion, whereas in the clinical setting chronic lameness can be presumed to have more influence. Chronic lameness is, however, much more difficult to mimic in an experimental situation.

Performance

In an in-depth longitudinal study on the effects of early training on jumping ability and the early detection of jumping potential, Santamaría [53] used many kinematic parameters, among which were kinematics of the back. It was shown that jumping technique, including the use of the back, to a large extent persisted from foal to adult age [54]. At the end of the 5-year study period, performance was judged by way of a puissance competition. Although back motion in itself did not discriminate between good and bad jumpers, the degree of hindlimb retroflexion (i.e. backward extension of the hindlimbs relative to the back when clearing the jump) was one of the kinematic parameters that were different between the good and the bad jumpers [55].

Saddlery

De Cocq et al. [56] investigated the effect of a saddle with and without added extra weight on back kinematics. They compared four conditions: no tack, a girth, a saddle, and a saddle with 75 kg of lead attached to it in horses walking, trotting and cantering on a treadmill. The weighted saddle appeared to have, at all three gaits, an overall extending effect on the back, but ROM remained the same (Figure 5.10). At canter, the same was true for the saddle-only condition. There was change in limb kinematics too, with forelimb retraction increasing. This observation is nice indirect evidence for the bow-and-string concept: the added weight on the back tends to extend the bow and the horse tries to counteract this influence by more retraction of the forelimbs, which has a flexing effect.

Head and neck position

Rhodin et al. [57] and Gómez Álvarez et al. [58] studied the influence of the position of head and neck on back kinematics. The item is of interest from an equestrian viewpoint. The rules of the Fédération Equestre Internationale (FEI) describe the desired position of head and neck for most dressage activities as follows: "The neck should

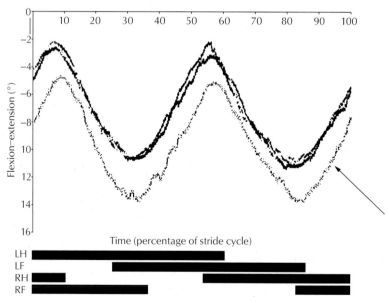

Figure 5.10 A diagram to show the range of motion (ROM) during a single stride cycle of T13 in four conditions: without a saddle, with only a tightened girth, with saddle and tightened girth, and with loaded saddle (75 kg) and tightened girth. Only the last condition (arrow) differed significantly and resulted in an overall increase in extension. However, ROM (maximal flexion minus maximal extension) remained the same. LH: left hind; RH: right hind; LF: left fore; RF: right fore. (Adapted from de Cocq et al. [56] with permission from *Equine Veterinary Journal* Ltd.)

be raised, the poll high and the head slightly in front of the vertical." This is a position that is considerably more upright than the position that the horse will assume by nature. Most classic training systems, that date back hundreds of years [59], use this position, or positions close to it, also during training. However, in the early 1970s it became en vogue in show jumping to train horses with a hyperflexed neck and a much lower and deeper position of the head, which is to a certain extent rolled up against the chest. This position was later named "Rollkur" in the German literature [60]. The technique was taken over by a number of dressage riders, some of whom became extremely successful, but the technique became heavily disputed because of an alleged impact on animal welfare. This has led to much debate in the lay press [61–63]. In an attempt to objectify the effect of head and neck position, Rhodin et al. [57] compared the free or natural position with a higher and lower position, effected by side reins, in unridden horses on a treadmill. They showed a significant reduction of FE and LB ROM of the lumbar back with the head in a high position. Also, AR was reduced. The low position, in which the head and neck were not as hyperflexed as in the Rollkur position, did not differ significantly from the free position, but showed a tendency towards a restriction of movement as well.

Gómez Álvarez et al. [58] studied the item more extensively as part of a large international collaborative project in which horses at Grand Prix level were measured while walking and trotting, ridden and unridden, on a treadmill with an inbuilt force plate under simultaneous motion capture by a 12-camera ProReflex system. Six head and neck positions (HNPs) were studied (Figure 5.11), of which HNP2 resembled the position as defined by the FEI rules, and HNP4 came as close as possible to the Rollkur position. The result was that differences in HNPs predominantly affected the vertebral angular motion patterns in the sagittal plane (i.e. FE). The positions in which the neck was extended (HNP2, -3, -5) increased extension in the anterior thoracic region, but flexion in the posterior thoracic and lumbar regions. For HNP4 the pattern was the opposite. Flexion–extension ROM was reduced at walk in the lumbar region in HNP2 and -5, and at trot

also in HNP3. In HNP5 (extremely high head) the effect was largest and this was the only position in which intravertebral pattern symmetry was negatively affected and hindlimb protraction reduced. In the low and deep position (HNP4) there was an overall increase in FE ROM, in both the thoracic and the lumbar areas (Figure 5.12). It was concluded that a very high position of the head seems to greatly disturb normal kinematics, but that the increased mobility of the back at HNP4 lends some credibility to the statement of a number of trainers that a low position of head and neck may be a useful aid in the gymnastic training of a horse [62].

The analysis system for thoracolumbar kinematics developed by Pourcelot et al. [17], and first applied by Audigié et al. [16], was used to try to discriminate between good and bad jumpers on the basis of back kinematics. Several differences between the groups were found, among which was an increased flexion of the thoracolumbar and lumbosacral junction before take-off in the bad jumpers, which might indicate a less efficient strutting action when forward movement is converted into upward movement [64]. During the airborne phase, lumbosacral extension was less in the bad jumpers.

Robert et al. [65] used the same technology to analyse the effect of treadmill speed on back kinematics (and muscle activity using surface EMG). Horses were trotted at speeds from 3.5 m/s to 6 m/s. It was shown that the amplitude (ROM) of FE and the maximal flexion angles decreased with increasing speed, whereas the extension angles remained the same. Muscle activity increased also, confirming the view that the large trunk muscles (longissimus dorsi and rectus abdominis) act to restrict back movement, rather than actively enhancing or inducing it.

An entirely different approach was chosen by Keegan et al. [66]. They used skin markers, some of which were located on the back, in 12 normal and 12 atactic horses, and analysed the data by computer-assisted, fuzzy clustering techniques that are based on the calculation of signal uncertainty. It appeared that the movement of the lumbar marker (with respect to both LB and FE) was among the few markers that were able to discriminate between normal horses and horses suffering from ataxia.

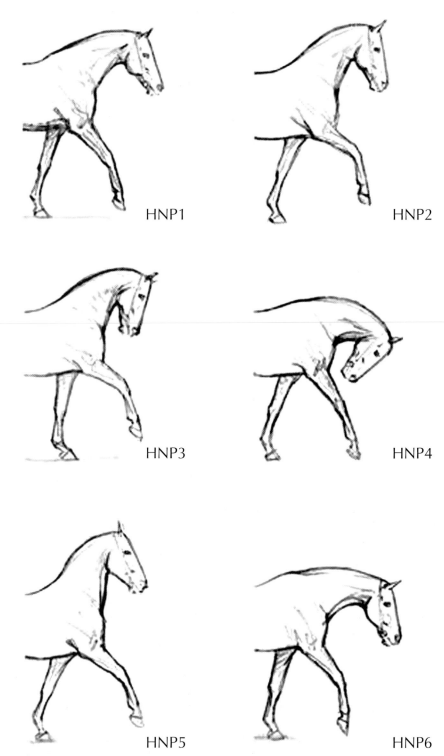

Figure 5.11 A diagram to show head and neck positions (HNPs). HNP1: control (head and neck unrestrained); HNP2: neck raised, bridge of the nose in front of the vertical; HNP3: as HNP2 with bridge of the nose behind the vertical; HNP4: head and neck lowered, nose behind the vertical; HNP5: head and neck in extreme high position; HNP6: head and neck forward downward. (From Gómez Álvarez et al. [58] with permission from Equine Veterinary Journal Ltd.)

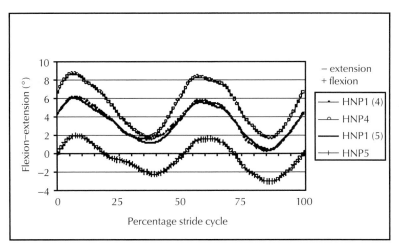

Figure 5.12   A diagram to show flexion–extension angular motion pattern (AMP) of one horse (T10 at walk). The curves represent head and neck positions 4 (HNP4) and 5 (HNP5). HNPs were compared with speed-matched trials with the head and neck in natural position, indicated as HNP1 (4) and HNP1 (5). The stride cycle starts with the left front limb. (From Gómez Álvarez et al. [58] with permission from *Equine Veterinary Journal* Ltd.)

Conclusions and possible future developments

Much has happened in the field of back kinematics since Jeffcott spoke the following words during the fourth Sir Frederick Hobday Memorial Lecture in 1979: "The biomechanics of the equine thoraco-lumbar spine have been considered to some extent, but it requires much greater study if the pathogenesis of the various thoracolumbar disorders are to be properly understood" [35]. We have since learnt much about the maximal ranges of motion of various segments of the equine thoracolumbar spine and the anatomical constraints that limit these motions through both *ex vivo* and *in vivo* research. The clinical evaluation of the motion pattern of the equine back is as difficult as it was in the 1970s, but kinematic analysis techniques have improved vastly and we are now able to document the kinematics of the equine back in a reliable and repeatable way in terms of ROMs and angular motion patterns of individual vertebrae, even if these values are not greater than a few centimetres or a couple of degrees. We should, however, recognise that the general drawbacks of kinematic analysis when used for diagnostic purposes still apply. Aberrant kinematic patterns are in most cases not very specific indicators of back

pathology because there are many more possible pathological conditions than ways that horses can alter their locomotion pattern. Furthermore, there is a large grey area between normal and pathological locomotion patterns. As in patients almost invariably no kinematic data are available that were captured before the onset of the problem, and individual variation in gait patterns is large, it is often impossible to draw conclusions based on a single measurement [67]. It has become clear that the item of individual variation is important particularly in the case of thoracolumbar kinematics, especially at the walk and canter and with respect to LB [26, 30].

The measurement of back kinematics has now become a standard element of various analysis protocols for equine kinematics and back kinematics have been used very successfully to assess the effect of a number of conditions and interventions on equine motion. As the back bridges the gap of the four extremities and back kinematics reflect, through the bow-and-string principle, what happens to the trunk, back kinematics are an excellent parameter to study the influence of any intervention on the animal as a whole. There is a need for hard, scientific data in this area, as has been demonstrated by the discussion on the use of the Rollkur, "over-bent" or "hyperflexed" position of the head in dressage training, which was based on emotion and prejudice rather than on scientifically proven facts. It should be realised, however, that, in items where the ethical acceptability of certain practices is questioned, a more comprehensive approach is required and biomechanical data will have to be complemented by facts from entirely different disciplines.

Telling the future is a hazardous undertaking, but it takes little imagination to predict that, as in any branch of kinematics, modelling will become more important in the study of equine thoracolumbar kinematics. Preliminary studies have already been published by the group from Vienna, who presented a segmental model of the back and simulated a regional increase in stiffness to study the effect on back motion as a whole [68, 69] and compared the outcome with data generated by ex vivo measurements on dissected spines [70]. As with any model, there is a risk that these models are going to lead a life of their own and validation with data acquired *in vivo* remains essential. Generating good quality input data on equine back movement for these models is not very easy, and nor is refining the model to approach real-life conditions, given the complex structure of the back. However, more and more input data on back kinematics, force distribution under the saddle and muscle activity are becoming available, and developments in the modelling and animation area, partly driven by the entertainment industry, happen fast. There is little doubt that much progress will be made in the next few years.

Models may teach us more about the general reaction pattern of the equine back, but are less suitable for use in individual cases. Monitoring and coaching of (top) performance horses with state-of-the-art technology, including the analysis of thoracolumbar kinematics, may be an important development in the near future. Currently cheap, easy-to-use devices are being developed that can register hoof acceleration patterns under field conditions and may help in fine-tuning shoeing practices of racing thoroughbred to the needs and specific requirements of an individual horse [71–73]. Similar developments are possible that will take the analysis of back kinematics out of the lab into the field. Combining data generated by the capture of back kinematics with data from other new technologies, such as saddle pressure measurement devices [74], may allow for the monitoring of subtle changes in the motion pattern of the equine athlete. Such an individualised monitoring programme, which may include other aspects of health and soundness, may lead to the early detection of abnormalities and hence permit timely and adequate preventive measures. In humans, such an individualised approach to peculiarities of gait [75] or to the adaptation of gait to, for example, special shoes [76] is not uncommon. Pattern recognition has been applied to horse–rider interaction as well [77]. These coaching and monitoring programmes for performance horses will never be a substitute for good horsemanship. However, they may support the good horseman or -woman in his or her decisions and they may be of help in the frequent cases of bad horsemanship, thus promoting the well-being of the horse for the benefit of the horse itself and its users.

References

1. van Weeren, P.R. History of locomotor research. In: Back W. and Clayton, H. (eds), *Equine Locomotion*. London: Saunders, 2001:1–35.
2. Slijper, E.J. Comparative biologic–anatomical investigations on the vertebral column and spinal musculature of mammals. *Proceedings of the koninklijke Nederlandse Akademie van wetenschappen series C – Biological and Medical Sciences* 1946;**42**:1–128.
3. Bergmann, C. Über die Verhältnisse der Wärme-Ökonomie der Thiere zu ihrer Grösse. *Göttinger Studien* 1847;**3**:595–708.
4. Krüger, W. Über Schwingungen der Wirbelsäule – insbesondere der Wirbelbrücke – des Pferdes während der Bewegung. *Berliner und Munchener tierarztliche Wochenschrift* 1939;**13**:129–133.
5. Zschokke, E. *Untersuchungen über das Verhältnis der Knochenbildung zur Statik und Mechanik des Vertebraten-skelettes*. Zurich: Orell Fussli, 1892.
6. Barthez, P.J. *Nouvelle mécanique des mouvements de l'homme et des animaux*. Paris: Carcassonne, 1798.
7. Koch, T. *Lehrbuch der Veterinär-Anatomie. Bd. I. Bewegungsapparat*. Berlin: VEB Gustav Fischer Verlag, 1970.
8. Jeffcott, L.B. and Dalin, G. Natural rigidity of the horse's backbone. *Equine Veterinary Journal* 1980;**12**: 101–108.
9. Townsend, H.G.G., Leach, D.H. and Fretz, P.B. 1983; Kinematics of the equine thoracolumbar spine. *Equine Veterinary Journal* **15**:117–122.
10. Townsend, H.G.G. and Leach, D.H. Relationship of intervertebral joint morphology and mobility in the

equine thoracolumbar spine. *Equine Veterinary Journal* 1984;**16**:461–466.

11. Denoix, J-M. Kinematics of the thoracolumbar spine in the horse during dorsoventral movements: a preliminary report. In: *Second International Conference on Equine Exercise Physiology*. Davis, CA: ICEEP Publications, 1987.

12. Denoix, J.M. Aspects fonctionnels des régions lombo-sacrale et sacro-iliaque du cheval. *Pratique Veterinaire Equine* 1992;**24**;13–21.

13. Degueurce, C., Chateau, H. and Denoix, J.M. In vitro assessment of movements of the sacroiliac joint in the horse. *Equine Veterinary Journal* 2004;**36**:694–698.

14. Goff, L.M., Jasiewicz, J., Jeffcotte, L.B. et al. Movement between the equine ilium and sacrum – in vivo and in vitro studies. *Equine Veterinary Journal* 2006;**36**(suppl):457–461.

15. Fredricson, I. and Drevemo, S. A new method of investigating equine locomotion. *Equine Veterinary Journal* 1971;**3**:137–140.

16. Audigié, F., Pourcelot, P., Degueurce, C., Denoix, J-M. and Geiger, D. Kinematics of the equine back: flexion–extension movements in sound trotting horses. *Equine Veterinary Journal* 1999;**30**(suppl): 210–213.

17. Pourcelot, P., Audigié, F.C.D., Denoix, J-M. and Geiger, D. Kinematics of the equine back: a method to study the thoracolumber flexion–extension movements at the trot. *Veterinary Research* 1998;**29**:519–525.

18. Tokuriki, M., Nakada, A. and Aoki, O. Electromyographic activity of trunk muscles in the horse during locomotion and synaptic connections of neurons of trunk muscles in the cat. In: *First ESB Workshop on Animal Locomotion*. Utrecht: S. Karger, 1991.

19. Licka, T.F., Peham, C. and Frey, A. Electromyographic activity of the longissimus dorsi muscles in horses during trotting on a treadmill. *American Journal of Veterinary Research* 2004;**65**:155–158.

20. Licka, T.F. and Peham, C. An objective method for evaluating the flexibility of the back of standing horses. *Equine Veterinary Journal* 1998;**30**:412–415.

21. Peham, C., Frey, A., Licka, T.F. and Scheidl, M. Evaluation of the EMG activity of the long back muscle during induced back movements at stance. *Equine Veterinary Journal* 2001;**33**(suppl):165–168.

22. Fick, R.A.G-u.M.B. Allgemeine Gelenk- und Muskelmechanik. In: Bardeleben, K. von (ed.), *Handbuch der Anatomie des Menschen*. Jena: Gustav Fischer, 1910.

23. Denoix, J.M. Lesions of the vertebral column in poor performance horses. In: *World Equine Veterinary Association symposium*. Pullman: WEVA Publications, 1999.

24. Haussler, K.K., Bertram, J.E.A., Gellman, K. and Hermanson, J.W. Dynamic analysis of in vivo segmental spinal motion: An instrumentation strategy. *Veterinary and Comparative Orthopaedics and Traumatology* 2000;**13**:9–17.

25. Haussler, K.K., Bertram, J.E.A., Gellman, K. and Hermanson, J.W. Segmental in-vivo vertebral kinematics at the walk, trot and canter: A preliminary study. *Equine Veterinary Journal* 2001;**33**(suppl): 160–164.

26. Faber, M., Schamhardt, H.C., van Weeren, P.R. et al. Basic three-dimensional kinematics of the vertebral column of horses walking on a treadmill. *American Journal of Veterinary Research* 2000;**61**:399–406.

27. Faber, M., Schamhardt, H.C. and van Weeren, P.R. Determination of 3D spinal kinematics without defining a local vertebral co-ordinate system. *Journal of Biomechanics* 1999;**32**:1355–1358.

28. Faber, M., Johnston, C., Schamhardt, H. et al. Basic three-dimensional kinematics of the vertebral column of horses trotting on a treadmill. *American Journal of Veterinary Research* 2001;**62**:757–764.

29. Faber, M., Schamhardt, H., van Weeren, P.R. and Barneveld, A. Methodology and validity of assessing kinematics of the thoracolumbar vertebral column in horses based on skin-fixated markers. *American Journal of Veterinary Research* 2001;**62**:301–306.

30. Faber, M., Johnston, C., Schamhardt, H.C. et al. Three-dimensional kinematics of the equine spine during canter. *Equine Veterinary Journal* 2001; **33**(suppl):145–149.

31. Faber, M., Johnston, C., van Weeren, P.R. and Barneveld, A. Repeatability of back kinematics in horses during treadmill locomotion. *Equine Veterinary Journal* 2002;**34**:235–241.

32. Johnston, C., Holmt, K., Faber, M. et al. Effect of conformational aspects on the movement of the equine back. *Equine Veterinary Journal* 2002;**34**(suppl): 314–318.

33. Johnston, C., Roethlisberger-Holm, K., Erichsen, C., Eksell, P. and Drevemo, S. Kinematic evaluation of the back in fully functioning riding horses. *Equine Veterinary Journal* 2004;**36**:495–498.

34. Faber, M., van Weeren, P.R., Scheepers, M. and Barneveld, A. Long-term follow-up of manipulative treatment in a horse with back problems. *Journal of Veterinary Medicine Series A* 2003;**50**:241–245.

35. Jeffcott, L.B. Radiographic examination of the equine vertebral column. *Veterinary Radiology* 1979;**20**:135–139.

36. Haussler, K.K., Hill, A.E., Puttlitz, C.M. and McIlwraith, C.W. Effects of vertebral mobilization and manipulation on kinematics of the thoracolumbar region. *American Journal of Veterinary Research* 2007; **68**:508–516.

37. Sullivan, K.A., Hill, A.E. and Haussler, K.K. The effects of chiropractic, massage and phenylbutazone on spinal mechanical nociceptive thresholds in

horses without clinical signs. *Equine Veterinary Journal* 2008;**40**:14–22.

38. Gómez Álvarez, C.B., l'Ami, J.J., Moffatt, D., Back, W. and van Weeren, P.R. Effect of chiropractic manipulations on the kinematics of back and limbs in horses with clinically diagnosed back problems. *Equine Veterinary Journal* 2008;**40**:in press.

39. Haussler, K.K. and Erb, H.N. Mechanical nociceptive thresholds in the axial skeleton of horses. *Equine Veterinary Journal* 2006;**38**:70–75.

40. Haussler, K.K. and Erb, H.N. Pressure algometry for the detection of induced back pain in horses: a preliminary study. *Equine Veterinary Journal* 2006;**38**: 76–81.

41. Wennerstrand, J., Johnston, C., Roethlisberger-Holm, K. et al. Kinematic evaluation of the back in the sport horse with back pain. *Equine Veterinary Journal* 2004;**36**:707–711.

42. Jeffcott, L.B. Disorders of the thoracolumbar spine of the horse – a survey of 443 cases. *Equine Veterinary Journal* 1980;**12**:197–210.

43. Roethlisberger-Holm, K., Wennerstrand, J., Lagerquist, U., Eksell, P. and Johnston, C. Effect of local analgesia on movement of the equine back. *Equine Veterinary Journal* 2006;**38**:65–69.

44. San Juan, J.G., Yaggie, J.A., Levy, S.S. et al. Effects of pelvic stabilization on lumbar muscle activity during dynamic exercise. *Journal of Strengthening and Conditioning Research* 2005;**19**:903–907.

45. Stubbs, N.C., Hodges, P.W., Jeffcott, L.B. et al. Functional anatomy of the caudal thoracolumbar and lumbosacral spine in the horse. *Equine Veterinary Journal* 2006;**36**(suppl):393–399.

46. Landman, M.A., de Blaauw, J.A., van Weeren, P.R. and Hofland, L.J. Field study of the prevalence of lameness in horses with back problems. *Veterinary Record* 2004;**155**:165–168.

47. Dyson, S.J. The interrelationships between back pain and lameness: a diagnostic challenge. In: *Annual Congress of the British Equine Veterinary Association*. Harrogate: Equine Veterinary Journal Publications, 2005.

48. Jeffcott, L.B., Dalin, G., Drevemo, S. et al. Effect of induced back pain on gait and performance of trotting horses. *Equine Veterinary Journal* 1982;**14**:129–133.

49. Buchner, H., Savelberg, H., Schamhardt, H. and Barneveld, A. Head and trunk movement adaptations in horses with experimentally induced fore- or hind limb lameness. *Equine Veterinary Journal* 1996;**28**:71–76.

50. Stashak, E. *Adams' Lameness in Horses*, 4th edn. Philadelphia: Lea & Febiger, 1976.

51. Gómez Álvarez, C.B., Wennerstrand, J., Bobbert, M.F. et al. The effect of induced forelimb lameness on the thoracolumbar kinematics in riding horses. *Equine Veterinary Journal* 2007;**39**:197–201.

52. Gómez Álvarez, C.B., Bobbert, M.F., Lamers, L. et al. The effect of induced hindlimb lameness on thoracolumbar kinematics during treadmill locomotion. *Equine Veterinary Journal* 2008; in press.

53. Santamaría, S. From foal to performer: development of the jumping technique and the effect of early training. Thesis, Utrecht University, 2004.

54. Santamaría, S., Bobbert, M.F., Back, W., Barneveld, A. and van Weeren, P.R. Evaluation of consistency of jumping technique in horses between the ages of 6 months and 4 years. *American Journal of Veterinary Research* 2004;**65**:945–990.

55. Bobbert, M.F., Santamaría, S., van Weeren, P.R., Back, W. and Barneveld, A. Can jumping capacity of adult show jumping horses be predicted on the basis of submaximal free jumps at foal age? A longitudinal study. *The Veterinary Journal* 2005;**170**:212–221.

56. de Cocq, P., van Weeren, P.R. and Back, W. Effects of girth, saddle and weight on movements of the horse. *Equine Veterinary Journal* 2005;**37**:231–234.

57. Rhodin, M., Johnston, C., Holm, K.R., Wennerstrand, J. and Drevemo, S. The influence of head and neck position on kinematics of the back in riding horses at the walk and trot. *Equine Veterinary Journal* 2005;**37**:7–11.

58. Gómez Álvarez, C.B., Rhodin, M., Bobbert, M.F. et al. The effect of head and neck position on the thoracolumbar kinematics in the unridden horse. *Equine Veterinary Journal* 2006;**36**(suppl):445–451.

59. Decarpentry, A.E. *Academic Equitation: A preparation for international dressage tests.* Tonbridge: J.A. Allen & Co., 1971.

60. Meyer, H.R.S.G. Rollkur. *St Georg* 1992:70–73.

61. Balkenhol, K., Müller, H., Plewa, M. and Heuschmann, G., 2003; Zur Entfaltung kommen – statt zur Brust genommen. *Reiter Revue* **46**, 46–51.

62. Janssen, S. Zur Brust genommen. *Reiter Revue* 2003;**46**:41–45.

63. Schrijer, S. and van Weeren, P.R. Auf dem falschen Rücken ausgetragen. *Reiter Revue* 2003;**46**:13–15.

64. Cassiat, G., Pourcelot, P., Tavernier, L. et al. Influence of individual competition level on back kinematics of horses jumping a vertical fence. *Equine Veterinary Journal* 2004;**36**:748–753.

65. Robert, C., Audigié, F., Valette, J.P., Pourcelot, P. and Denoix, J-M. Effects of treadmill speed on the mechanics of the back in the trotting saddlehorse. *Equine Vet Journal* 2001;**33**(suppl):154–159.

66. Keegan, K.G., Arafat, S., Skubic, M. et al. Detection of spinal ataxia in horses using fuzzy clustering of body position uncertainty. *Equine Veterinary Journal* 2004;**36**:712–717.

67. van Weeren, P.R. The clinical applicability of automated gait analysis systems. *Equine Veterinary Journal* 2002;**34**:218–219.

68. Peham, C. and Schobesberger, H. Influence of the load of a rider or of a region with increased stiffness on the equine back: a modelling study. *Equine Veterinary Journal* 2004;**36**:703–705.
69. Peham, C. and Schobesberger, H. A novel method to estimate the stiffness of the equine back. *Journal of Biomechanics* 2006;**39**:2845–2849.
70. Schlacher, C., Peham, C., Licka, T.F. and Schobesberger, H. Determination of the stiffness of the equine spine. *Equine Veterinary Journal* 2004;**36**:699–702.
71. Dallap Schaer, B., Ryan, C.T., Boston, R.C. and Nunamaker, D.M. The horse–racetrack interface: a preliminary study on the effect of shoeing on impact trauma using a novel wireless data acquisition system. *Equine Veterinary Journal* 2006;**38**:664–670.
72. Dyson, S., Murray, R., Branch, M. and Harding, E. The sacroiliac joints: evaluation using nuclear scintigraphy. Part 2: Lame horses. *Equine Veterinary Journal* 2003;**35**:233–9.
73. Ryan, C.T., Dallap Schaer, B. and Nunamaker, D.M. A novel Wireless Data Acquisition System for the measurement of hoof accelerations in the exercising horse. *Equine Veterinary Journal* 2006;**38**:671–674.
74. von Rechenberg, B. Saddle evaluation; poor fit contributing to back problems in horses. In: Auer, J.A. and Stick, J.A. (eds), *Equine Surgery.* St Louis, MO: Saunders, 2006:963–971.
75. Schöllhorn, W.I., Nigg, B.M., Stefanshyn, D. and Liu, W. Identification of individual walking patterns using time discrete and time continuous data sets. *Gait and Posture* 2002;**15**:180–186.
76. Nigg, B.M., Khan, A., Fisher, V. and Stefanshyn, D. Effect of shoe insert construction on foot and leg movement. *Medicine and Science in Sports and Exercise* 1998;**30**:550–555.
77. Schöllhorn, W.I., Peham, C., Licka, T.F. and Scheidl, M. A pattern recognition approach for the quantification of horse and rider interactions. *Equine Veterinary Journal* 2006;**36**(suppl):400–405.

Section 2

The Investigation of Back Pathology

6 The Clinical Examination

Graham A. Munroe

Introduction

A thorough clinical examination is the absolute foundation of good veterinary practice and its use in the diagnosis of equine back pathology is no exception. The process of the clinical examination involves collection of information about normal, as well as abnormal, function of the back, pelvis and limbs of the horse. In general, the steps followed during the clinical evaluation of horses with suspected back pathology include the following:

- Determination and clarification of the presenting problem.
- Determination of the temporal course of the problem. When did the problem start? Is the problem getting worse/better or staying the same?
- Performance of a thorough physical examination.
- Establishment of a list of possible differential diagnoses that can affect or cause disease in this particular area of the back or pelvis.
- Determination of which diagnostic test(s) will establish whether the disease is present and its extent.

Factors that might complicate the clinical examination

The cause of back pain can be very difficult to pinpoint in some cases and requires a thorough and systematic approach to the clinical examination along with advanced diagnostic aids in specific cases. On many occasions a definitive diagnosis can be made only by eliminating other conditions that may present as possible back pain.

An example of a condition that must be recognised and ruled out is whether or not the horse is "cold backed". "Cold backed" is a term used to describe cases in which there is an apparent marked hypersensitivity over the back. These horses show transient stiffness and marked dipping of the spine after the rider mounts the horse and sits in the saddle. These horses often have no other clinical signs and a source of pain is rarely found, although some may have had previous back pain.

The diagnosis of back pain in the horse is further confused in that some animals appear to be "thin skinned" or naturally sensitive, and resent palpation of the back in the apparent absence of genuine pathology. It must be appreciated that assessment of the degree of pain in a case is complicated by the marked individual variation in the response to pain, and this can certainly be affected by the animal's breeding and temperament. Anecdotally draft horses and ponies appear to tolerate pain very stoically and show few clinical signs, whereas some other breeds such as thoroughbred and warmblood horses are more likely to react to a painful stimulus. However, every horse is an individual and it is well recognised that some horses seem to be better able to cope with pain than others and apparently perform at very high levels, despite the presence of clearly evident back pathology and its associated pain.

The purpose of the clinical examination

Information collected during the clinical examination is used for two main purposes:

1. To determine if abnormalities exist in the back or pelvis
2. To determine the most suitable way of definitively diagnosing the pathology present.

Background to the clinical examination of a horse with suspected back pain

Back pain is a common presenting complaint from owners and riders in a variety of horses but particularly in performance horses, such as show jumpers and dressage horses. One of the most important factors to be aware of when dealing with horses with suspected back pain is that the owner/rider/trainer usually becomes aware of a problem due to a lack of or poor performance of the animal rather than actual thoracolumbar pain.

Miscellaneous cases of perceived back pain

Although many horses that present to the veterinary surgeon for back pain do have a genuine problem, there are a number of cases that do not. In some of these latter cases the problems that are considered by the owner/rider/trainer to be due to back pain are due instead to faulty or poorly fitting saddlery or poor riding. Sadly it is also true

that in other cases inadequately or poorly schooled horses may present with an owner's complaint of "back pain" subsequent to their perceived abnormal movement or inability to perform dressage movements or jump large enough fences. Close questioning usually reveals that these horses have simply never performed at the levels expected and are usually insufficiently athletic to do so. This is in contrast to the proven competition horse that is clearly unable to perform at its previous level of athletic function – these horses are far more likely to have genuine pathology. Finally, and somewhat controversially, there are the apparent or alleged back problems, which are popular with owners, trainers and various "back people", and which have limited anatomical or pathophysiological evidence for their existence. Such problems include the horse having "put its back out" or having a "trapped or pinched nerve". Such diagnoses contribute nothing to a proper understanding of genuine back pathology.

Primary back pain versus secondary back pain

There are a considerable number of clinically significant osseous and soft tissue-related primary back problems which are discussed in detail elsewhere in this book, but in many cases back pain arises secondary to other problems. Horses with back pain as a secondary consequence often have primary orthopaedic conditions. In most cases orthopaedic problems with the hindlimbs (often bilateral pathology) [1] are the cause of secondary back pain. However, on some occasions back pain can be also associated with forelimb lameness. These lamenesses have been proposed to lead to major changes in the gait of the horse that result in secondary pain in the pelvic and back regions as a consequence of using these structures.

The clinical examination

The complete clinical examination includes the following:

- Clinical history
- Clinical examination at rest

- Initial inspection
- Symmetry of pelvis and hindquarter muscles
- Palpation of the thoracolumbar spine and sacrum
- Manipulation
- Examination of fore- and hindlimbs
- Examination of the neck
- Rectal examination
- Oral examination
- Clinical examination at exercise
- Ridden exercise
- Neurological examination (see Chapter 7).

Clinical history

Acquiring a good, comprehensive history is particularly important in those horses presenting with back pain. The clinical signs of back pain are varied and multiple, and easily confusable with a number of other clinical problems. Both a general clinical history and a specific clinical history should be taken (Boxes 6.1 and 6.2).

Box 6.1   Important data to be gathered when taking a *general* clinical history of a horse with suspected back pathology

Date of acquisition
Pre-purchase examination
Onset and duration of clinical signs
Type of work
Have clinical signs improved or worsened?
Any treatment given?
Response to treatment
Details of saddlery
Rider's capability

Box 6.2   Important data to be gathered when taking a *specific* clinical history of a horse with suspected back pathology

Any falls or trauma?
Difficulty urinating/defecating?
Does the horse lie down and/or roll?
Reluctant to be rugged or groomed?
Difficulty with farrier?

After the basic signalment (age, breed and sex of the horse) is taken, in the author's opinion the starting point for the history should be the date of acquisition of the horse, which may be associated with a pre-purchase veterinary examination. Although back problems may pre-exist this point, and it is important to ascertain any prior history, this will have been a comprehensive veterinary examination at a definite point in time from which the clinician can work. It is important to question the owner about the time of onset of the clinical signs and the duration of the clinical signs to ascertain whether the problem is acute or chronic. Information on the management of the horse and the problems regarding performance are all extremely important. The type of work that the horse performs and how this has changed, as well as whether the horse shows the signs during free exercise, can be helpful. Detailed information about the horse's performance before and after the point of any deterioration is useful, particularly close questioning to determine whether the signs may have been occurring earlier than the owner has noticed them. It is also important to ascertain whether the clinical signs are improving, worsening or remaining the same, and to note any treatment given, medication, physiotherapy or manipulation, and any response seen.

Details about the saddle, and whether pads or numnahs are used, and whether these were fitted by a qualified person or have been changed recently, are essential. It is important to assess (tactfully!) the rider's size and skill because these will have a direct effect on how the horse is ridden and the forces to which the horse's back will be subjected. It is vital during the history taking and the examination to assess the quality of the schooling and equitation of the horse and the experience of the rider, because many problems supposedly related to back pain are in fact due to poor schooling of the horse or poor ability of the rider, as has been noted above. If the horse has been ridden by other, perhaps more experienced, riders, it is useful to find out how this affected the clinical signs.

Further information regarding the clinical history should be focused on previous falls or any acute traumatic incident that may have led to damage to the back. At rest, there may be a history, in severe cases, of horses having difficulty in straddling to urinate or defecate, or reluctance to lie down or roll, especially in its stable. The owner may have noted resentment to placement of rugs over the loins or quarters, or during grooming. The farrier may have commented that the horse shows reluctance to having the legs lifted or shod. In some cases there is a history of the horse responding unusually to weight on its back and these horses are sometimes termed "cold backed", as discussed above. This can be learned behaviour, possibly following back pain, and can be a misleading sign that should be viewed with caution. The horse may collapse or roach (arch the back upwards) when backed or ridden, occasionally bucking/rearing on mounting or when ridden, and there may be problems during saddling up or girth tightening.

The history of any problems occurring at exercise is extremely important, particularly in helping to differentiate primary from secondary back problems. There may be a history at exercise of unilateral or bilateral hindlimb or multiple leg lameness. On many occasions these are missed by the owner and not picked up until there is a veterinary examination or when the horse is presented to a more experienced owner or trainer.

At exercise there may be a resistance to moving backwards or reining back when ridden, and changes in general attitude of the horse during exercise. This can manifest as signs of a lack of enthusiasm for work with a poor and restricted gait, particularly at faster paces. The owner may complain of poorly defined gait changes when ridden, suggesting hindlimb stiffness or decreased impulsion, or, particularly in dressage animals, lack of bend or suppleness in the back. There may be a marked difference between in-hand and ridden gaits.

In the jumping horse disinclination to jump, particularly over combination-type fences, may be a feature. When they do jump they may jump with a fixed back, making the horse very flat through the jumps and leading to an increased chance of hitting the jumps. A loss of jumping fluidity, timing and confidence with decreased performance is a common complaint. In horses undertaking dressage or other flat work there may be problems in movement, a history of decreasing scores during dressage competitions, a failure to stop or yield to aids, a lack of bend or resistance to collection, a developing sour attitude and poor impulsion. Finally, back pain can give rise to clinical signs of head shaking and tail swishing and, when seen, these signs should always be considered as a possible indicator of back pain.

Clinical examination at rest

The clinical examination at rest needs to be carried out carefully with examination of the whole horse for other causes of lameness and loss of performance problems. Signs of back pain are often varied, subtle and inconsistent between individuals, and therefore it is important that there is a systematic and logical approach to examination.

Initial inspection

The author prefers to have the horse stood "four square" (Plate 4) on a flat, hard surface, preferably outside, but alternatively in a large box, or occasionally in stocks. This is used to carry out a general appraisal of the conformation of the fore- and hindlimbs, as well as assessing general condition and muscling of the horse. Specific note is made of whether the horse is subjectively "long" or "short" in its back (Plate 5), with regard to conformation, and whether there are any spinal curvatures, such as lumbar kyphosis, thoracic lordosis (Plate 6) or scoliosis (Table 6.1, and see Chapters 8 and 15).

Table 6.1 The nomenclature of abnormal spinal conformation

Term	Origin	Explanation
Kyphosis	Greek: "hump"	Upward (dorsal) curvature of the back. Usually lumbar
Lordosis	Greek: "bent backwards"	Downward (ventral) curvature of the back. Usually thoracic
Scoliosis	Greek: "crooked"	Lateral and rotational curvature of the spine

Scoliosis is best diagnosed by viewing the dorsal midline of the back from behind the horse (Plate 7a), standing on a raised stool or chair as necessary, with the horse straight and aligned through its neck, back and quarters. Lateral curvature may also occur due to spastic sclerosis from long-term pain in the back leading to changes in muscle tension. Epiaxial muscle atrophy may also occur due to areas of pain or inadequate suitable work. At this stage in the clinical examination the symmetry of gluteal and pelvic muscles should also be carefully assessed (Plate 7b). Any lumps, scars or saddle marks on the withers or saddle region should be noted and examined further at the palpation stage. During this visual inspection, it is important to start to assess the animal's temperament and general behaviour and whether it is well schooled and disciplined. Some clinicians believe that there is a correlation between nervous or temperamental animals and the incidence of back pain, although many horses with a chronic back problem may alter their behaviour or change temperament in response to the pain. In some cases with severe back pain the horse may assume abnormal conformations such as standing with the front limbs out in front of it, in a similar manner to a laminitic horse, or commonly tucking its limbs and hind quarters underneath it and assuming a rather "humped" hindlimb and lower back posture.

Symmetry of pelvis and hindquarter muscles and bones

Assessment of the symmetry of the pelvis and hindquarter muscles is extremely important in differentiating a pelvic or hindlimb lameness problem. It should be carried out as subjectively as possible by standing the horse on a level surface and by using assistant's fingers or tape markers on both prominences of the *tubera coxae*. The significance of any asymmetry observed must be considered in the light of other clinical signs and the history (Table 6.2).

Slight deviations from pure symmetry are certainly detectable but may not be clinically significant. Unilateral muscle wastage, particularly of the gluteals, over the quarters without any bony asymmetry of the pelvis is common in hindlimb

Table 6.2   The clinical interpretation of pelvic asymmetry

Clinical sign	Most likely interpretation
Unilateral gluteal muscle wastage	Hindlimb lameness
Elevation of 1 *tuber sacrale* ± muscle wastage	Dorsal sacroiliac thickening/sacroiliac disease/fractured ilial wing
Lowered *tuber sacrale* + muscle wastage	? Chronic sacroiliac disease
Lowered *tuber coxae*	*Tuber coxae* damage, e.g. fracture
Lowered *tuber ischii*	*Tuber ischii* damage, e.g. fracture

lameness, with the muscle wastage indicating the most lame limb. Elevation of one *tuber sacrale*, with or without gluteal muscle wastage (Plate 7b), can be seen in problems involving thickening and damage to the dorsal sacroiliac ligament (see Chapter 17), sacroiliac joint disease (see Chapter 18) and in some race horses with stress fractures of the wing of the ilium (see Chapters 13 and 22). Lowered *tuber sacrale* and/or *tuber coxae* on one side, along with muscle wastage, has been suggested to indicate chronic sacroiliac disease, although Dyson and Murray [2] (2003) noted that only 5% of their confirmed cases of sacroiliac disease had pelvic asymmetry, challenging such dogma. This study certainly indicates that chronic sacroiliac disease is not associated with pelvic asymmetry. However, pelvic asymmetry elsewhere in the pelvis can be useful diagnostically. Lowering of one of the *tuber coxae*, without any associated lowering of the *tuber sacrale* or tuber ischii, is associated with *tuber coxae* damage such as old fractures at this site. Lowering of the *tuber ischii* with no alteration to the *tuber sacrale* or *tuber coxae* may suggest a fractured *tuber ischii*.

Palpation of the thoracolumbar spine and sacrum

Palpation of the thoracolumbar spine and sacrum is one of the most important parts of the clinical examination and if carried out carefully can be a surprisingly accurate technique for detecting pain [3]. It is important to have the horse standing square on a hard surface, e.g. in a quiet box with plenty of time allowed for the horse to relax, or to have the horse in stocks to restrict evasive movements. A start is usually made at the withers, working caudally towards the base of the tail. The fingers are gently, but firmly, run along the back, first in the midline (Plate 8a) and then on either side. The process should be repeated a number of times to allow the horse to become accustomed to the examination. There should be symmetry and balance in the horse's reaction to palpation. It is important to assess the feel of the back and the horse's reaction to palpation, and to try to decide whether any reaction is due to pain or behavioural. In cases of back pathology the horse may guard or splint its back or neck when palpated, or even when just approached. There may be muscle fasciculation in the local area or more generally, with prolonged (>2 seconds) time to the muscles relaxing. The horse with back pathology may try to move away from the palpation and show abnormal behaviour such as tail swishing, head and ear movement, and even kicking actions. It is important to palpate the tips of the dorsal spinous processes and the interspinous spaces. This is most easily achieved in the lumbar region. Any protrusion or displacement of the summits should be noted and marked on the horse with a small clipped area of hair. Spasm or guarding of the longissimus dorsi muscles can be part of a primary problem or an indicator of deeper pain.

Any skin lesions (see Chapter 22), white hairs, loss of hair especially asymmetrically, or scars or swellings in the thoracolumbar region should be noted.

The tips of the sacral spinous processes should also be noted. The dorsal sacroiliac ligament should be assessed for any swelling or pain, as should the tendinous insertions of longissimus dorsi on to the spinous processes of S2 and S3. The area around the *tuber sacrale* and the areas lateral to the *tuber sacrale* should be carefully palpated for any evidence of pain, fibrosis or thickening (Plate 8b). Pain here may be associated with ilial stress fractures in racehorses and also sacroiliac joint disease (Plate 8b). The tail and croup region should be assessed for flaccidity (Plate 9), any asymmetry of the tail and any evidence of cauda equina neuritis.

Manipulation

Careful manipulation can give a considerable amount of information to the examining clinician regarding the source of any back pain. Usually the author starts by running a blunt instrument, such as a pen top, from the lateral side of the withers caudally to the tail head. This is repeated on both sides on a number of occasions to note the normal reaction. Alternatively pinching or pressing can be carried out at various points. In the normal horse pressure on to the caudal thoracic area leads to extension of the spine (dorsi-flexion or dip, Plate 10a), whereas pressure above the tail head leads to flexion of the spine (ventro flexion or arching, Plate 10b), and pressure laterally over the *longissimus dorsi* muscles causes lateral flexion (Table 6.3). It is important to assess the amount of movement and whether there are any signs of pain or altered behaviour.

In the normal horse the movements of the thoracolumbar spine are smooth movements that are easily repeated without any resentment by the horse. Any change in the degree and smoothness of these movements, or a response from the horse such as limb flexion or movement of the tail, kicking, rearing or grunting, may be significant. It is important, however, to make sure that these responses are repeatable. After manipulation the horse with back pathology may become reluctant to move and assume a rather rigid back conforma-

Table 6.3   The response of the horse to manipulation of the back

Site of pressure	Result	Movement
Caudal thoracic	Dorsiflexion	Dipping of spine
Tail head or sternum	Ventroflexion	Arching of spine
Longissimus dorsi	Lateroflexion	Lateral movements of spine

tion. Pain or discomfort may be evident as spasm or guarding of *longissimus dorsi*, locally or generally, which can be palpated or sometimes visually noted. By applying pressure in the caudal lumbar region, and over the entire pelvic region including the *tubers sacrale*, *coxae* and *ischii*, damage to muscles, ligaments and bones of the sacroiliac region and pelvis may be revealed as resentment by the horse and dropping of the hindquarters on that side. Specific pelvic manipulation tests have been described but the author has found these of limited use. Degree of movement on manipulation may reflect the type of horse. Ponies and cobs, which often have a thicker coat and less reactive behaviour, often show a lesser response than thoroughbreds or warmbloods.

Examination of fore- and hindlimbs

After assessment of the back and pelvis, the conformation and stance of the fore- and hindlimbs should be carefully examined. Any areas of muscle atrophy may suggest long-term chronic lameness or neurological dysfunction. The limbs should be examined individually for swellings, particularly of the joints and other synovial structures. The feet should be examined in detail for shape, symmetry and balance, and hoof testers used carefully to help rule out foot pain. All four limbs should be palpated, in a logical sequence, in both a flexed and a standing mode. During this phase the legs and joints should be manipulated, in both flexion and extension.

Examination of the neck

The neck from poll to withers should be palpated on both sides and assessed for symmetry, swelling, muscle spasm and sites of pain. The ability of the horse to lower and raise its head and neck, and flex laterally to left and right, should be examined using either a carrot or small bowl of food (Plate 11). Horses with neck pain will show abnormality of movement and may not be able to eat from the floor or graze. In many cases the horse with neck pain will move its body to obtain the offered edible prize rather than move the neck.

Rectal examination

If there is a history of trauma and possible damage to the pelvic canal, or the clinician is concerned about the sacroiliac region, sublumbar muscle pain or vertebral body fractures, a rectal examination may be helpful in detecting the site of pain in these areas. It is useful to carry out a rectal examination before and after exercise to ascertain whether there is any pain after exercise.

Oral examination

A basic oral examination is useful in all suspected back cases because problems with oral pain will affect the control and movement of the horse. If sedation is required for the use of an oral gag, this part of the overall examination should be carried out after all exercise has finished.

Evaluation of saddlery

Any skin lesions involving the withers or the area immediately under the saddle may indicate historical or current problems of saddle fitting or a rider who is riding incorrectly (see Chapter 24 for a detailed discussion of saddle fit). Swelling and oedema under the saddle may be only transient and should be checked immediately after the saddle is removed. If problems with the saddle are suspected, the saddle should be checked by a master saddler or other expert saddler for a proper fit to the individual horse, and that there are no abnormalities of the saddle, such as incorrect stuffing and damaged tree. It is important also to check the girth in terms of its type and fit. There should not be any sores or skin lesions where the girth sits around the thorax.

Clinical examination at exercise

Initially the horse should be examined in-hand, on a loose rein, on a flat surface and with a competent handler. The horse should be viewed at the walk and trot in a straight line from the back, front and both sides (Plate 12). Careful observation of the gait is important in determining if there is any unilateral or bilateral fore- or hindlimb lameness. Primary back problems rarely lead to hindlimb or forelimb lameness but occasionally there may be signs of a shifting lameness or unlevelness. Chronic back pain tends to lead to a restricted hindlimb action with poor hock flexion and, occasionally, unilateral or bilateral dragging of hindlimb toes. If there is more severe pain there may be a wide, straddling, hindlimb gait. Occasionally horses with low-grade back pain develop a very close hindlimb gait or "plaiting", although this may occur for other reasons.

Flexion tests of the fore and hind limbs may also be performed. Hindlimb flexion tests are often negative if there is a purely back problem, although they may be positive if there is an underlying hindlimb lameness. Of particular interest in the context of the diagnosis of back and pelvic pathology is the observation that flexion tests of one hindlimb may lead to lameness on the opposite hindlimb in sacroiliac disease. In addition, affected horses show resentment during the procedure, which can be a useful initial indicator of a problem in this region.

After an examination in a straight line and flexion tests the horse should be turned tightly in both directions while in-hand to assess how well the horse bends its spine laterally and flexes. When the horse has serious back pain there is a loss of suppleness and there may be back spasm leading to difficulty in turning. Horses with hindlimb lameness, cervical pain and neurological deficits may find this difficult. The horse should also be backed up. In some cases of back pain there may be an initial reluctance to backing with raising of the head and arching of the back, followed by back muscle spasm and occasionally dragging of the forelimbs. The horse should also be backed up and down a slope and in some cases of sacroiliac disease there may be evidence of increased resentment to this.

After the in-hand examination the horse should be lunged for 10–15 minutes on both reins, i.e. to the left and right, and the horse's gait assessed as previously during this exercise. The straight-line in-hand examination should be repeated after this exercise period. On the lunge it is important to carefully evaluate the hindlimb action initially at the trot for evidence of a shortened stiff hindlimb gait, poor tracking up, toe dragging, plaiting, lack

of bend in the back with a tendency for the horse to lean out of the circle, head elevation and positioning of the head outside the circle, and finally for any evidence of spasm in longissimus dorsi while at exercise.

Lunging at the canter may show marked signs in horses with back pain but again these are not exclusive. The horse may find it difficult to transfer from one gait to another, particularly from a canter to a trot and a trot to a walk. The horse may have an inability to lead off on the correct leg (disunited gait) and show evidence of poor hindlimb impulsion with a "bunny-hopping" hindlimb gait. The horse may tend to pull its body forward using excessive forelimb action and there may be signs of lack of concentration in the horse's head and tail swishing. These changes may be accentuated by placing a surcingle or saddle on the horse and repeating the exercise.

Ridden exercise

It is essential to try to observe the horse either ridden or, if it is a driven horse, driven to note what changes during this period of work. The horse should be carefully observed from saddling, when there may be evidence of pain or resentment on girth tightening, through mounting to being ridden. The fit of the saddle pad or numnah can be carefully checked at this stage and, if necessary, a qualified saddler should also be involved. The horse should have ridden/driven exercise carried out with the usual saddlery/harness and the usual rider/driver. It is important to assess the horse's action at the walk, trot and canter and, if the horse is a jumping horse, also while jumping. In a driven horse the horse should be observed while the harness is put in place and throughout its normal work programme. It is important to assess the qualifications of the rider/driver for the horse. Gait changes should be assessed further with particular attention paid to any abnormality that occurred on the lunge. In many cases with back pain the changes are exaggerated when ridden/driven, particularly at the canter, the sitting trot or on the turn. It is useful to observe the position of the saddle and rider during exercise and afterwards, because in a horse with back pain the saddle often becomes twisted to one side away from the painful side.

The horse should be allowed to cool down after exercise and then be re-examined in-hand afterwards to assess its action. In some cases there is increased stiffness that may be related to low-grade myopathies or to joint disease elsewhere in the limbs.

During the whole exercise process it is important to talk to the rider/driver to ascertain their feelings and what they are noticing about the horse's action.

Neurological examination

Horses with suspected back pain should always have a basic neurological examination (see Chapter 7), because back pain, altered gait or unusual lameness can all be consistent with a primary neurological problem. Horses with low-grade neurological disease may present with low-grade hindlimb incoordination, weakness or lameness, which is easily confused with orthopaedic limb disease, back problems or just plain immaturity of the horse.

Further management of the case

At the end of this clinical examination the examining veterinary surgeon should have some indication as to whether she or he is dealing with a primary or secondary back problem, and whether there is any evidence of fore- or hindlimb lameness or behavioural issues. In some cases there is a clear indication of which direction to pursue; in others there is not.

In cases when it is difficult to be absolutely clear as to whether the horse has genuine back pain, re-examination on a separate occasion repeating the methodical examination as before may be helpful in clarifying the position (Plate 13). Using the skills and opinions of other clinicians at the same time can also be very enlightening. In general, the author holds the view that a horse that has undergone a behavioural change *may* be suffering from back pain, but there are occasions when one has to conclude that the only problem the horse has is a primary behavioural problem and the services of a qualified behavioural consultant are required. On other occasions the services of a fully qualified animal physiotherapist can be most useful in determining whether there are any other sources of pain or stiffness in other areas of the body (see Chapters 22–24).

In some cases where there is an issue as to whether pain is present it is possible and acceptable to use up to 10 days of non-steroidal analgesic administration followed by re-examination to see whether the horse's clinical signs are altered. Clearly horses with a behavioural problem will not show any improvement during the period of anti-inflammatory administration, whereas a horse with back pathology and pain will respond. It is also useful to have the horse's rider/driver to work the horse during this period to assess whether the horse's clinical signs change.

Ancillary clinical aids

Additional clinical aids to diagnosis include muscle stimulation by faradic stimulator, often by an animal physiotherapist, and assessing the horse's subsequent response. Horses with muscle soreness and guarding may show increased resentment. Full haematology and biological profiles can be useful to eliminate other causes of poor performance. Back pain and pathology due to a primary muscle problem are recognised (see Chapter 16). In order to diagnose muscle disorder a standard exercise test can be carried out by assessing the levels of serum aspartate aminotransferase (AST) and creatine kinase (CK) at rest, immediately post-exercise and 18–24 hours after exercise. The exercise regimen used in this standard exercise test is lunging of the horse for 10–15 minutes. Active muscle damage is indicated when there is a rise of two to five times the resting levels of the muscle enzymes on the post-exercise samples.

Other clinical aids include the use of local anaesthetic infiltration of suspected sites of back pathology. This is usually carried out after identification of specific sites of pain clinically, or evidence of pathology on radiographs or bone scintigraphy. Most commonly, local anaesthetic infiltration is carried out where there is crowding or overriding of dorsal spinous processes evident on radiographs or nuclear scintigrams, but it is not clear if these bony changes are clinically significant (Plate 14) (see Chapters 8 and 14). In order to perform this test the horse's performance signs are recorded before and after injection of a small amount of local anaesthetic into specific sites under radiographic or ultrasonographic guidance. Individual periarticular facet joints of the adjoining thoracolumbar vertebrae have also been injected, under ultrasonographic guidance, with local anaesthetic and/or corticosteroids (see Chapter 10), and the clinical response of the horse assessed thereafter. The interpretation of this technique is difficult because these injections are effectively intramuscular and may affect the dorsal and ventral rami of the spinal nerves [4]. More recently there has been use of "sacroiliac joint local anaesthesia techniques" to assess pain in the sacroiliac joint region (see Chapter 18). These have been noted to have impressive results on horses with pain in this area [2], but are not universally accepted as specific enough to be diagnostic.

On many occasions horses with back pain are treated on the basis of clinical examination only and their response to symptomatic treatment is used to assess how much further to investigate the problem. Some horses respond positively to symptomatic treatment and require no further examinations. On other occasions the horse does not respond to treatment, in the short or long term, and these cases require further clinical examination. Subsequent examination may determine the need for further diagnostic techniques such as scintigraphic examination, often followed by radiography and ultrasonography of the identified region of interest.

References

1. Landman, M.A., de Blaauw, J.A., van Weeren, P.R. and Hofland, L.J. Field study of the prevalence of lameness in horses with back problems. *Veterinary Record* 2004;**155**:165–168.
2. Dyson, S. and Murray, R. Pain associated with the sacroiliac joint region: a clinical study of 74 horses. *Equine Veterinary Journal* 2003;**35**:240–245.
3. Ranner, W., Gerhards, H. and Klee, W. Diagnostic validity of palpation in horses with back problems. *Berliner und Munchener tierarztliche Wochenschrift* 2002;**115**:420–424.
4. Denoix, J-M. and Dyson S.J. Thoracolumbar spine. In: Ross, R.W and Dyson, S.J. (eds), *Diagnosis and Management of Lameness in the Horse*. Philadelphia: Sounders, 2003: 509–521.

7

The Neurological Examination

Constanze Fintl

Introduction

A general neurological assessment, including that of the back and pelvis, is usually performed while doing the routine physical examination. Further evaluation may be necessary if the clinician is alerted to apparent neurological deficits or if a lesion must be ruled out as part of a clinical investigation. In some cases of back or pelvic pathology gait abnormalities or neurological deficits similar to those seen in neurological cases are detected. Therefore a sound knowledge of the neurological examination of the horse and some of the normal variations that can be expected is very important. Although this chapter is predominantly concerned with the examination of the back and pelvis, it is important that these findings are not interpreted in isolation but included in the overall neurological evaluation of the horse. The aim of the neurological examination is to localise the lesion anatomically. Once the lesions have been localised, a list of differential diagnoses can be generated and further diagnostic tests targeted. The following description of a neurological examination is based on that described by Mayhew [1].

History

A systematic approach is essential to any clinical investigation and a natural starting point is obtaining a full history containing relevant information such as age, breed and use of the animal. An attempt should be made to establish the time of onset and progression of the perceived abnormality and clearly any history of trauma may be relevant. Immunisation history may also be of relevance, particularly if more than one animal is affected or new arrivals have recently been introduced into a yard. A number of important infectious diseases of horses are recognised to cause neurological deficits; these include equine herpesvirus type 1 (EHV 1), equine protozoal myeloencephalitis (EPM), West Nile virus, and eastern, western and Venezuelan equine encephalitis (EEE, WEE and VEE) virus. Infectious causes should be considered a differential diagnosis particularly if asymmetrical focal or multifocal neurological deficits are evident.

Examination at rest

Once a thorough history has been obtained, the neurological examination begins with assessing the horse at rest. In addition to observing behaviour and posture, this examination assesses simple and complex reflex pathways testing both afferent sensory and efferent motor fibres, which will help the examiner localise the anatomical site of the lesion(s).

Palpation assessing evidence of localised pain, muscle wastage and asymmetry as well as feeling for areas of patchy sweating or areas of reduced skin sensitivity should also be performed. Hypalgesia and analgesia of cutaneous areas of the skin are good indications of a primary neurological lesion [2]. In contrast, although increased sensitivity or pain may be indicative of a primary neurological lesion, it is more likely to result from inflammation at the level of pain receptors in peripheral tissues, e.g. muscles, ligaments and joints [1, 2].

Head

The head of the horse should be carefully examined and the behaviour and demeanour assessed. Some broad observations can be made about clinical signs that are seen associated with the brain. Such clinical signs include circling, head turning, head pressing or excessive yawning. Alterations in behaviour or mentation may be associated with forebrain diseases and head pressing is often seen in metabolic conditions such as hepatic encephalopathy.

Assuming that there is no evidence of a forebrain or brain-stem lesion resulting in abnormal behaviour or posture, cranial nerve function is evaluated assessing functional reflexes such as the menace response and pupillary light reflexes, rather than examining each of these nerves individually. Table 7.1 summarises the variety of tests that may be useful in establishing cranial nerve function and the parts of the nervous system that are involved in each test.

Local reflexes

Evaluation of reflex arcs, some of which also involve higher centres, is an important part of the neurological examination and can be very useful in localising a lesion to a certain area of the central or peripheral nervous systems.

Laryngeal adductor reflex ("slap test")

The laryngeal adductor reflex was first described by Greet et al. [3]. However, although the reflex is described here for completeness, it must be recognised that it is not considered a significantly sensitive or specific test for cervical or brain-stem lesions.

The reflex test is performed by slapping the skin just caudal to the dorsal part of the scapula with a flattened hand, while the other hand is used to palpate the contralateral dorsal and lateral laryngeal musculature over the muscular processes of the arytenoid cartilage. In normal horses the response to the slap is to briefly adduct the contralateral arytenoid cartilage, which can be felt as a gentle flutter under the fingers. In some cases it is difficult to palpate the response and endoscopy may be necessary to visualise the arytenoids during the test.

The laryngeal adductor reflex tests both afferent and efferent pathways. The afferent pathway is via the sensory receptors of somatic sensation and pain that send nerve fibres to the spinal cord. These fibres ascend to the medulla, where they send branches to the vagal nuclei as they ascend towards the somatosensory cortex and pain recognition areas. The efferent pathway is through the vagal nerve which runs in an extremely circuitous route to get to the laryngeal musculature. The vagus descends to the cranial thorax; the laryngeal branch then ascends back to the larynx in the recurrent laryngeal nerve. Damage to any part of this pathway can lead to failure of the horse to respond to the laryngeal adductor reflex.

Cervicofacial and local cervical reflexes

The exact anatomical pathways for the cervicofacial and local cervical reflexes are not precisely determined, but it is likely that they involve sensory afferents and motor efferents of the particular local cervical spinal nerves, as well as the facial nucleus in the medulla and facial nerve [1, 4, 5]. These reflex pathways are assessed by stimulating the neck with an instrument (such as a pen tip), which should result in contraction of facial muscles (seen as a lower lip curl of withdrawal) and the cutaneous colli respectively. Suppression of these two reflexes may suggest a lesion at any of these points, although it is worth noting that there is individual variability in the degree of

Table 7.1   Summary of the tests that may be useful in establishing cranial nerve function and the parts of the nervous system that are involved in each test

Test or observation	Cranial nerves / parts of CNS involved	Comments
Pupillary light reflex	II (sensory) and III (motor)	Direct – light causes reflex constriction in same eye. Consensual – light causes constriction in other eye. Assesses both optic and oculomotor nerves
Blink reflex	V (sensory) and VII (motor)	
Corneal reflex	V (sensory) and VI (motor)	
Tongue tone	XII (motor)	
Jaw tone	V (motor)	Mandibular branch of V innervates muscles of mastication, in particular masseter and temporalis muscles
Drooping of face	VII (motor)	'Muscles of facial expression' innervated by VII. Lip droop and/or muzzle deviation (towards normal side)
Pharyngeal and laryngeal dysfunction	IX, X and XI	
Spontaneous nystagmus	VIII	Unilateral VIII lesions – head tilt to the side of the lesion, fast phase of nystagmus away from lesion. In central vestibular disease nystagmus is variable. In chronic lesions nystagmus can resolve
Abnormal pupil position	May involve III, IV, VI and VIII	Elongated pupil makes assessment of strabismus easy, e.g. raise head, eye moves ventrally
Dilated pupil	II and III	May also involve midbrain compression
Constricted pupil	Sympathetic supply to eye	May also involve diffuse forebrain disorders
Menace response	II (sensory) and VII (motor)	A learned response not a reflex, >90% optic nerve fibres cross at optic chiasm in the horse. Assesses both visual pathways and facial nerve
Fixation response	II and higher pathways including visual cortex	
Response to noise	VIII detects noise, auditory cortex locates position of noise	
Sensation to face	V	Mandibular, maxillary and ophthalmic branches

response to this test so some caution in interpretation is warranted. Some very stoical horses will not show any response to stimulation.

Cutaneous sensation

Cutaneous, i.e. somatic afferent, sensation is best assessed using a so-called "two-step" test described by Bailey and Kitchell [6]. In this test a fold of skin is grasped between a pair of artery forceps and, once the horse has adjusted to this, a short, sharp squeeze should be performed in order to elicit a response. Cutaneous areas for the equine thoracic limbs have been electrophysiologically mapped and areas of single nerve supply (autonomous zones) have been determined [6], hence sensory deficits of this region may sometimes be precisely located.

Panniculus reflex

Examination of the trunk (including the back and pelvis) also involves assessing reflex pathways. Prodding the side of the trunk should elicit contraction of the *cutaneous trunci* muscle. This reflex relies on sensory information travelling to the spinal cord through thoracospinal nerves where the impulse is continued cranially to the C8–T1 segment of the spinal cord. This segment is the principal supply of the lateral thoracic nerve, stimulation of which results in contraction of cutaneous trunci [7]. A spinal cord lesion interfering with this reflex must therefore be located cranially to the area being tested. Due the presence of segmental afferents (from T1 to L1) and a single efferent, the lesion site can sometimes be quite accurately localised. This reflex may not occur caudal to the mid-lumbar region and again there may be individual differences in the degree of response to this test.

Further sensory evaluation of the caudal part of the trunk and hindlimbs should also be made. Unlike in the thoracic limb, electrophysiologically mapped cutaneous areas and autonomous zones have not yet been described in the pelvic limb and assessment of the individual nerve supply is based on the topographical anatomy of the individual peripheral nerves [8, 9] (see Figure 4.5 in Chapter 4).

Vertebra prominens reflex

Further assessment of the back and pelvis is performed by assessing the *vertebra prominens* reflex [10]. Pinching and pressing down on the thoracolumbar or lumbosacral paravertebral muscles causes a normal animal to dorsiflex 'dip' the thoracolumbar vertebral column (see Chapter 6). Hyperextension and buckling should not occur unless there is abnormal weakness present. Pressure applied at the lumbosacral junction elicits the same reflex but with more obvious tilting up of the pelvis due to enhancement of the supporting reaction in the hindlimbs [10]. If pressure is applied over the croup, flexion of the lumbosacral joint occurs as well as flexion in other limb joints. The afferent limb of this reflex is through the dorsal branches of the sacral nerves but that of the efferent limb is not known [10]. In clinical cases, failure

to move the back appropriately in response to stimulation may be due to a neurological problem, but is usually considered to be due to be pain secondary to back pathology.

Vertebral flexion test

The ability of the horse to laterally flex the thoracic and lumbar vertebral column can be assessed by firmly stroking the skin overlying the longissimus dorsi musculature with a blunt instrument [11]. Contraction of this muscle should result in lateral flexion. Failure to do so may indicate a neurological deficit, especially if severe muscle atrophy is present. However, as described above, reluctance in flexing the spinal column is usually considered to result from back pathology. Lesions affecting the thoracolumbar grey matter cause muscle atrophy, and asymmetrical myelopathies may result in scoliosis of the thoracolumbar vertebral column with initially the concave side opposite the site of the lesion [1].

Perineal reflex

The perineal reflex is a relatively easy reflex to evaluate, with contraction of the anal sphincter muscle and clamping down of the tail in response to brisk stimulation of the anal area [1]. This reflex tests both sacral and caudal segments and nerves. When evaluating this reflex, it is important to observe whether the horse is able to perceive the sensation centrally and is not just performing a segmental reflex action, in order to differentiate sensory and motor deficits if the reflex response is reduced or absent. This can be achieved by simply observing the head of the horse while the anal area is stimulated, to see whether it turns or shows other signs of central perception of the stimulus such as laying the ears back.

Anal and tail tone

A normal tail hangs in a relaxed fashion. However, when handled or grasped the normal horse will clamp the tail down, making the application of a tail bandage difficult, for example. Horses with reduced or absent tail tone will have a more 'floppy' tail, although vast individual variation in the degree of tone and how easily the tail can be manipulated in different horses can make interpretation difficult. A loss of tail tone implicates a lesion involving the caudal nerves or spinal cord segments.

Areas of sweating

Areas of localised sweating may also be of help when attempting to determine the anatomical site of a lesion, hence any such abnormalities should be carefully documented in terms of the precise anatomical location. Ipsilateral sweating caudal to the lesion indicates involvement of descending sympathetic tracts in the spinal cord, whereas lesions involving specific pre- or postganglionic peripheral sympathetic fibres (second- or third-order neurons) cause patchy sweating at the level of the lesion [1].

Examination of posture and gaits

Evaluation of posture and gait is an essential part of the neurological examination. It aims to reveal signs of paresis (weakness) and/or ataxia (abnormalities of proprioception) and to determine which limbs are affected. Paresis may involve flexor or extensor muscle groups and ataxia can be characterised as having components of hypermetria (high striding) or hypometria (spasticity). These abnormalities of gait may be associated with brain-stem, cerebellar, spinal cord, lower motor neuron (LMN) or peripheral neuromuscular lesion(s) [1].

Although this discussion focuses on evaluating the posture and gait of the pelvic limbs, it is again important to emphasise that these findings must be incorporated into the overall neurological assessment. As part of this assessment it is clearly essential also to evaluate the posture and gait of the thoracic limbs. The following discussion is based on the assumption of no detectable abnormalities of these.

Evaluation of weakness

The examination should begin with assessment of the gait when the horse is walked in-hand. Evi-

dence of flexor weakness may be evident if the horse has a low arc of foot flight, easily stumbles or is noted to be scuffing its toes. Extensor weakness may be evident if the horse is easily pulled to the side while walking (Plate 15). This may be caused by lesions affecting descending upper motor neuron (UMN) tracts, ventral grey matter or peripheral nerves to the main extensor muscles. If extensor weakness is evident only while walking it is suggestive of a UMN lesion. Typically when a tail pull is performed with the horse standing, the extensor reflex is exacerbated as the UMN is no longer able to dampen down this reflex. No evidence of weakness during this test also suggests that the LMNs, as well as the peripheral nerves and neuromuscular endplates, are all intact. If there are lesions present in the latter, it is usually easy to pull the horse to the side while both walking and standing still. If only one limb is affected it is reasonable first to assume that the horse has a peripheral nerve or muscle (LMN) lesion in that limb [1], with the exception of EPM cases, in which multifocal pathology is seen.

Subtle signs of weakness in both pelvic and thoracic limbs may be exacerbated by pulling on the tail and head collar at the same time while circling the horse (Plate 16), although thoracic limb weakness may be further assessed by performing a hopping test.

Evaluation of ataxia

When evaluating possible signs of ataxia, the stride length should be assessed for asymmetry or irregularity. This is best performed with the examiner walking parallel with the horse. The gait should also be evaluated for signs of hypo- or hypermetria or a combination of these (dysmetria). Subtle signs may be made more evident if the horse is made to suddenly stop or back up as well as by making these manoeuvres from trot. Raising the head while walking can also exaggerate the clinical signs (Plate 17). In addition, making the horse perform more complicated tasks, such as walking up and down slopes with the head elevated, will alter the visual, vestibular and proprioceptive input, and may exacerbate deficits in conscious proprioception. Making the horse circle tightly around the handler may also exacerbate signs of ataxia. Horses with pelvic limb ataxia will typically pivot on the inner foot whereas pivoting on the outer foot may display a wide swinging motion.

Another test that is routinely performed to assess proprioceptive deficits in the horse is placing the limbs in abnormal positions. These positions include, for example, placing the foot out to the side of the horse or underneath the horse, and assessing whether and how long it may take for the horse to correct itself to a normal weight-bearing position (Plate 18). However, although this can be a useful test it may not always produce consistent and reliable results. There does appear to be a wide individual variation in this response, as was observed in the tail tone, with some stoical horses being apparently quite happy to stand with a leg in an abnormal position for a prolonged period of time, particularly a hindlimb. It may be of more use to observe how long the horse takes to correct the position of its limbs after a sudden stop from a trot or from backing up, and the way in which a horse just stands in the stable can often give very useful information on whether there is a proprioceptive deficit.

Proprioception can also be evaluated dynamically. Walking horses up and down curbs may give additional information on whether there are proprioceptive deficits. However, the results of this test are often influenced by the temperament of the horse and an animal that is not concentrating or is distracted may appear excessively clumsy whereas a horse with neurological deficits may be particularly careful when placing its limbs and so may not make any deficit more evident.

If there is only pelvic limb involvement, the neurological lesion must be located caudal to T2 [7]. However, in the case of mild cervical spinal cord lesions, particularly when very chronic, signs of weakness and ataxia may be evident only in the pelvic limbs and in these cases it may be safer to conclude that the horse has a lesion between C1 and S3 [12].

The tests described may have to be repeated in order to reveal more subtle abnormalities that may not have been apparent during the initial examination.

Conclusion

Depending on the suggested anatomical site of the lesion(s) further diagnostic procedures may be performed such as radiography, scintigraphy, ultrasonography and electromyography which may help the clinician reach a diagnosis to aid treatment and prognosis.

References

1. Mayhew, I.G. Neurological evaluation. In: Mayhew, I.G. (ed.), *Large Animal Neurology: A handbook for veterinary clinicians*, Baltimore, MD: William & Wilkins, 1989: 15–49.
2. Blythe, L.L. and Engel, H.N. Neuroanatomy and neurological examination. *Veterinary Clinics of North America* 1999;**15.1**:71–85.
3. Greet, T.R.C., Jeffcott, L.B. and Whitwell, K.E. The slap test for laryngeal adductory function in horses with suspected spinal cord damage. *Equine Veterinary Journal* 1980;**12**:127–131.
4. Mayhew, I.G. The equine spinal cord in health and disease. In: *Annual Convention of the American Association of Equine Practitioners*. Albuquerque: American Association of Equine Practitioners, 1999.
5. Rooney, J.R. Two cervical reflexes in the horse. *Journal of the American Veterinary Medical Association* 1973;**162**:117–118.
6. Bailey, C.S. and Kitchell, R.L. Cutaneous sensory testing in the dog. *Journal of Veterinary Internal Medicine* 1982;**1**:128–135.
7. De Lahunta, A. *Veterinary Neuroanatomy and Clinical Neurology*. Philadelphia: W.B. Saunders Co., 1983: 318.
8. Blythe, L.L. Neurologic examination of the horse. *Veterinary Clinics of North America Equine Practice* 1987;**3.7**:255–281.
9. Grau, H. Die Lautinnervation an den Gliedmassen des Pferdes. *Archiv für Wissenschaftliche und Praktische Tierheilkunde* 1935;**69**:96–116.
10. Rooney, J.R. *Clinical Neurology of the Horse*. Philadelphia, PA: KNA Press Inc., 1971.
11. Jeffcott, L.B. Back problems in the horse. In: *Annual Convention of the American Association of Equine Practitioners*. Toronto: American Association of Equine Practitioners, 1985.
12. Mayhew, I.G. The diseased spinal cord. In: *Annual Convention of the American Association of Equine Practitioners*. Albuquerque: American Association of Equine Practitioners, 1999.

8 Radiography

Frances M.D. Henson

Introduction

Radiography is an extremely important diagnostic imaging technique for use in the diagnosis of back pathology in the horse. Radiographic images can be obtained in both the standing animal and under general anaesthesia, although standing radiography is used almost exclusively in clinical practice. This chapter describes the equipment required for radiography of the equine back, the technique for acquiring radiographic images of the back, the normal radiographic anatomy of the equine spine and an introduction to the radiographic appearance of pathology in the equine spine.

Indications for radiography of the back and/or pelvis

The indications for radiography of the back and pelvis include the following:

- The presence of specific areas of suspected pathology. An example of this would be finding heat, pain and swelling in the withers region on a clinical examination which might indicate a fracture of the dorsal spinous processes (DSPs) of the vertebrae.
- When indicated by another diagnostic imaging technique. An example of this would be where

a nuclear scintigraphic examination has identified an area of increased radionuclide uptake in a vertebra.
- As part of a general investigation into back pain.

Technical difficulties with radiography of the equine back and pelvis

In the horse, unlike the situation in humans and small animals, radiography is limited to specific areas of the back and pelvis. This limitation is due to the large size of the adult horse and the amount of soft tissue overlaying most of the thoracolumbar spine and pelvis. Both of these factors necessitate the use of extremely high exposures and cause a high amount of scatter, which degrades the radiographic image.

Structures that can be readily imaged in the standing horse

In the standing horse thoracic vertebra T1 is readily imaged on lateromedial projections; however, the scapula overlies the vertebral bodies and DSPs of T2 and -3, and the vertebral bodies of T4–8. In this region only the DSPs of T4–8 are imaged. From approximately T9 to L3–4, the entire vertebral body and DSPs can be seen. From L3 caudally it is extremely difficult to get satisfactory pictures of the vertebral body and DSPs; the lumbosacral spine and iliac wings are superimposed and only in foals and small, thin ponies can different structures be visualised. The sacrum cannot be visualised in the standing horse and the pelvis visualised only grossly in comparison to the detail obtained at other sites. In order to obtain images of these areas radiography under general anaesthesia is recommended, although this is expensive and may cause a deterioration in the clinical condition.

Radiographic technique

Patient preparation

The horse should be brushed over to check that there is no mud or other substance in the coat that might lead to radiographic artefacts. Before starting the radiographic examination, intravenous sedation is recommended. This has a number of advantages: first it minimises movement of the patient and second it means that the horse needs less close restraint, and the handler can move further away from the horse and hence the X-ray beam. Sedation can, however, cause truncal swaying at high doses. The use of stocks to restrain the horse is a matter of individual veterinarian preference; however, they can be extremely useful where available to minimise movement. Whether or not stocks are available, the horse must be standing straight and must be weight bearing evenly on all four limbs in order to reduce rotational artefacts.

To help placement and orientation of radiographs adhesive labels can be used on the coat of the skin to aid the radiographer in spacing out the film series. Alternatively lead markers can be used to assist in the localisation of specific areas of pathology. This is particularly useful in the pre-surgical planning stage when considering surgical removal of clinically significant DSPs.

Equipment

Radiography of the back requires radiographic equipment with an output of up to 150 kV and 250–500 mA. As mentioned above the large soft tissue mass of the horse and the subsequent scattering of radiation are a limitation to the acquisition of high-quality equine back radiographs. A number of different measures can be taken to help reduce the effect of scatter [1].

First it is recommended that rare-earth film/screen systems are used – this allows the exposure factors to be reduced. A grid (preferably a cross-hatched parallel grid with a ratio of 12:1) is necessary for most radiographs, apart from the summits of the DSPs, to reduce the effect of scattered radiation. In addition, for exposures over 100 kV it is recommended that a lead sheet should be placed behind the cassette to prevent backscatter.

Due to the extensive soft tissue mass of the equine back and the position of the vertebrae and the DSPs, there is a considerable difference in tissue attenuation between the main regions of interest, i.e. the vertebral bodies and the summits of the DSPs. Thus, to image these two different anatomical sites, either two radiographs with different exposures must be taken, or a beam filtration device used. With traditional, non-digital radiography it is usually necessary to have a device that permits a higher exposure to be set for the deeper structures of the back while filtering the beam for the summits of the DSPs. There are different ways of achieving this; some clinics have a "Dodger" beam filter that uses aluminium wedges to achieve beam filtration [2]; other clinics have constructed devices that perform essentially the same function. However, with digital radiography becoming increasingly widespread throughout equine clinics, such filters are not necessarily needed because it is possible to alter the contrast of the radiographs in post-acquisitional processing. Regardless of the method of controlling exposures, close collimation to the region of interest is always recommended in order to enhance image quality if a lesion is detected on survey films.

To obtain standing radiographs of the horse there are a number of ways in which the equipment can be utilised but ideally the X-ray tube is mounted on an overhead gantry with a linked cassette holder to ensure that the X-ray beam and the film are aligned (Figure 8.1a). The cassette holder can be mounted on the opposite wall or any other suitable upright structure (Figure 8.1a). Large cassettes are required (35 × 43 cm recommended) to hold the large radiographic films.

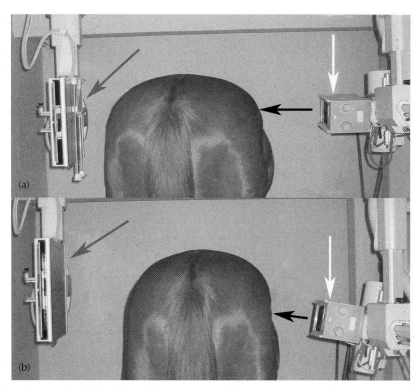

Figure 8.1   Photographs to show the position of the tube head (white arrow), cassette holder (grey arrow) and direction of X-ray beam (black arrow) when acquiring: (a) lateromedial images of the back of the horse and (b) DM20°VL oblique images. (a) Tube head is positioned horizontal to the ground and the beam travels horizontally. (b) Tube head is angled proximally and the beam travels upwards from the tube head. Note, in both photographs, that the cassette holder is aligned with the direction of the tube head angulation and X-ray beam.

Table 8.1   Radiographic exposures for different areas of the thoracolumbar spine using X-ray machine in an average 500 kg thoroughbred horse

Radiographic view	Peak (kV)	(mA)	Grid?	Cassette
DSP T3–7 (withers)	75	15	No	Rapid
DSP T8–13 (mid-thoracic)	80	25	No	Rapid
DSP T13–15 (caudal thoracic)	85	25	No	Rapid
DSP T16–18, L1–4 (thoracolumbar)	90	35	No	Rapid
Thoracic articular facets (oblique)	110	220	Yes	Rapid
Lumbar articular facets (oblique)	110	250	Yes	Rapid
Sacroiliac joint under general anaesthetic	96	500	Yes	Rapid

Exposure values

It is difficult to be prescriptive regarding exposure factors and times for radiography of the equine back because different machines, different techni-cal set-ups and different sizes of horse mean that what is correct for one situation is under- or over-exposed in another. The exposures detailed in Table 8.1 are intended as a rough guide for veteri-narians beginning to acquire images of the equine back. They should be altered according to individual situations, and use of a detailed record of exposure values used and the outcome is considered good clinical practice.

Positioning and radiograph acquisition

Essentially two sets of radiographs are acquired in a "back series": a set of slightly overlapping *lateromedial radiographs* obtained in order to highlight the DSPs and to allow assessment of the ventral surfaces of the vertebral bodies (usually taken from one side only), and a set of slightly overlapping *oblique radiographs* obtained primarily in order to highlight the articular facet articulations (taken from both the left and right of the horse in order to highlight left and right facet joints).

Lateromedial radiographs

To acquire lateromedial radiographs the beam should be centred 10–15 cm ventral to the dorsal skin surface in order to be centred on the DSP (in an average-sized 500 kg horse, this distance should be adjusted for the size of the horse). The beam is angled horizontally (Figure 8.2a). Three to four radiographs are usually required to image the spine from the withers region to approximately L2–3; these radiographs should be positioned so that they overlap in order to ensure that no pathology is missed by being marginalised on the edge of a radiograph. The first radiograph is taken of the withers region and subsequent radiographs follow on caudally. In order to image the DSP of T1 a lateromedial radiograph is taken centred over the vertebral body of C6–7 with the X-ray beam angled horizontally.

Oblique radiographs

To acquire radiographs of the articular facets the beam is centred 20–25 cm below the dorsum and angled upwards (ventral to dorsal) at an angle of 20–30° (dorsomedial 20° ventrolateral oblique [DM20°VLO]; Figure 8.2b). The DM20°VLO view reduces the superimposition of the articulations

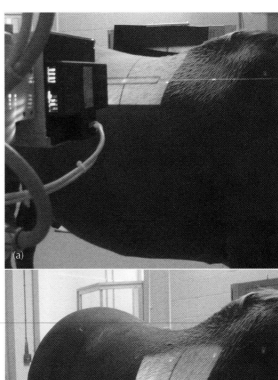

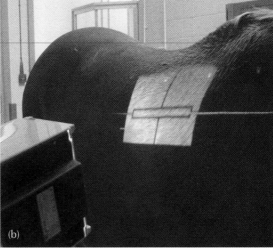

Figure 8.2   Photographs to show the centring of the beam and the collimation of the beam used to acquire (a) lateromedial and (b) DM20°VLO radiographs. (a) Beam is centred just above the vertebral bodies of the horse (10–15 cm below the dorsum); (b) beam is centred 20 cm distal to this point. The small white markers seen to run from cranial to caudal on the side of the horse are stickers applied to identify where different images have been centred.

and, in the lumbar region, reduces superimposition of the transverse processes. Three radiographs on each side (total six) are usually required to image the articular facets (three radiographs to highlight left-hand-side articular facets, and three to highlight right-hand-side ones); again these radiographs should be positioned so that they overlap.

Radiography under general anaesthesia

Although standing radiography is very useful in most clinical cases, the technique does have its limitations. To obtain optimum lateral views of the caudal lumbar spine, ventrodorsal views of the thoracolumbar spine (in all but the smallest ponies and foals) and ventrodorsal views of the sacroiliac joints, radiography under general anaesthesia is indicated. General anaesthesia is needed because all these views require use of very high exposures; rendering the horse immobile during the acquisition of the images produces diagnostic films because it reduces the movement blur that would otherwise occur.

To obtain radiographs under general anaesthesia the horse should be anaesthetised and positioned with the aid of a hoist. Care must be taken with this positioning and padding/support to ensure that the horse is positioned precisely and that there is no rotation of the spine. For lateromedial radiographs, supports under the proximal fore- and hindlimbs are required to ensure that the limbs are parallel with the trunk. To obtain ventrodorsal views the horse should be positioned carefully in dorsal recumbency, again ensuring that there is no rotation of the spine, with the hindlimbs flexed in a neutral ("frog-legged") position.

Of the views that can be obtained under general anaesthesia, radiography of the sacroiliac joint has been well described. To obtain radiographs of the sacroiliac region, the horse is positioned in dorsal recumbency with the legs in a neutral position as described above, with the X-ray beam centred on the midline at the level of the tuber sacrale. This radiographic approach ensures that the X-ray beam strikes the pelvis either perpendicular or slightly caudocranial (no more than $10°$ angle) to the sacroiliac joint.

Exposures of 96 kV and 500 mA for 5 seconds have been recommended to image the sacroiliac region in warmblood horses of approximately 500 kg [3]. To produce a radiographic image that can be interpreted, Gorgas et al. [3] described a radiographic technique in which active ventilation was performed during the exposure, in order to cause movement and radiographic blurring of superimposed gastrointestinal structures, followed by digital enhancement of the images obtained.

Radiography of the pelvis – standing technique

Standing radiography of the pelvis in the horse is not difficult technically but, due to the large size of the horse, the overlying muscle mass in the pelvic region and the movement that occurs, the resultant images are of poor quality and difficult to interpret. Pelvic radiography is usually performed when a fracture of the ilial shaft is suspected.

A number of different techniques have been described as follows.

Lateromedial radiography

To obtain lateromedial radiographs, the tube head is positioned lateral to the pelvis and the cassette positioned on the other side of the pelvis, adjacent to the musculature. This approach is rarely performed because it provides little information except in the smallest of ponies, although it has been described as useful in identifying fractures of the tuber sacrale.

Ventrodorsal radiography

To obtain ventrodorsal radiographs, the tube head is positioned ventrally to the abdomen, just cranial to the hindleg, and the cassette is positioned dorsal to the sacrum (Figure 8.3). The disadvantages of this technique are that centring of the beam and collimation are difficult and imprecise. In addition there is considerable risk to the tube head because it is positioned underneath the horse [4]. However, it is possible to get acceptable quality radiographs using this technique and to identify gross disruptions in the pelvic symmetry or bony displacement.

Lateral–oblique radiography (lateral–dorsal 30° lateroventral obliques)

To obtain lateral-oblique radiographs, the tube head is angled approximately $30°$ ventrally from

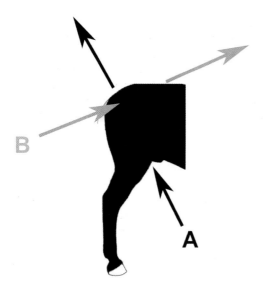

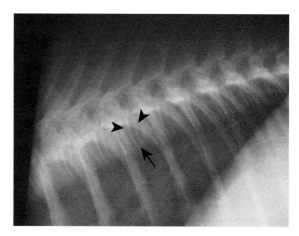

Figure 8.4   A lateromedial radiograph of the vertebral column of a 6-week-old miniature horse. Intervertebral disc space can be seen (arrow) and the open growth plates of the vertebrae are visible (arrowhead).

Figure 8.3   A drawing to demonstrate two different radiographic angles for acquiring pelvic radiographs in the standing horse. (a) The direction of the X-ray beam to acquire ventrodorsal radiographs. (b) The direction of the X-ray beam to acquire lateral–oblique radiographs.

the horizontal, centred between the level of the greater trochanter and the base of the tail, approximately two-thirds of the way along the craniocaudal distance between the palpable landmarks of the tuber sacrale and the tuber ischii (Figure 8.3). The cassette is positioned vertically against the side of the pelvis under examination and the rectum is emptied of faeces in order to provide an air-filled region within the pelvis. It is recommended that a rare-earth screen and stationary parallel grid be used. The radiographic exposure required to image the pelvis depends on the size of the horse and the muscle mass; however, a range of between 90 and 130 kV and between 124 and 400 mA has been described [5].

Normal radiographic appearance of the back

Skeletally immature horses

The thoracolumbar spine changes in angulations from birth to about 6 months, with the thoracolumbar spine having a dorsal curvature (kyphosis) that straightens out at 6 months. As discussed in Chapter 1, the cranial and caudal physes of the vertebrae are visible in foals up to approximately 6 months of age (Figure 8.4). From this age they begin to close; the cranial physes begin to close from 6 months onwards, and the caudal physes from 24 months onwards. The separate centres of ossification of the cranial thoracic DSPs (except T1) begin to develop at approximately 12 months of age; the centres of ossification have a very irregular outline and remain separate from the parent bone throughout life.

Skeletally mature radiographic anatomy

The normal structure of the vertebrae is discussed in Chapter 1 and a working knowledge of the normal anatomy should be acquired before radiographic interpretation.

Dorsal spinous processes

The DSP of T1 is usually visible on a lateromedial radiograph of the base of the neck; it has a triangular shape and is approximately the height of the vertebral body. T1 has no separate centre of ossification (Figure 8.5). Advancing caudally, the DSP of T2 is not usually visible radiographically, but the DSPs of T3–8 are readily visible on radiography. Each of these DSPs has a clearly visible separate centre of ossification throughout life, which must not be mistaken for a fracture or osteolysis (Figure 8.6). In the withers region T4–6 have the

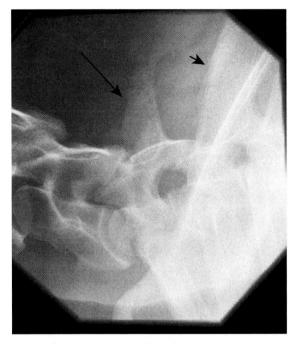

Figure 8.5 A lateromedial radiograph of the vertebral column obtained at the base of the neck to show the radiographic appearance of the first thoracic vertebra (T1; arrow). Note that the dorsal spinous process is markedly enlarged compared with cervical vertebrae (cranial). However, note the cranial edge of the scapular rising up to obscure the dorsal spinal process of T2 (arrow head).

longest DSPs. The DSPs gradually reduce in length caudally from T6, with the cranial thoracic DSP angled slightly caudal and the caudal thoracic DSP angled slightly cranial. The anticlinal vertebra is usually either T15 or T16 (Figure 8.7). Using the standard standing lateromedial radiographic technique described, the DSPs of vertebrae up to L1–2 are visible in most horses.

Vertebral bodies and discs

The vertebral bodies and related structures of approximately T11 to L1–2 can be visualised on standing lateromedial radiographs. The cranial and caudal extremities of the vertebral body, articular facets, ventral aspect of the vertebrae, angulation of the vertebrae relative to each other and articulations of the ribs must all be carefully examined.

In mature horses the intervertebral disc spaces are uniform in width from dorsal to ventral, following the curve of the cranial border of the vertebral body (Figure 8.8). The disc spaces are relatively narrow compared with other species. The cranial and caudal extremities of the vertebrae are smooth, with the caudal extremity appearing sclerotic relative to the cranial extremity. Ventrally the vertebrae are smooth in the normal horse, with no evidence of new bone formation around the intervertebral disc.

Vertebral body articulations

The articular facets of the thoracolumbar vertebrae and the articulations of the ribs are clearly seen on the oblique views. The articular facets are

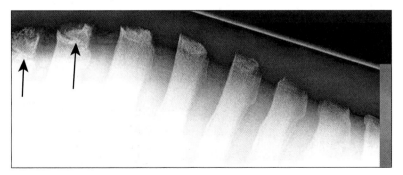

Figure 8.6 A lateromedial radiograph of the dorsal spinous processes obtained in the withers region (thoracic vertebrae T4–11) to show the radiographic appearance of the summits of these vertebrae. The summits of the more cranial vertebrae show separate centres of ossification (arrow).

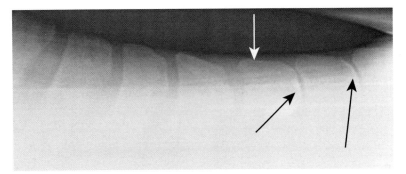

Figure 8.7   A lateromedial radiograph of the dorsal spinous processes obtained in the mid-thoracic region (thoracic vertebrae T12–18) to show the direction of angulation of these vertebrae and the radiographic appearance of the summits of these vertebrae. The anticlinal vertebra (T16) is indicated with a white arrow. Cranial to the anticlinal vertebra the dorsal spinous processes (DSPs) point caudally; caudal to the anticlinal vertebra the DSPs point cranially. Cranial to the anticlinal vertebra the DSPs have space between them, caudal to the anticlinal vertebra the DSPs are close together (but not touching). However, there is evidence of remodelling of the adjacent bony surfaces, indicated by sclerosis of the bone (black arrows).

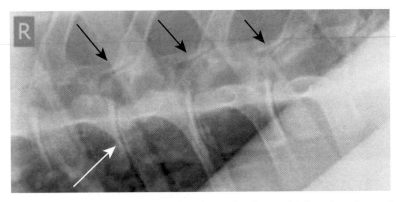

Figure 8.8   A DM20°VLO radiograph of the vertebral bodies obtained in the caudal thoracic region to show the radiographic appearance of the intervertebral discs and the articular facets of the vertebrae. The intervertebral disc spaces are uniform in width from dorsal to ventral (white arrow). The articular facets are seen as radiolucent dog-legged or "inverted L" shapes at the base of the articular with the rib on this radiograph (black arrows). The two cranial facets indicated are normal articular facet articulations; the most caudal facet has sclerosis associated with the joint edges.

identified as inverted "L" or dog-legged radiolucent lines dorsal to the vertebral canal (Figure 8.8). The morphology and positioning of the articular facets alter depending on the position of the facet within the spine. The angulation of the facets changes from nearly horizontal in the cranial thoracic spine to almost vertical more caudally and, radiographically, the lumbar articular facets are more radio-opaque and more irregular in structure than in the thoracic region.

The articulations of the ribs are also seen on the oblique projections. The ribs initially course back dorsally and caudally in the cranial thoracic region; more caudally they course ventrally.

Lumbar, sacral and coccygeal vertebrae

It is extremely difficult to obtain diagnostic radiographs of the lumbar and sacral vertebrae in the standing horse, although it can be attempted using a lateromedial technique centred on the region of interest in smaller horses and ponies. The coccygeal vertebrae are more readily imaged and either lateromedial or dorsoventral views can be obtained of this area if required.

Sacroiliac region

Using the technique described above for radiography of the sacroiliac region, some of the anatomical features of the sacroiliac joints have been described. The cranial sacral borders and the sacral wings are the most readily visible features. Radiographically the cranial sacral borders have been described as having either a "T" or a "Y" appearance, and the sacral wings as having a butterfly, wing, horn or leaf configuration. However, the significance of these morphological descriptions has not been demonstrated [3].

Pelvis

In the normal pelvis standing radiography reveals the outline of the ilial shaft and the outline of the acetabulum (Figure 8.9). General anaesthesia is required to visualise the full extent of the pelvis,

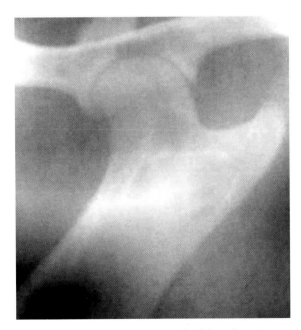

Figure 8.9 A lateromedial radiograph of the pelvis obtained in a standing horse. The quality of the image is relatively poor, reflecting the difficulty in obtaining radiographs at this site. The radiograph shows the proximal femur and its articulation with the acetabulum. The ilial shaft runs cranial and caudal to the acetabulum.

where the ilial wings, ilial shaft, acetabula, pubis and ischial tuberosities can all be imaged.

An introduction to radiographic abnormalities of the back and pelvis

Radiographic abnormalities are commonly seen in the equine back; indeed, it is rare to examine a set of radiographs from a horse and detect no radiographic changes. The challenge to the veterinarian who is investigating the cause of back pain in a horse is, first, to identify the radiographic changes present and, second and more importantly, to understand the clinical significance of these changes. In this section a brief introduction to the radiographic changes that may be encountered is given. For more specific changes please refer to the specific individual chapters referred to in the text.

Congenital defects

As discussed in detail in Chapter 15, a number of congenital disorders can affect the back of the horse. These can be divided into conditions that are readily detectable clinically (lordosis, scoliosis and kyphosis) and defects that are more usually detected radiographically (hemivertebrae and congenital fusion of the thoracolumbar vertebral bodies or articular processes).

Lordosis may be caused by congenital hypoplasia of the articular processes but may also be acquired. Radiographically lordosis is recognised as a ventral convexity of the thoracolumbar spine. Kyphosis, in contrast, is recognised as a dorsal convexity of the thoracolumbar spine. Scoliosis (a twisting of the spine) is best diagnosed on dorsoventral radiographs. In these radiographs scoliosis is recognised radiographically as a deviation of the spine from a normal, straight appearance (Figure 8.10). In addition wedge-shaped vertebral bodies may be seen. On lateromedial radiographs there is an asymmetry in the positioning of the ribs and an alteration in the length of the vertebral bodies.

Radiographically diagnosed congenital defects may be incidental findings on routine radiographic examination or they may be severe, causing back weakness and clinical signs.

Radiographic abnormalities of the DSP

Radiography of the equine back is most commonly performed in order to identify whether or not the horse is showing evidence of over-riding DSPs

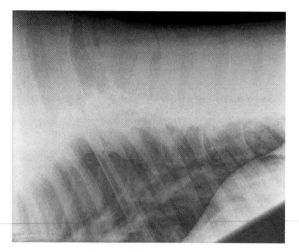

Figure 8.10 A lateromedial radiograph of the thoracic spine of a yearling filly to show marked scoliosis (lateral deviation of the vertebral column). Note the abnormal shape and position of the dorsal spinous process and vertebral bodies. (Image courtesy of Mr R. Pilsworth.)

(ORDSPs); however, there are many radiographic abnormalities that can be detected in the region of the DSPs in the horse. These include fractured DSPs (see Figure 13.1, Chapter 13). In cases of fractured DSPs the long DSPs are usually noted to be displaced either cranially or caudally. Usually the fractured summit is seen distal to its predicted site on the radiograph. Care must be taken not to confuse separate centres of ossification in the cranial thoracic DSPs (see Figure 8.6) with fractures of the DSPs, as discussed earlier.

The radiographic signs of ORDSPs are basically evidence of two DSPs either being closer together than normal or overlapping/making contact. It must be recognised that many clinically normal horses have DSPs that are in close apposition, particularly in the caudal thoracic and lumbar regions. Indeed, it has been shown that, in one study of normal horses, 34% showed some degree of DSP impingement [2]. *The diagnosis of clinically significant ORDSPs cannot, therefore, be made on radiographic signs alone.* Abnormalities of the DSPs range from DSPs that are close at their summits to overlapped DSPs that have clear radiographic signs of remodelling. The spectrum of changes seen in the DSPs ranges, therefore, from the mildly affected to severely affected. In mildly affected

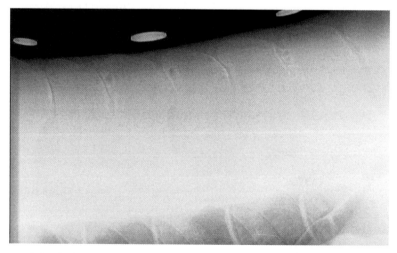

Figure 8.11 A lateromedial radiograph of the dorsal spinous processes (DSPs) obtained in the thoracic region to show the radiographic appearance associated with over-riding DSPs. There is sclerosis associated with the bones that are in contact, remodelling of the DSPs and areas of radiolucency associated with this remodelling. The white, radiodense markers above the bones are markers placed upon the skin to identify the location of individual DSPs before surgical removal of the DSPs. (Image courtesy of Dr J. Kidd.)

cases the DSPs are close but not in apposition. However, changes at the cranial and caudal cortical borders of the proximal aspect of the DSPs are seen (see Figure 8.7), indicating that contact is occurring, probably when the horse is moving, being ridden or jumping.

This category of ORDSPs can be considered *dynamic ORDSPs*. The changes seen in the DSPs are areas of sclerosis on the cranial and caudal borders of the DSPs, running along their edge (see Figure 8.7) but rarely affecting the central section

of the bone. It is of note that it is extremely rare to see sclerosis in the distal portion of the DSPs. More advanced radiographic signs of ORDSPs include marked sclerosis and remodelling of the cranial and caudal borders of the DSPs, and the development of cyst-like lucencies within the bones where they are in contact (Figure 8.11). In addition, at the summits of the DSPs new bone formation can occur (Figure 8.12). In severe cases the DSPs are clearly in apposition or even overlapping (*static ORDSPs*) (Figure 8.13).

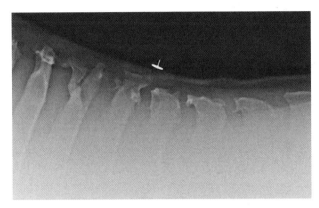

Figure 8.12   A lateromedial radiograph of the dorsal spinous processes (DSPs) obtained in the mid-thoracic region to show the radiographic appearance associated with marked remodelling of the DSPs. The summits of these DSPs are dramatically remodelled and, in one case, appear to have split. The cause of this remodelling is not known but it may be due to direct trauma to this site. The white, radiodense marker above the bones is placed to identify the location of individual DSPs. (Image courtesy of Dr J. Kidd.)

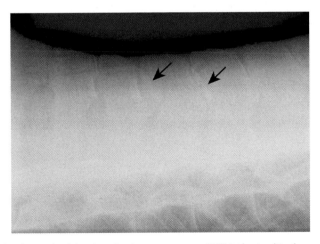

Figure 8.13   A lateromedial radiograph of the dorsal spinous processes (DSPs) obtained in the caudal thoracic region to show the radiographic appearance associated with overlapping DSPs. In this horse the DSPs do not have sufficient room within the back and have overlapped each other (arrows). (Image courtesy of Dr J. Kidd.)

Table 8.2 The radiographic grading systems for overriding dorsal spinous processes (DSPs) of Denoix and Dyson [7] and Desbrosse et al. ([8])

Grade	Radiographic appearance [7]	Radiographic appearance [8]
1	ISS narrowing, mild sclerosis of the cortical margins of the DSPs	Enthesiopathies of the supraspinous ligament
2	Loss of ISS, moderate sclerosis of the cortical margins of the DSPS	Enthesiopathies of the interspinous ligament
3	Severe sclerosis of the caudal margin of the DSPs (can be due to transverse thickening), radiolucencies	Impingement of the DSPs
4	Severe sclerosis of the caudal margin of the DSPs, change in shape of DSPs	Impingement with bone sclerosis and/or osteolysis

ISS, interspinous space.

The radiographic changes seen in ORDSPs have been the subject of a number of grading systems including those of Petersson et al. [6], Denoix and Dyson [7], and Desbrosse et al. [8] (Table 8.2). However, there are no published studies correlating the severity of the radiographic changes with clinical pain.

In addition to bony changes caused by ORDSPs, other radiographic abnormalities can be detected. These include enthesiophyte formation on the cranial and caudal borders of the DSPs, presumed to be due to new bone formation within or at the origin/insertion of the interspinous ligament. Similarly damage to the superspinous ligament (SSL) can lead to periosteal reaction and new bone formation on the summit(s) of the DSPs. In rare cases avulsion of the SSL is diagnosed radiographically by the presence of a detached piece of bone from the summit of the DSPs.

Radiographic abnormalities of the vertebral bodies

New bone formation on the ventral aspect of the vertebrae is an uncommon finding in the horse compared with cats and dogs. This new bone formation is termed "ventral spondylosis" in the horse (see Chapter 15). The new bone formation that is observed on the ventral aspect of the vertebrae forms a spectrum of changes (Figure 8.14). In some cases small osteophytes are noted on the ventral surface of the vertebral bodies close to the intervertebral disc. In more advanced cases,

the new bone formation is sizeable and can fuse beneath the disc space. The clinical significance of ventral spondylitis in the horse is not known (see Chapter 15) but it is recognised that it can be seen occasionally as an incidental finding in some horses.

Radiography is important in the diagnosis of osteomyelitis or neoplasia of the vertebrae, both of which are relatively rare conditions in the horse (see Chapter 15). Osteomyelitis leads to new bone formation around the vertebral body, areas of radiolucency in the vertebrae and, in advanced cases, pathological fractures. A distinct disease entity is that of 'fistulous withers' – osteomyelitis of the withers region (T4–7) – which can occur secondary to the primary soft tissue infection (often a *Brucella* species). On lateromedial radiographs remodelling and new bone formation are seen on the affected DSPs.

Radiography is also extremely used to detect fractures of the vertebral bodies. The most common sites for fractures are the cranial thoracic region (T1–3), the mid-thoracic region (T9–16) and the lumbar vertebrae [1]. Radiographic signs of a fractured vertebra include ventral displacement of the vertebrae, apparent shortening or tilting of a DSP and alterations in the angulation of the vertebral bodies. Other radiographic abnormalities that have been reported include poor definition of the articular facets due to callus formation [1]. However, it should be noted that radiography can prove disappointing in the identification of vertebrae fractures and is, of course limited to T1 and T9 to L1–2 in its extent. Other imaging

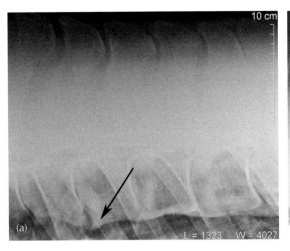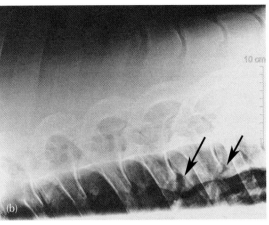

Figure 8.14   (a) A lateromedial radiograph and (b) a DM20°VLO radiograph of the vertebral bodies obtained in the thoracic region to show the radiographic appearance of ventral spondylosis. (a) Ventral spondylosis is seen on the ventral aspect of the vertebra (arrow) (compare with the same normal anatomical site in Figure 8.8). (b) The obliquity of the radiograph demonstrates the extent of the ventral new bone formation and the spondylosis on the vertebra caudal to the one originally identified (arrows).

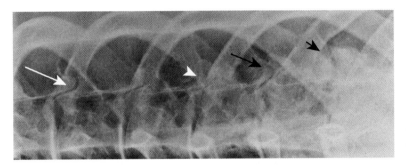

Figure 8.15   A DM20°VLO radiograph of the vertebral bodies obtained in the caudal thoracic region to show the radiographic appearance of osteoarthritis of the articular facets of the vertebrae. A normal articular facet is present cranially in this radiograph (white arrow). A facet that has lost the joint space (ankylosis) is present (white arrowhead). More caudally a moderate amount of new bone formation is seen at one facet (black arrow) and a marked amount of new bone formation is seen in the next facet (black arrowhead). (Image courtesy of Dr J. Kidd.)

modalities, e.g. nuclear scintigraphy, should be considered to confirm the diagnosis or if radiography does not identify a lesion in a horse with clinical signs indicating presence of a fracture (see Chapter 9).

Radiographic abnormalities of the articular facets

In contrast to radiography of DSPs, radiographs of the articular facets of the mid-thoracic to cranial lumbar spine are difficult to obtain and, in the normal horse, it is not usual to detect radiographic abnormalities. When abnormalities are detected then, at the current time, they are considered to be likely to be clinically significant (see Chapter 15), especially if there is evidence of active bone remodelling demonstrated by nuclear scintigraphy. Evidence of degenerative joint disease of the articular facets of the thoracolumbar spine can be detected on the DM20°VLO view. Articular facet osteoarthritis is recognised on radiography by new bone formation around the facets, loss of joint space (ankylosis) and sclerosis around the joint margins (Figure 8.15). The appearance of affected facets can be compared with the appearance of the facets cranial and caudal to the suspected lesion and to the DM20°VLO of the other side of the horse. Denoix [9] has described eight different types of pathology at the articular facets of the thoracolumbar spine (Table 8.3).

When radiographic changes consistent with a diagnosis of articular facet osteoarthritis are seen,

a nuclear scintigraphic examination is recommended (see Chapter 9), to provide more detail about active remodelling at this site (see Chapter 15).

Radiographic abnormalities of the pelvis

The only conditions of the pelvis that may be investigated reasonably with radiography are

Table 8.3 Classification of the radiographic signs of articular facet pathology [9]

Type of pathology	Grades	Radiographic signs	Observations
Asymmetry	1	Double joint space or no clear joint space	Rarely pathological
Changes in articular process opacity	2, 3	Subchondral bone sclerosis (2) and/or radiolucent areas (3), increased opacity of the intervertebral articulations (2) and articular processes (3)	Two mainly found T16–L3
Periarticular proliferation	4, 5	Dorsal (4) and ventral (5) new bone formation, increased size of the intervertebral articulations (4)	Four mainly found T16–L3, five lumbar area
Ankylosis	6, 7	Adjacent vertebrae connected by dorsal bridge (6), no joint space (7)	Six mainly found T16–L3, seven lumbar area
Fracture	8	Presence of radiolucent lines on articular processes	Located at any site

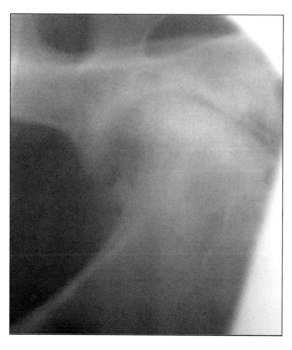

Figure 8.16 A lateromedial radiograph of the pelvis obtained in a standing horse. The radiograph shows the proximal femur and its articulation with the acetabulum. This is an example of a non-acute pelvic fracture through the acetabulum. There is an incongruity in the acetabulum and marked new bone formation associated with the proximal femur due to osteoarthritis in response to the fracture.

pelvic fractures or sacroiliac pathology. Pelvic fractures can be detected either in the standing horse or under general anaesthesia, as described above, and are seen as marked incongruencies in the ilial shaft or wing (Figure 8.16). Radiography of the sacroiliac region is technically possible, but due to a number of factors the radiographs obtained can be difficult to interpret. These factors include the large soft tissue mass overlying the area, the presence of ingesta in the pelvis and the orientation of the sacroiliac joints relative to the direction of the X-ray beam. Radiographic changes described in sacroiliac disease include smooth new bone on the caudal aspect of the joint or widening of the sacroiliac joint [10].

References

1. Weaver, M.P., Jeffcott, L.B. and Novak, M. Radiology and scintigraphy. In: Haussler, K.K. (ed.), *Veterinary Clinics of North America Equine Practice: Back problems*. Philadelphia: W.B. Saunders Co., 1999: 113–130.

2. Jeffcott, L.B. Radiographic examination of the equine vertebral column. *Veterinary Radiology* 1979;**20**:135–139.

3. Gorgas, D., Kircher, P., Doherr, M.G., Ueltschi, G. and Lang, J. Radiographic technique and anatomy of the equine sacro-iliac region. *Veterinary Radiology and Ultrasound* 2007;**48**:6501–6506.

4. May, S.A., J, P.L., Peacock, P.J. and Edwards, G.B. Radiographic technique for the pelvis in the standing horse. *Equine Veterinary Journal* 1991;**23**:312–314.

5. Barrett, E.L., Talbot, A.M., Driver, A.J., Barr, F.J. and Barr, A.R.S. A technique for pelvic radiography in the standing horse. *Equine Veterinary Journal* 2006;**38**:266–270.

6. Pettersson, H., Stromberg, B. and Myrin, I. Das thorkolumbe, interspinale Syndrom (TLI) des Reitpferdes – Retrospektiver Vergleich konservativ und chirurgisch behandelter Falle. *Pferdeheilkunde* 1987;**3**:313–319.

7. Denoix, J-M. and Dyson, S.J., Thoracolumbar spine. In: Ross, M.W. and Dyson, S.J. (eds), *Diagnosis and Management of Lameness in the Horse*, Philadelphia: Saunders, 2003: 509–521.

8. Desbrosse, F.G., Perrin, R., Launois, T., Vanderweerd, J-M.E. and Clegg, P.D. Endoscopic resection of dorsal spinous processes and interspinous ligaments in ten horses. *Veterinary Surgery* 2007;**36**:149–155.

9. Denoix, J.M. Lesions of the vertebral column in poor performance horses. In: *World Equine Veterinary Association symposium*. Pullman: WEVA Publications, 1999.

10. Jeffcott, L.B. Radiographic appearance of equine lumbosacral and pelvic abnormalities by linear tomography. *Veterinary Radiology* 1983;**24**:204–213.

9 Nuclear Scintigraphy

Alastair Nelson

Introduction

Nuclear scintigraphy, or "bone scanning", has become an established part of the clinical work-up of back and pelvic problems in the horse since it was first described by Ueltschi in 1977 [1]. Nuclear scintigraphy has long been used in the investigation of back pain in humans and the ability to use nuclear scintigraphy in the investigation of equine back pain was a major breakthrough in diagnostic imaging of this difficult region. As described in Chapter 8, radiography of the back and pelvis is limited due to the large size of the patient, the overlying soft tissue structures and the need for high-power X-ray machines. Nuclear scintigraphy, in contrast, permits visualisation of the whole back and pelvis and allows identification of active bone remodelling.

Indications for nuclear scintigraphy of the back and/or pelvis

The indications for nuclear scintigraphy of the back and pelvis include the following:

- The presence of specific areas of pathology. An example of this would be a suspected fracture of the lumbar vertebrae.
- When indicated by another diagnostic imaging technique. An example of this would be when

there is radiographic evidence of overriding dorsal spinous processes (DSPs) on radiography, and nuclear scintigraphy is needed to provide information about the activity of the pathology.
- When used as the sole method of imaging the back, pelvis and proximal hindlimb regions, where it can be extremely difficult, or even impossible, to obtain good quality diagnostic radiographs, e.g. the sacral vertebrae.
- As part of a general investigation into back pain or unexplained lameness.

Mechanism of action

Nuclear scintigraphy is a measure of function of an organ or tissue, rather than an anatomical imaging modality. Thus scintigraphy relies on the metabolism of an organ in order to be effective, so nuclear scintigraphic images reflect physiological function rather than anatomical structure [2]. Although scintigraphy does not provide the anatomical resolution to enable the specific cause of the altered radionuclide uptake to be determined, different patterns and locations of uptake can predict certain pathological findings [3, 4].

The principle of nuclear scintigraphy is that a radiolabelled agent (radionuclide) is introduced into the body, chemically bound to a tracer agent.

The tracer agent is bound within the organ of interest with the radiolabelled agent therefore also bound. The location of the radiolabelled agent is then imaged using a gamma camera or point probe. The tracer agent is specifically chosen, according to which target tissue the technique is seeking to evaluate, e.g. iodine-131 (^{131}I)-labelled meta-iodobenzylguanidine (MBG) is used to diagnose neural crest tumours, whereas gallium-67 (^{67}Ga) citrate and *in vitro* labelled leukocytes are routinely used to identify and localise infectious and inflammatory conditions. At the current time the standard agents used in obtaining bone-phase scintigraphic images in the horse are technetium-99m (^{99m}Tc)-labelled methylene diphosphonate (MDP) or hydroxymethylene diphosphonate (HDP). The disintegration of the isotope results in the emission of gamma rays with an energy peak of 140 keV. The isotope has a half-life of 6 hours, making it an ideal agent for use in a clinical setting.

To obtain scintigraphic images of the horse the ^{99m}Tc-labelled MDP/HDP is injected intravenously, usually through a previously placed intravenous catheter. The agent is then distributed around the body via the bloodstream. It attaches to exposed hydroxyapatite within osseous structures, so the uptake of the radionuclide is relative to the osteoblastic activity and/or metabolism of the bone and the blood flow to the bone [3]. This results in active uptake of radioactivity into the metabolically active parts of the skeleton, recognised as a "hot spot" on the scintigraphic image. Thus, the amount of radioactivity in a part of the skeleton is related in the main to the specific activity of the region, but also partly to the general metabolic activity and blood flow to that region.

Procedure for scintigraphy of the back and pelvis

The protocol used for back scintigraphy is similar to that used for other parts of the body. A few differences must, however, be noted. When acquiring images of the limbs in lameness cases, it is customary to exercise the horse before injection of the radionuclide, to ensure good uptake of tracer agent into the limb. In contrast, when evaluating radionuclide uptake in the equine back, this exercise is less critical, because blood flow to the back is unlikely to be a rate-limiting step in the level of uptake. In fact over-exercise of a horse that has been rested before scintigraphy for clinical reasons may lead to exercise-induced rhabdomyolysis, which can lead to marked uptake of radioactivity into the soft tissues. Although this may be a clinically significant finding relating to the horse's clinical problems, it also has the effect of superimposing soft tissue uptake over bone uptake, which may mask any abnormal uptake in the bone itself.

As described above the horse is injected with 10 MBq/kg ^{99m}Tc-labelled MDP through an intravenous catheter, ensuring appropriate safety of the handler and injector. An intravenous catheter is recommended because it prevents inadvertent spillage of the radiolabel during the intravenous injection in non-cooperative patients. After the injection the horse is usually left in the stable before taking the bone phase images. If venous and/or soft tissue (pool) phase images are required, the horse may be immediately moved to the scintigraphic imaging suite. In all cases it is recommended that a diuretic should be administered intravenously between 15 and 60 minutes after radionuclide injection to promote evacuation of the bladder before scintigraphic evaluation. The benefits of this are twofold: first, the bladder shadow is less likely to mask uptake within the bony structures of the pelvis (Plate 19) and, second, it may reduce the radiation dose to handlers of the horse.

The three phases of the scintigraphic examination

As mentioned above there are three phases during which scintigraphic images can be acquired (Table 9.1). The first or *vascular* phase occurs immediately after injection and lasts for 1–3 minutes. During this time the radionuclide is circulated round the body in the bloodstream. In the imaging of the back and pelvis of the horse, there are very few occasions when the vascular phase is useful. One of these occasions is, however, in cases of suspected aortic thromboembolism. Flow phase images can allow identification of an obstructive thrombus and may give some quantitative infor-

Table 9.1 The three phases of the scintigraphic examination of the back and pelvis: the time at which the images are acquired, the anatomical structures imaged and examples of the pathology that may be detected in each phase

Phase	Time image acquired after injection (min)	Anatomical structures imaged	Example of pathology detected
Vascular	1–3	Blood vessels	Aortic thromboembolism
Soft tissue	3–15	Muscles and other soft tissue structures	Exertional rhabdomyolysis
Bone	120–180	Bone	Fractures, osteoarthritis

mation as to the reduction in blood flow due to the thrombus.

The second phase of imaging is the *soft tissue* (pool) phase, which occurs 3–15 minutes after injection into the horse [5]. This is the time when the radiolabel is distributed in a relatively even fashion throughout the soft tissues, and is rarely useful in cases of equine back and pelvis pathology. However, the soft tissue phase may be useful in cases of equine rhabdomyolysis, in which muscle retention of MDP has been reported in some cases, although in the author's opinion this is often best seen on the bone phase (see below).

Bone phase imaging is the most commonly performed of the three phases in the examination of the back and pelvis in the horse. Imaging of the bone phase of the scintigraphic examination takes place between 120 and 180 minutes after injection. This time delay allows clearance of radioactivity from the soft tissues. In the bone phase the radionuclide is clearly detected within the bones and areas of increased uptake are detectable as "hot spots". In a very few cases, an area of photopenia (decreased radionuclide uptake) is detected (e.g. in septic osteomyelitis, bone sequestrum) [6].

Image acquisition of the spine

There are a number of different techniques described to ensure comprehensive imaging of the spine. The most thorough imaging technique described is that the horse should be imaged from both left and right sides using a gamma camera. The initial scintigrams should be obtained with the camera perpendicular to the ground (lateromedial) for views of the cranial thoracic spine

(withers region). For mid-thoracic, caudal thoracic and lumbar vertebrae, dorsolateral 45° ventromedial oblique (DL45°VMO) views should be obtained. The DL45°VMO views are preferable to lateromedial scintigrams at this site because the camera can be brought nearer to the skin surface, reducing the distance between the camera and the spine and decreasing scatter. Ideally, the horse should be imaged from both the left and the right, otherwise subtle asymmetrical lesions may be missed. If an area of increased radionuclide uptake is detected appropriate lesion-oriented views can then be obtained, e.g. dorsoventral views.

However, such a detailed examination can be extremely time-consuming in a busy clinic situation. If a rapid screen of the patient is required the author recommends that DL45°VMO images are obtained from the right-hand side of each horse from T1 to L6. Additional left DL45°VMO views and dorsal views can be taken of the thoracolumbar spine as required, which may help with lateralisation of a lesion within the spine.

Image acquisition of the pelvis

A routine examination of the pelvis includes a DL45°VMO view of both ilial wings to include the *tuber coxae* (obtained by angling the camera head over the gluteal region), a dorsoventral view of the paired *tubera sacrale*, a dorsoventral view of the sacral region and lateromedial views of the ilial shaft/acetabular/femoral head region. Additional oblique images to highlight the tail head, tail and *tuber ischii* region can be obtained as deemed clinically necessary, and the author recommends that a second dorsal oblique view centred on the hips is also very helpful.

Technical aspects

It is recommended that the scintigraphic images are acquired using a 128 × 128 or a 256 × 256 matrix. Although the 256 matrix will give a less pixelated image, the image counts must be high enough to ensure an adequate signal-to-noise ratio. This will usually require counts of at least 500 000 per image.

Motion correction is frequently used and highly recommended in the acquisition of scintigrams from the equine back and pelvis, in order to reduce blurring of the image as a result of horse movement. In "motion correction" essentially a number of short (2- or 3-second) static images are obtained and then these images are stacked together to produce the final image. This final image is corrected for movement by the processing computer. Movement correction is carried out as routine in many practices, although this will not eliminate the movement associated with respiration.

A variety of post-processing tools can be used to optimise the image for viewing. These include altering the display window levels, and the use of filters such as smoothing or Metz. Regions of interest (ROIs) can be used to mask out areas of high uptake not related to the back, such as the kidneys and bladder, as well as areas of physiological high uptake within the back and pelvis, such as the *tuber coxae*, to allow better visualisation of other areas within the image. ROIs can also be drawn around anatomical structures to give uptake ratios as discussed later in this chapter.

Considerations in the analysis of scintigrams

When reading nuclear scintigrams, it must be recognised that the amount of radioactivity detected by the gamma camera is proportional not only to the amount of radioactivity in the bone but also to the thickness of the soft tissues interposed between the bone and the gamma camera. It is particularly important to be aware of these attenuating effects of the overlying soft tissue when examining scintigrams of the back, because soft tissue thickness can vary widely over different anatomical regions and from left to right, e.g. in a horse with marked one-sided gluteal atrophy. Other variables to be taken into account when assessing the scintigram are the age of the horse and the angle of the camera relative to the back at acquisition. The age of the horse affects the pattern of radionuclide uptake because the growth plates will be visible on the scintigrams as areas of increased radionuclide uptake – these must not be confused with pathological remodelling. The angle of the camera affects the scintigram – increasing the laterality of the image will lead to fewer counts being registered from the spinous processes.

The normal scintigraphic appearance of the back and pelvis in the horse

The acquisition of many images from the back and pelvis of normal horses has allowed a "normal" pattern of radionuclide uptake to be recognised and described (Table 9.2).

Scintigraphic abnormalities of the back and pelvis

Before any discussion of scintigraphic abnormalities of the back and pelvis, it is crucial to realise that an increase in radionuclide uptake does not necessarily equate with pathology. An increase in radionuclide uptake can be due either to *physiological* remodelling or to *pathological* remodelling, and it is vital that a thorough clinical examination and other diagnostic imaging techniques be employed by the veterinarian before a diagnosis is made.

Scintigraphic abnormalities of the spine

Scintigraphic abnormalities of the dorsal spinous processes

A number of conditions can cause abnormally increased radionuclide uptake in the dorsal spinous processes (DSPs) including a fracture of the DSP, overriding DSP (ORDSPs) and remodelling at the insertion of the supraspinous ligament on the summit of the DSP.

Table 9.2 The scintigraphic appearance of the back and pelvis in the routinely obtained scintigraphic views in a normal horse

Region	View	Scintigraphic description
Cranial thoracolumbar spine	Lateromedial (Plate 20a)	The DSPs of T3–8 seen dorsally and caudally. There are marked areas of increased uptake on the caudal border of the scapula (S) and associated with the summits of the dorsal spinous processes of T3–8. These are normal "hot spots". It has been suggested that the increased radionuclide in these summits is because these areas retain separate centres of ossification (SCOs) and thus remodelling continues to occur throughout life. In addition higher counts will be seen in the tips of the DSP in the withers region due to the lack of soft tissue coverage
Mid-thoracolumbar spine	Lateromedial (Plate 20b)	In this view the vertebral bodies (V) are visible and show uniform uptake of radionuclide in a dorsal and ventral plane. There is a mild increase in uptake in the last four or five thoracic vertebrae. The ribs (R) are also clearly visible, running ventrocaudally from the vertebral column. The ribs have an even distribution of radionuclide uptake throughout their length. The summits of the T9 DSP caudally do not show significant increases in radionuclide uptake in the normal horse, and can be difficult to distinguish from the soft tissue background
Mid-thoracolumbar spine	DLVMO (Plate 20c)	This view is used in order to obtain information about the articular facets (AF) of the spine. Camera angulation means that the facets are no longer superimposed as they are in the lateromedial view. The articular facets of the vertebral column are seen to form a parallel line of radionuclide uptake above the vertebral bodies (VBs). This uptake is continuous with no focal areas of increased uptake visible
Mid-thoracolumbar spine		A straight vertebral column with uniform radionuclide uptake throughout the VBs
Caudal thoracolumbar spine	Lateromedial (Plate 20d)	The scintigraphic uptake is similar to that seen in the mid-thoracic region with the vertebral column dominating in the cranial aspect of the image. There is uniform radionuclide uptake in the vertebral bodies, ribs and DSPs as seen more cranially. Caudally in the image, however, the kidney (K) will be revealed as a large area of increased radionuclide uptake just distal to the vertebral column overlying ribs 16–18
Caudal thoracolumbar spine	DLVMO	As in the mid-thoracolumbar spine view this view separates the articular facets. However, in this region care must be taken to identify both kidneys on the oblique views of the cranial lumbar region because they may be superimposed over the vertebrae and give a false impression of increased uptake in the bone (see Plate 17)
Caudal thoracolumbar spine	DV	This view reveals a straight vertebral column with uniform radionuclide uptake throughout the vertebral bodies. The kidneys are seen as areas of increased radionuclide uptake either side of the midline
Cranial pelvis	DV (Plate 21a)	In this view the *tuber sacrale* (TS) is always seen as an area of increased radionuclide uptake. In the normal horse the TSs appear as paired comma-shaped "hot spots" just either side of the midline. The bladder shadow is often seen as a large area of increased radionuclide uptake just behind the TS, usually in the midline, although the bladder shadow can be very asymmetrical and mimic pelvic pathology. In some cases, where there is a significant amount of radionuclide retained in the bladder, it is not possible to ascertain whether or not there is any pathology in the pelvis and it is recommended that a repeat scintigraphic examination be made 6 hours later/after urination. Alternatively, angulation of the camera head in a craniocaudal direction can help distinguish between uptake within the bladder and genuine uptake within the pelvis itself

Table 9.2 *Continued*

Region	View	Scintigraphic description
Cranial pelvis	DLVMO (Plate 21b)	This view highlights the iliac wings. Dorsally the TSs are seen as "hot spots", whereas ventrally the *tubera coxae* (TCs) are marked areas of increased uptake. Uptake in the iliac wing (IW) is relatively low and should be evenly distributed
Cranial pelvis	Lateromedial	The TSs are seen as a focal area of increased radionuclide uptake in the dorsocranial aspect of the view and the hip joint is seen in the middle of the view. The hip joint is an area of relatively poorly defined increase in uptake. In this view some detail of the proximal femur can be seen, e.g. the greater trochanter
Caudal pelvis	DV	In this view the paired TSs are still present and the sacrum is seen in the midline. To either side of the sacrum the hip joint is seen as a focal area of increased uptake
Caudal pelvis	Lateromedial (Plate 21c)	In this view the hip joint is seen as an area of relatively poorly defined increase in uptake. Again, in this view some detail of the proximal femur can be seen, e.g. the GT. The *tuber ischii* (TI) can be seen as an area of increased uptake caudal to the hip
Caudal pelvis	Caudal view	This view is obtained by positioning the camera behind the horse. The coccygeal vertebrae are seen in the midline of the image and the paired TIs are seen either side of the midline

These descriptions should be read together with Plates 20 and 21. DLVMO view, dorsolateral–ventromedial oblique; DSPs, dorsal spinous processes; DV view, dorsoventral view.

DSP fracture

Fractures of the DSPs cause a marked focal increase in radionuclide uptake at the site of the fracture. If a fracture is suspected on the basis of the radionuclide uptake, radiography is recommended to confirm the diagnosis. However, as noted in Chapter 13, it is important not to undertake a scintigraphic examination too close to the point of injury because insufficient time will have elapsed to allow significant radionuclide uptake at the fracture site. It is therefore advised that at least 5–7 days are left between the time of the injury and nuclear scintigraphy in order to maximise the specificity of the technique, although no studies have been carried out to determine this experimentally [3].

Overriding DSPs

Following the introduction of nuclear scintigraphy as a diagnostic technique of considerable use in the diagnosis of back pathology, several assumptions were made about the "normal" scintigram. One of these assumptions was that in the "normal" horse no radionuclide uptake is detected in the region of the DPSs. However, a small number of recent studies have demonstrated that an increase in radionuclide uptake can be demonstrated in horses without overt back pain, including, in one study, 50 out of 78 horses showing such uptake [7]. Erichsen et al. [8] demonstrated that low-grade increases in radionuclide uptake were common between T12 and T18 in her study group (Swedish warmbloods). In addition, this group [9] reported on the radiographic and nuclear scintigraphic findings in groups of normal riding horses and horses with back pain, and showed that these modalities did not distinguish between horses with and horses without back pain. To be more specific about the amount of radionuclide detected in an area, the use of a DSP ratio (ratio of uptake of DSPs and rib 15 or 16) has also been described, although not in clinical cases [8]. At the current time therefore it is important to realise that increased radionuclide uptake in the DSPs may not always indicate pathology at this site, so it is vital to use other diagnostic modalities, e.g. local anaesthetic techniques to confirm the diagnosis (see Chapter 14) [10].

Abnormally increased radionuclide uptake in the dorsal tip of the DSPs can be seen associated with damage to the attachment of the supraspinous ligament; this is often generalised throughout the thoracolumbar region. An ultrasonographic evaluation of the supraspinous ligament and DSP summits is warranted in order to identify pathology at this site (see Chapter 10). Increased radionuclide uptake is often seen in the DSPs in the mid- to caudal thoracic spine (Plate 22) and in these cases more than one DSP is usually affected. This increased radionuclide uptake is often interpreted as a positive indicator of impingement of DSPs, especially when interpreted with clinical and radiographic signs (Plate 22).

Scintigraphic abnormalities of the vertebral region

Increased radionuclide uptake in the vertebral region can be due to vertebral body fractures, osteoarthritis of the dorsal articular facets, stress fractures, ventral spondylosis, vertebral body osteomyelitis and rarely neoplasia.

Vertebral body fractures

Vertebral body fractures (traumatic or stress) lead to marked areas of focally increased radionuclide uptake at the site of the fractures. Often the "hot spot" is so intense that the other structures on the scintigram are markedly reduced in contrast. The diagnosis of a traumatic fracture is confirmed on clinical signs and radiography (if in an anatomical place that can be visualised radiographically; see Chapter 13), although stress fractures may be diagnosed on the basis of the scintigram and history alone (see Chapter 15). Occasionally a marked focal increase in uptake will be seen in a single dorsal articular facet or in the adjacent dorsal part of the vertebral body, often due to a stress fracture of dorsal articular facet or vertebral body (Plate 23).

Osteoarthritis

Osteoarthritis (OA) of the dorsal articular facets of the thoracolumbar spine is characterised by increased radionuclide uptake in the region of the articular facets. This is often best visualised on oblique scintigrams (see Chapter 15). This increase in uptake is seen just above the midline of the vertebral body uptake. The uptake may be asymmetrical between left and right because the OA may be unilateral. This increased uptake is usually associated with radiographic signs of OA (see Chapter 8) within dorsal articular facets, but is not always necessarily associated with clinical signs of back pain.

Miscellaneous conditions

Osteomyelitis and neoplasia are very rare in the equine spine but focal areas of increased radionuclide uptake may be suggestive of such pathology. Again a radiographic evaluation of the area will provide further diagnostic detail. Ventral spondylitis is occasionally seen as an area of increased radionuclide uptake on the ventral surface of the vertebrae (see Chapter 15).

Scintigraphic abnormalities of the sacroiliac region

Nuclear scintigraphy is widely used in the diagnosis of sacroiliac dysfunction (SID). Indeed, given the difficulties of radiography at the site and the limitations of ultrasonography to provide images deep in the pelvis, nuclear scintigraphy may be the only imaging modality that can be used to image this region. Nuclear scintigraphy of the sacroiliac joint (SIJ) can be performed in the standing horse and under general anaesthesia. It is recommended that dynamically acquired, motion-corrected images are the best scintigrams to obtain of the SIJ region and that the dorsoventral view is the most useful, with oblique views of the ilial wing (lateral oblique projection [11]) also helpful in the identification of the location of areas of increased radionuclide uptake associated with the ilial wing and SIJ.

Regardless of the method of acquisition there are three described ways of acquiring information about the radionuclide uptake at the SIJ:

1. **Visual assessment**: the scintigrams should, first, be assessed visually to look for bilateral symmetry, radionuclide uptake and any obvious asymmetries or abnormalities. As described in Table 9.2, a normal dorsoventral scintigram of the SIJ region has increased radionuclide uptake at the site of the paired *tubera sacralae*, with minimal uptake along the ilial wing until the *tuber coxae* is reached (see Plate 21a). In some horses a small amount of radionuclide uptake is seen between the *tubera sacralae*, which is uptake associated with a sacral DSP. The SIJ region is seen adjacent and abaxial to the *tuber sacralae*. In horses in which there is increased radionuclide uptake in the SIJ, increased radionuclide may be seen to extend abaxially to as far as the midpoint between the *tuber coxae* and the *tuber sacralae*. The exact site of the SIJ, when imaged using nuclear scintigraphy, has been a subject of some discussion among researchers. However, it is generally accepted, by most researchers and clinicians, that the region abaxial to the *tuber sacrale* represents the region of the SIJ (Plate 24a), although it is not immediately adjacent.

2. **Profile analysis**: profile analysis gives a subjective evaluation of the pattern of radionuclide uptake, allowing an assessment of the symmetry of the uptake within the ilial wing region [12]. Profile analysis is performed by using a computer program first to draw a line through the *tuber sacrale* perpendicular to the vertebral column on the dorsoventral scintigram, and then to create a horizontal profile of the number of scintillation counts along the line. The results are displayed as a graph (see Plate 21d). In normal horses the SIJ profile is approximately bilaterally symmetrical. The slope of the profile has been reported to be steeper in young horses, than in older animals [12], reflecting a bigger contrast in radionuclide uptake between the wing of the ilium and the *tuber sacrale* in the younger animal, or perhaps more activity at the *tuber sacrale* before the separate centre of ossification fuses to the parent bone. In horses with pathology at this site there is an asymmetry of the plotted profile and/or widening and flattening of the profile on the affected side (see Figure 18.4 in Chapter 18).

3. **Region of interest (ROI) analysis**: identification of an ROI and determining a ratio between the SIJ ROI and another anatomically fixed ROIs permits the quantification of radionuclide uptake. A number of different scintigraphic ratios for the SIJ have been described, including comparison of the SIJ region with the fifth lumbar vertebra [12] and the sixth lumbar vertebra [13]. Using ROIs it has been shown that there is significant variation in the uptake of radionuclide uptake at the tuber sacrale with age, but not in the SIJ. However, overriding opinion is that the symmetry of the scintigraphic image of the dorsoventral pelvis is the most important feature to assess.

The effect of lameness on the scintigraphic image of the SIJ has also been investigated. Lameness in one hindlimb causes increased radionuclide uptake at the SIJ on the affected side, regardless of whether or not the lameness is due to SIJ pathology [14]. This may be a consequence of reduced muscle mass on the affected side, although this was not demonstrated by the authors of this study. In both normal and lame horses tuber sacrale radionuclide uptake decreased with increasing age. In lame horses there was a trend towards decreased SIJ uptake with increasing age, not seen in normal horses. Increased radionuclide uptake in SIJ overlaps among normal, lame and SIJ horses, and should not be used in isolation.

Scintigraphic abnormalities of the pelvis

The usefulness of nuclear scintigraphy in the diagnosis of back and pelvic injuries was demonstrated early in the development of this clinical technique, when it was shown to be highly accurate in identifying stress fractures in the pelvis [15]. However, when interpreting scintigrams of the pelvis region, it is important to recognise the "hot spots" that are seen associated with bladder activity and the previously mentioned artefacts caused by unilateral (usually gluteal) muscle wasting. It is recommended that motion correction programmes and quantitative methods of analysis should be used to assist interpretations of scintigrams in this region, because in this area subtle pathology can often be missed [16]. As discussed above it is recommended that post-processing image masking be used to remove bladder and/or kidney activity. A number of different scintigraphic conditions can be detected scintigraphically, as follows.

Ilial wing stress fractures (see Chapter 13)

These are the most common pelvic fracture [17] and are seen as markedly focal uptake in the wing of the ilium, most often in the axial third of the bone (Plate 24b).

Traumatic pelvic fractures (see Chapter 13)

Fractures of all parts of the pelvis can be detected by nuclear scintigraphy and are seen as focally increased uptake at the affected site. The scintigraphic views discussed above are the standard views used to identify pathology, but bilateral fractures and fractures close to the tuber sacrale may require additional oblique views [11].

Although nuclear scintigraphy is excellent at identifying pelvic fractures, previous comments about the time between initial damage and the scintigraphic examination should be noted [17]. Nuclear scintigraphy can be particularly helpful in identifying not only the presence of a fracture but also the *site* of the fracture, e.g. in traumatic fractures of the ilial shaft, it is important, prognostically, to ascertain whether or not the acetabulum is involved in the damage and this can be identified on the scintigram.

Tuber ischii damage (see Chapter 13)

Increased radionuclide uptake associated with the tuber ischii is occasionally seen. In some cases mild increases in uptake have been hypothesised to be caused by avulsion of muscles off the lateral edge of the tuber ischii and can be associated with increased uptake and lameness. In cases of tuber ischii fracture, marked focal increase in radionuclide uptake is seen, usually unilaterally.

Coxofemoral joint pathology (see Chapter 13)

Coxofemoral pathology is detected by an increase in radionuclide uptake in the hip joint region (Plate 24c). However, as stated above the hip joint in normal horses is not always seen as a precise, focal articulation and the hip joint has a low degree of uptake in normal horses. Fractures of the acetabulum or femoral neck often have relatively mild increases in uptake due to a relatively low percentage increase in uptake, and there is marked soft tissue attenuation of the radionuclide signal at this site.

Sacral trauma (see Chapter 13)

Increased radionuclide uptake in the sacrum is usually seen associated with traumatic fracture or, in rare cases of mild increases in uptake, with damage to the dorsal sacroiliac ligament.

Tail trauma

Uptake within the coccygeal vertebrae is occasionally detected and usually reflects a fracture at this site.

Miscellaneous uptake in the back and pelvis

Increased radionuclide uptake is also detected in other conditions in the back and pelvis. Soft tissue uptake is occasionally seen within the *longissimus dorsi* muscles and gluteal muscles, and is considered an indication of exertional rhabdomyolysis. Linear uptake may also be seen in the muscles of the pelvis in isolation or associated with increased uptake in the bone at insertion of the muscle.

In addition to increased uptake in soft tissues, marked focal increases in uptake are occasionally seen in the paravertebral structures such as the facet joints of the rib or focal marked uptake within the body of the rib (see Figure 22.9 in Chapter 22). An ultrasonographic examination often confirms these as fractures. More subtle increases in uptake may be seen at the tips of the transverse processes of the lumbar vertebrae where false joints can form. The clinical significance of these scintigraphic changes can be assessed using local anaesthesia.

Limitations in the use of nuclear scintigraphy in the vertebral column and pelvis

In the initial enthusiasm that greeted the arrival of nuclear scintigraphy into the equine veterinarians' diagnostic imaging array, it was all too easy to acquire an image, find a "hot spot" and make a diagnosis. However, the validity of the technique remains, in many clinical situations, unproven. There are a number of different reasons that make determining this validity difficult: first, postmortem studies of normal equine athletes have demonstrated that a high prevalence of subclinical pathological changes exist in the vertebral column and pelvis, e.g. in the lumbosacral region [18]. Thus finding a "hot spot" in the back or pelvis cannot be assumed to be the cause of perceived pain. Second, there are few opportunities to prove the precision of nuclear scintigraphy because this requires pathological examination of the bones at postmortem examination. In many cases this opportunity does not exist. In human medicine advanced imaging technologies such as magnetic resonance imaging (MRI), computed tomography (CT) and single photon emission CT (SPECT) are used in the evaluation of the back and pelvis [3]. Until these imaging modalities are available to the equine veterinarian and more postmortem studies are reported, the validity of the scintigraphic examination remains unproven.

References

1. Ueltschi, G. Bone and joint imaging with ^{99m}Technetium labelled phosphates as a new diagnostic aid in veterinary orthopaedics. *Journal of the American Radiological Association* 1977;**18**:80–84.
2. Weaver, M.P., Jeffcott, L.B. and Nowak, M. Radiology and scintigraphy. *Veterinary Clinics of North America Equine Practice* 1999;**1**:113–129.
3. Archer, D.C., Boswell, J.C., Voute, L.C. and Clegg, P.D. Skeletal scintigraphy in the horse: current indications and validity as a diagnostic test. *Veterinary Journal* 2007;**173**:31–44.
4. Twardock, A.R. Equine bone scintigraphic uptake patterns related to age, breed, and occupation. *Veterinary Clinics of North America Equine Practice* 2001;**17.1**:75–94.

5. Ross, M.W. and Stacy, V.S., Nuclear medicine. In: Ross, M.W. and Dyson, S.J. (eds), *Diagnosis and Management of Lameness in the Horse*. Philadelphia: Saunders, 2003: 198–212.
6. Levine, D.G., Ross, B.M., Ross, M.W., Richardson, D.W. and Martin, B.B. Decreased radiopharmaceutical uptake (photopenia) in delayed phase scintigraphic images in three horses. *Veterinary Radiology and Ultrasound* 2007;**48**:467–470.
7. Ehrlich, P.J., Seeherman, H.J., O'Callaghan, M.W., Dohoo, I.R. and Brimacomhe, M. Results of bone scintigraphy in horses used for show jumping, hunting, or eventing: 141 cases (1988–1994). *Journal of the American Veterinary Medical Association* 1998 **213**:1460–1467.
8. Erichsen, C., Eksell, P., Widstrom, C. et al. Scintigraphy of the sacroiliac joint region in asymptomatic riding horses: scintigraphic appearance and evaluation of method. *Veterinary Radiology & Ultrasound* 2003; **44**:699–706.
9. Erichsen, C., Eksell, P., Holm, K.R., Lord, P. and Johnston, C. Relationship between scintigraphic and radiographic evaluations of spinous processes in the thoracolumbar spine in riding horses without clinical signs of back problems. *Equine Veterinary Journal* 2004;**36**:458–465.
10. Walmsley, J.P., Pettersson, H., Winberg, F. and McEvoy, F. Impingement of the dorsal spinous processes in two hundred and fifteen horses: case selection, surgical technique and results. *Equine Veterinary Journal* 2002;**34**:23–28.
11. Hornof, W.J., Stover, S.M., Koblik, P.D. and Arthur, R.M. Oblique views of the ilium and the scintigraphic appearance of stress fractures of the ilium. *Equine Veterinary Journal* 1996;**28**:355–358.
12. Dyson, S., Murray, R., Branch, M. et al. The sacroiliac joints: evaluation using nuclear scintigraphy. Part 1: The normal horse. *Equine Veterinary Journal* 2003;**35**:226–232.
13. Tucker, R., Schneider, R., Sondliof, A.H., Ragle, C.A. and Tyler, J.W. Bone scintigraphy in the diagnosis of sacroiliac injury in twelve horses. *Equine Veterinary Journal* 1998;**30**:390–395.
14. Dyson, S., Murray, R., Branch, M. and Harding, E. The sacroiliac joints: evaluation using nuclear scintigraphy. Part 2: Lame horses *Equine Veterinary Journal* 2003;**35**:233–239.
15. Pilsworth, R.C., Sheperd, M.C., Herinckx, B. and Holmes, M.A. Fracture of the wing of the ilium, adjacent to the sacroiliac joint, in Thoroughbred racehorses. *Equine Veterinary Journal* 1994;**26**:94–99.
16. Davenport-Goodhall, C.L. and Ross, M.W. Scintigraphic abnormalities of the pelvic region in horses examined because of lameness or poor performance: 128 cases (1993–2000). *Journal of the American Veterinary Medical Association* 2004;**224**:88–95.

17. Pilsworth, R.C., Holmes, M.A. and Shepherd, M. An improved method for the scintigraphic detection of acute bone damage to the equine pelvis by probe point counting. *Veterinary Record* 1993;**133**:490–495.

18. Haussler, K.K. and Stover, S.M. Stress fractures of the vertebral lamina and pelvis in Thoroughbred racehorses. *Equine Veterinary Journal* 1998;**30**:374–381.

10 Ultrasonography of the Thoracolumbar Region

Luis P. Lamas and Marcus J. Head

Although radiography and nuclear scintigraphy are excellent diagnostic imaging techniques for imaging bony back and pelvis pathology, ultrasonography is the imaging modality of choice for the superficial soft tissues of this region. Ultrasonography can be performed in the thoracic spine, as described in this chapter, and in the lumbar spine, sacroiliac region and pelvis as described in Chapter 11.

Ultrasonography of the thoracic spine is performed:

- when specifically indicated on the basis of the clinical examination, i.e. a swelling is detected in the region of the supraspinous ligament
- when indicated by other diagnostic imaging techniques, e.g. to further investigate articular facet osteoarthritis identified by radiography and nuclear scintigraphy
- as part of a general investigation into back pain and/or loss of performance
- to facilitate the administration of diagnostic analgesia or medication.

General considerations

The horse should be adequately restrained, preferably in stocks, and the hair clipped from the dorsal midline. The area to undergo ultrasonography is then cleaned and ultrasound coupling gel applied. Ultrasonography of this region can be done with linear, curvilinear and sector scanners using frequencies between 2.5 and 7.5 MHz depending on the structure to be viewed.

Ultrasonography of the thoracic spine allows assessment of the following important structures:

- Supraspinous ligament (SSL)
- Intraspinous ligament (ISL)
- Muscles
- Dorsal spinous processes (DSPs) of the vertebrae
- Articular facets of the vertebrae (AFs).

SSL and ISL ultrasonography

As outlined above, ultrasonography of the soft tissue of the thoracic spine is used to identify the structure or any abnormalities in the SSL, ISL and the muscles. As discussed in Chapter 2, the SSL is the continuation of the more elastic nuchal ligament, which originates at the occipital bone and has its most caudal insertion onto the last lumbar vertebra [1] (Figure 10.1). As it runs caudally it becomes progressively less extensible. It also is thicker in the cranial thoracic region and the lumbosacral area [2]. The SSL has multiple attachments to the tendinous portion of the longissimus

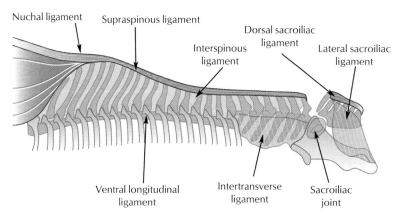

Figure 10.1   A line diagram to show the position of the significant soft tissue structures in the back (Courtesy of Professor L.B. Jeffcott.)

dorsi muscles, which are important for the stabilising function of this ligament. The SSL lies directly beneath the skin and a variable amount of subcutaneous adipose tissue. The ventral fibres of the ligament course downwards to become continuous with the ISL, which attaches to the cranial and caudal margins of adjacent DSPs.

Ultrasonographic technique

Ultrasonographic evaluation should be performed using a high-frequency linear ultrasound probe (7.5–12 MHz). A 7.5-MHz probe is most routinely used. The hair should be clipped with a no. 40 blade in a 3–4 cm wide strip. In most routine cases this clip is begun at the base of the withers because lesions of the SSL are uncommon cranial to this point [3]), and continued caudally to the caudal sacral region. Evaluation requires a systematic and thorough approach. It is important to image the entire thoracolumbar portion of the ligament using both longitudinal (long-axis) and transverse (cross-sectional, short-axis) images:

- Longitudinal section: in longitudinal section the ligament is seen as a horizontal structure with a prominent fibre pattern present on the midline (Figure 10.2a).
- Transverse section: in transverse section the ligament is seen as a small oval hyperechoic structure that is better identified in the spaces between adjacent DSPs (Figure 10.2b).

The ligament should be examined for the following characteristics.

Echogenicity

The normal SSL has a heterogeneous echogenicity (Figure 10.2a). The dorsal portion of the SSL is generally more hyperechoic than the ventral fibres and the ISL, which are more hypoechoic. The change in echogenicity occurs because of the difference in SSL fibre orientation between the dorsal and ventral parts of SSL. As the SSL fibres become deeper their angle becomes more acute, resulting in a decrease in echogenicity. Immediately adjacent to the dorsal margin of the DSPs there is a hypoechoic cap (1 mm approximately) formed by the fibrocartilaginous pad over each DSP. The normal echogenicity of the SSL can be altered in a number of ways. Both hyperechoic and hypoechoic regions may be detected on ultrasonography (Figure 10.2c, d). These may be clinically significant (see Chapter 17).

Fibre pattern

A linear fibre pattern should be present in the dorsal portion of the ligament. Fibre pattern scoring systems used in other structures [4] could theoretically be used for the SSL, although this is not currently in common use. Adjacent to the DSP and in the interspinous region the fibre pattern is difficult to assess because of the change in fibre direction as discussed previously (Figure 10.2a).

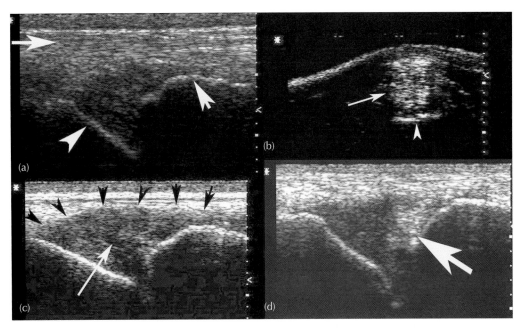

Figure 10.2   Ultrasonograms to show the ultrasonographic appearance of the supraspinous ligament (SSL): (a) longitudinal section; (b) transverse section. (a) The normal appearance of the ligament. The ligament runs over the summits of the dorsal spinous processes (DSPs, arrowheads) and is seen to be a horizontal structure. The fibre pattern is visible (arrow). (b) Transverse section through the SSL (arrow) as it runs over the summit of a DSP (arrowhead). (c) A hypoechoic lesion (blacker) within the SSL (arrow). This hypoechoic lesion extends dorsally into the body of the SSL (black arrowheads). (d) A hyperechoic lesion (whiter) within the SSL (arrow) adjacent to a DSP.

Objective measurements

A normal range of measurements of the SSL has not been determined. However, some generalisations about the size of the ligament can be made.

Longitudinal section

In longitudinal section the ligament thickness should be measured in the dorsoventral plane at the level of the middle of the DSP summit. Care must be taken to avoid misinterpretations caused by possible differences in the contour of adjacent DSPs. Comparing the dimensions of adjacent sections of the ligament is an acceptable method of size evaluation.

Transverse section

In transverse section the SSL is continuous with the thick echogenic thoracolumbar fascia on either side [2], and so accurate measurements are hard to make. Comparison of the dimensions of adjacent sections of the ligament is an acceptable method of size evaluation.

Enthesiopathy

Insertional desmopathy of SSL can be readily identified using ultrasonography. Insertional desmopathy occurs when the fibres of the SSL become pulled from the dorsal surface of the DSP; this is reflected in the alteration in the appearance of the DSP. On ultrasonography, the main characteristic of enthesiopathy is the irregular shape of the dorsal surface of the DSP (Figure 10.3a), although an increase in echogenicity of the SSL may also be seen. The presence of small hyperechoic detached fragments of bone from the dorsal margins of the DSP is associated with the more severe cases (avulsion fractures). When an avulsion fracture is suspected, low exposure radiographs of the area may be taken for further full evaluation. In the more cranial DSPs the incomplete centres of ossification should not be confused with avulsion fractures as noted in previous chapters.

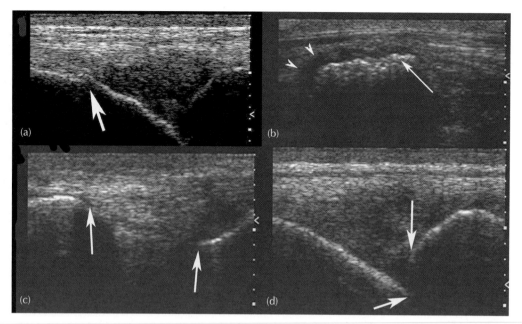

Figure 10.3 Ultrasonograms to show the ultrasonography of bone in the thoracic region. (a) Enthesiopathy: the supraspinous ligament (SSL) has been torn away from the summit of the dorsal spinous process (DSP) and a small piece of bone has become detached (arrow). (b) The normal appearance of the summit of the DSP of the sixth thoracic vertebra on a transverse (cross-section) scan. Note the roughened appearance of the secondary centre of ossification in the summit of this bone (arrow). Note also the cartilage cap overlying the summit, seen as a hypoechogenic region (arrowheads delineate the lateral margin), between the bone and the overlying SSL. (c, d) Ultrasonograms to identify the proximity of two DSPs in the longitudinal plane: (c) DSPs are clearly separate in this horse in the caudal thoracic region (the white arrows show the caudal edge of one DSP and the cranial edge of the next DSP). (d) DSPs are very close together (the white arrows show the caudal edge of one DSP and the cranial edge of the next DSP).

Ultrasonography of the muscles of the thoracic spine

Muscular ultrasonography is discussed in detail in Chapter 16.

Ultrasonography of the bone

Although the deeper structures of the vertebral column are not accessible, ultrasonography of some of the more superficial bony structures is possible. Ultrasonography of the summits of the DSPs and the articular facets of the thoracolumbar spine has been described. In addition it is possible to use ultrasonography of these regions to facilitate ultrasonographically guided injections, e.g. to medicate the articular facets in cases of osteoarthritis (see Chapter 15).

Ultrasonography of the DSPs

Ultrasonography can provide very useful information about the summits of the DSPs and their relationship with each other. In the normal horse the dorsal surfaces of the summits of the DSPs of T7–18 are smooth and seen as a hyperechoic line horizontal to the skin. In contrast the summits of T3–6, with their separate centres of ossification, have roughened summits (Figure 10.3b).

Ultrasonography can provide information on the interspinous spaces between the DSPs – the space can be seen in normal regions of the spine (Figure 10.3c), but in cases where there is contact between the DSPs this space is lost (see Chapter 14). Where overriding DSPs (ORDSPs) occur it is also possible to identify this overriding (Figure 10.3d), on both longitudinal and transverse views, and also to identify any remodelling that is associated with this anatomical abnormality. Desmitis of the SSL following impingement of the DSPs has not been recognised as a clinical entity, although an ultrasonographic appearance consistent with enthesiopathies is often present with ORDSPs due to the bone modelling that has occurred.

Ultrasonography of the DSP can also be used to identify fractures of the DSP, although these can usually be clearly seen on radiography (see Chapter 13) and other, far less common conditions, such as congenital malformations and developmental variations in the interspinous spaces [5].

Ultrasonography of the "articular facets" – the articular process–synovial intervertebral articulation

The articular facet complex is formed by the caudal articular facet of the cranial vertebra, the synovial intervertebral articulation and the cranial articular facet (AF) of the adjacent vertebra [6] (see Chapter 1). As discussed in Chapter 15 pathology at the articular facets is considered, at the current time, to probably be a significant cause of back pain in the horse [7]. In most cases radiographic examination and/or nuclear scintigraphic examination will have alerted the clinician to the possibility of a lesion at a specific region (see Chapters 8 and 9). Ultrasonographic examination of the affected area of the thoracolumbar area, and particularly the lumbar articular facet joints, is a very useful procedure, and with practice and good equipment it is a very sensitive way of detecting enlargement of the facet joints that are commonly affected by osteoarthritis and stress fractures. In addition this ultrasonography technique will also enable ultrasound-guided injection of the joints to be performed.

Technique

The AF are best imaged using a convex low-frequency (2.5–5 MHz) transducer. As described above the hair is clipped from the region to be imaged, extending 6–12 cm from the midline depending on the size of the horse, the skin cleaned and ultrasound coupling applied.

The AF are most usefully imaged in transverse views (perpendicular to the midline). To obtain images of the AF, place the probe a few centimetres (2–4 cm) to the side of midline of the back, and tilt the probe head back and forth (towards the head and then tail) until the joint is visible. The DSP can be used as a convenient reference point within the ultrasound scans. By starting cranially and moving slowly towards the tail, each joint will appear sequentially. The articular facets are located differently with respect to the DSP at different levels of the spine [6]. Denoix [6] describes that in the mid-thoracic region the AF are located in the middle of the apex of the cranial vertebra; by approximately T16 the AF are located at the level of the interspinous spaces and, in the caudal thoracic and lumbar areas, the AF are located in the middle of the apex of the caudal vertebrae.

The AF can be imaged on either transverse or longitudinal scans. On transverse sections the joints appear as the corner of a square at the junction of the DSPs and TPs (Figure 10.4). With a good quality scanner, it is possible to differentiate the cranial and caudal articular processes of each vertebra. It is useful to compare each joint with the ones immediately cranial and caudal to it and with the contralateral joint. In a normal horse the right and left AFs are symmetrical. Longitudinal scans also allow identification of the facets. On longitudinal scan the bone surfaces are regular and, again, the right and left AFs are symmetrical. The advantage of the longitudinal scan is that it permits a comparison of adjacent joints simultaneously.

A number of abnormalities of the AFs have been described. These abnormalities have been classified into eight types [6] (see Chapter 8). In many cases, however, it is not possible to see sufficient detail of the AF to be able to classify the lesion. This may be due to a number of factors, including the large size of the patient, the capabilities of the ultrasound machine and the operator's experience. It is usually possible to assess and identify any asymmetries of the AFs, loss of the facet joint space (indicative of AF osteoarthritis) and the presence of proliferative new bone formation. New bone formation is the most commonly identified ultrasonographic abnormality detected at this

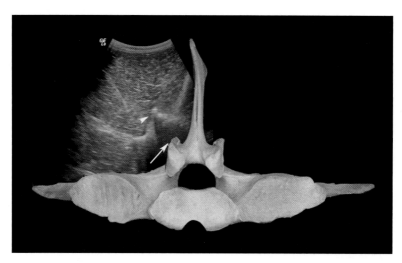

Figure 10.4 A postmortem specimen of a vertebra and a transverse ultrasonogram of the same region to demonstrate the ultrasonographic view of articular facets. The articular facet is seen at the base of the dorsal spinous process (DSP) in the postmortem specimen (arrow points to the angle of the joint). In the ultrasonogram the facet is seen to form a sharp, angled structure at the base of the DSP (arrowhead points to the angle of the joint). Note the elongated transverse processes extending from the vertebral body.

site and is identified by the production of an enlarged, irregular outline associated with the facet (see Chapter 22).

Ultrasound-guided injection in the thoracic spine

As mentioned above the technique of AF ultrasonography is extremely useful in that it permits ultrasound-guided injections of diseased facet joints as described by Denoix [8].

To medicate the region surrounding the facets, the skin should be clipped and prepared aseptically. Ultrasonography is used to identify the AF in the transverse plane as previously discussed. A spinal needle is then introduced through the skin and aimed towards the facet. The needle should be angled at 45° to the skin surface and the site of entry is between 2 and 6 cm from the midline depending on the size of the horse. The ultrasound image will allow the needle to be traced in real time as it passes through the soft tissues towards the joint. In most cases an intra-articular injection is not possible, due to the angle of the facet, poor image quality on the ultrasound, new bone formation or joint ankylosis. In these cases the medication is injected periarticularly in the region of multifidus (see Chapter 15). In addition an ultrasound-guided technique of injection of the nerves proposed to innervate the AFs has been described [9]. The AFs are innervated by the medial branch of the dorsal ramus (the spinal nerve splits into dorsal and ventral rami once it exits the intervertebral canal, see Chapter 4). This nerve branch runs in a groove on the base of the articular process of the caudal vertebra, in direct contact with the cranial aspect of the transverse process of that vertebra. To desensitise this nerve the ultrasound probe is placed 3 cm lateral to the median plane transversally and the AF identified. Once the characteristic AF has been identified the scanner is re-positioned 5 cm caudally and a needle introduced obliquely at an angle of 45° until it hits bone. Local anaesthetic solution can then be injected.

Conclusion

In conclusion, ultrasonography of the thoracic spine is an extremely important imaging technique in the horse. Pathology in the soft tissue structures of the thoracic spine is discussed in Chapter 17.

References

1. Getty, R., ed. *Sisson and Grossman's The Anatomy of Domestic Animals*. 5 edn. Philadelphia: W.B. Saunders, 1975.

2. Denoix, J.M. Ligament injuries of the axial skeleton in the horse: Supraspinal and sacroiliac desmopathies. In: Rantanen, N.W., Hauser, M.L., Matthew, R. (eds), *Proceedings of the First Dubai International Equine Symposium*. USA: Rantanen Design, 1996: 273–286.

3. Henson, F.M., Lamas, L., Knezevic, S. and Jeffcott, L.B. Ultrasonographic evaluation of the supraspinous ligament in a series of ridden and unridden horses and horses with unrelated back pathology. *BMC Veterinary Research* 2006;**3**:3.

4. Genovese, R.L., Rantanen, N.W., Simpson, B.S. and Simpson, D.M. Clinical experience with quantitative analysis of superficial digital flexor tendon injuries in Thoroughbred and Standardbred racehorses. *Veterinary Clinics of North American Equine Practice* 1990;**6**:129–145.

5. Haussler, K.K., Stover, S.M. and Willits, N.H. Developmental variation in lumbosacropelvic anatomy of Thoroughbred racehorses. *American Journal of Veterinary Research* 1997;**58**:1083–1087.

6. Denoix, J.M. Lesions of the vertebral column in poor performance horses. Presented at the World Equine Veterinary Association symposium, Paris, 1999.

7. Denoix, J.M. Ultrasonographic evaluation of back lesions. In: Haussler, K.K. (ed.), *Veterinary Clinics of North America Equine Practice*. Philadelphia: Saunders, 1999: 131–139.

8. Denoix, J.M. Apport des injections echoguidees pour les traitment locaux et intra-articulaires. Presented at the French Equine Veterinary Association, Angers, 1995.

9. Vandeweerd, J.M., Desbrosse, F., Clegg, P. et al. Innervation and nerve injections of the lumbar spine of the horse: a cadaveric study. *Equine Veterinary Journal* 2007;**39**:59–63.

11 Ultrasonography of the Lumbosacral Spine and Pelvis

Mary Beth Whitcomb

Introduction

Although nuclear scintigraphy and radiography are useful in the evaluation of horses with back or pelvic abnormalities, ultrasonography is frequently used as the primary imaging modality for soft tissue and osseous abnormalities at many referral hospitals. Such clinics are more likely to be equipped with the transducers necessary to perform a complete examination, but a standard tendon or rectal format transducer owned by most practitioners can be used to evaluate many of the structures presented in this chapter. It is recognised that examination and interpretation of some of the structures discussed in this chapter can be technically challenging to the beginner. Armed with a solid understanding of osseous and soft tissue anatomy, experience will provide the dedicated veterinarian with an adequate skill level to evaluate most horses.

The clinical presentation of horses undergoing lumbar/sacroiliac ultrasonography is typically quite different from that of horses presenting for pelvic ultrasonography. Therefore, the ultrasonographic techniques to evaluate the lumbar and sacroiliac regions are presented separately from those used to evaluate the pelvis in this chapter.

Lumbar spine and sacroiliac region

Most horses that present for examination of the lumbosacral region have a history or clinical finding of pain on palpation. Less frequently, horses present for diffuse or focal lumbar swelling or *tuber sacrale* asymmetry. Other indications include increased radiopharmaceutical uptake on nuclear scintigraphy, lameness not abated by diagnostic anaesthesia of the hindlimbs, a positive response to sacroiliac joint anaesthesia, behavioural changes perceived by the owner as related to back pain and known trauma to the region. Differentiation between lumbar and sacroiliac pain is difficult in most horses, and ultrasonographic investigation of both regions should be performed in all cases with transcutaneous and transrectal approaches.

Multiple transducers are required to perform a complete exam. A high-frequency (8–14 MHz), straight, linear transducer should be used for evaluation of the dorsal spinous processes and supraspinous ligament of the lumbar spine as well as the short dorsal sacroiliac ligaments. A midrange-frequency (4–8 MHz), microconvex transducer may be useful to visualise the sacroiliac ligaments in large horses or those with significant subcutaneous fat accumulation. This transducer is also useful for transrectal examination of the caudal lumbar and lumbosacral disc spaces, and right and left sacroiliac joints, although a standard rectal transducer set at its highest frequency can also be used. A low-frequency (2–5 MHz), curvilinear transducer is often necessary for evaluation of the lumbar articular facets and transverse processes, especially in large horses. Although the microconvex transducer can penetrate to the depths required to visualise these structures, diagnostic images are often obtained only in young or thin horses with this transducer. A program suitable for musculoskeletal use (tendon, small parts, etc.) should be selected, although an abdominal program may be helpful when using the low-frequency curvilinear transducer.

Alcohol saturation is often adequate in young or thin horses, but clipping the hair with no. 40 blades is necessary to obtain diagnostic images in many horses. Significant dorsal fat accumulation in well-fed or obese horses can significantly impede image quality. In such cases, clipping the hair will provide the examiner with the best opportunity to obtain a diagnostic examination. In addition, the skin of the back can be quite thick and an occasional horse or pony may require razor shaving in order to obtain images of the lumbar or sacroiliac region.

Transcutaneous evaluation

Lumbar spine

Evaluation of the lumbar spine should begin with the dorsal spinous processes (DSPs) and supraspinous ligament (SSL). Both are located along the dorsal midline and are evaluated using transverse and longitudinal techniques at a depth setting of 4–6 cm. The use of a standoff pad may help to maintain skin contact in thin horses with prominent DSPs. Each DSP should demonstrate a relatively smooth, flat-to-convex shape, although occasional small surface defects can be seen in horses without a history of back problems. The DSPs are more superficially located in the cranial lumbar spine and become deeper relative to the skin surface as the exam progresses caudally. DSPs should be regularly spaced and aligned along dorsal midline.

The SSL is located between the skin surface and the DSPs along the length of the lumbar spine. Its size and shape vary as it extends caudally from the DSPs of L1–6. At L1 and L2, it has a small, slightly crescent shape on transverse views, becomes progressively larger from L3 through L5 (Figure 11.1) and may show an undulating or "S"-shaped appearance at L6 (Figure 11.2). Echogenicity is somewhat variable, especially in the mid-to-caudal lumbar regions and between the DSPs due to the varying orientation of fibres as they insert onto the cranial aspect of each DSP. On longitudinal views, fibre pattern should appear relatively linear overlying each DSP but will appear somewhat irregular between DSPs.

The right and left articular facets of the lumbar spine are best visualised by placing the transducer (low-frequency curvilinear) perpendicular to the long axis of the spine, slightly to the right and left of midline, respectively. The facet joints are located 8–10 cm from the skin surface and therefore scanning depth should be set at 10–15 cm. Normal articular facets will show a step-like appearance on transverse views (Figure 11.3). Mild cortical irregularity may be present in horses without clinical signs. Longitudinal views are obtained by placing the transducer parasagittally approximately 4–5 cm to the right and left of midline. Facet joints should be regularly spaced and should not be contiguous with adjacent facets.

The transverse processes of the lumbar spine extend to the right and left of the vertebral bodies in an almost horizontal plane. They can be evaluated using transverse and longitudinal views by following their bony surfaces from midline to their abaxial extents, using the same transducer and machine settings as for the articular facets. All bony surfaces should be smooth. Although clinically significant abnormalities of the transverse processes are not common, evaluation should not be neglected. Interpretation is relatively straightforward, and the exam can be performed in a timely fashion.

Sacroiliac region

The short dorsal sacroiliac ligaments (DSILs) are paired structures that originate on the right and left tubera sacrale and course caudally alongside

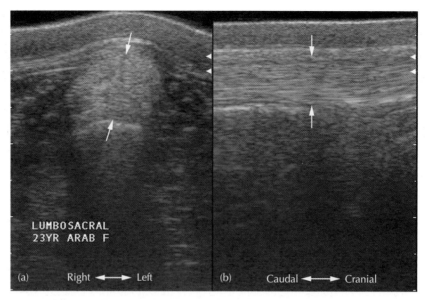

Figure 11.1 The ultrasonographic appearance of the supraspinous ligament in the lumbar region. Ultrasonograms to show the ultrasonographic appearance of the normal supraspinous ligament (arrows) at the level of the dorsal spinous process of L4. (a) Transverse and (b) longitudinal images. The ligament has a round-to-oval shape at this level with a slightly mottled echogenicity. Image obtained with 10.0 MHz linear transducer, scanning depth = 4 cm.

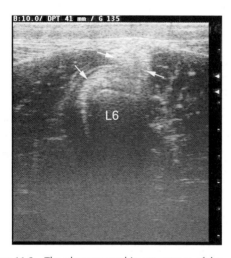

Figure 11.2 The ultrasonographic appearance of the supraspinous ligament in the lumbar region. Transverse ultrasonogram to show the ultrasonographic appearance of the normal supraspinous ligament (arrows) at the level of the dorsal spinous process of L6. The undulating appearance of the ligament at this level depends somewhat on the weight-bearing status of the horse and will change as the horse shifts weight between hind limbs. Image obtained with 10.0 MHz linear transducer, scanning depth = 4 cm.

the dorsal sacral processes to their insertions on the caudal sacral process. These ligaments are located relatively close to the skin surface and a shallow depth setting of 4–7 cm should be used. Large horses may require an increased depth setting and a decreased frequency setting for adequate penetration and visualisation. Each ligament should be evaluated individually by locating the tuber sacrale to the left and right of midline and then following each ligament caudally to its insertion. At the origin, the ligament has a thin crescent shape on transverse views (Figure 11.4), becomes somewhat round to oval shaped in the mid-ligament region (Figure 11.5) and is semicircular at its insertion onto the sacrum (Figure 11.6). Echogenicity is fairly homogeneous and fibre pattern is linear in most horses; however, some variability in both parameters will be seen in normal horses. Such variability can complicate detection of many mild and even moderate injuries. There is also considerable anatomical variation between horses due to caudal continuation of the thoracolumbar fascia (TLF) that joins the short DSIL caudal to the tuber sacrale. The TLF inserts

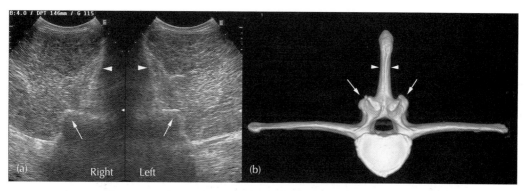

Figure 11.3   The ultrasonographic appearance of the articular facets of the lumbar vertebra. (a) A normal transverse ultrasonogram of the right and left articular facets (arrows). (b) A cranial view of an anatomical specimen of a lumbar vertebra. In (a) note the step-like appearance of each facet joint to the right and left of the dorsal spinous process (arrowheads). Image obtained with 4.0 MHz curvilinear transducer, scanning depth = 15 cm.

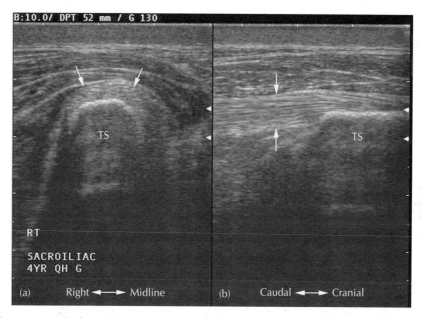

Figure 11.4   Ultrasonograms to show the appearance of the short dorsal sacroiliac ligament at its origin on the right tuber sacrale (TS): (a) transverse and (b) longitudinal ultrasonographic images of the right short dorsal sacroiliac ligament (arrows). Note the smooth bony surface of the TS in this adult horse. Image obtained with 10 MHz linear transducer, scanning depth = 5 cm.

along the medial border of each short DSIL in most horses. Less commonly, the TLF is located dorsal to the short DSIL before their confluence, creating an almost bipartite appearance. Such an appearance will be bilaterally symmetrical and should not be confused with injury (Figure 11.7).

Although clinical abnormalities of the *tubera sacralae* are uncommon, they should be evaluated together with the short DSIL. Each *tuber sacrale* should demonstrate smooth bony contours in adult horses; however, minor surface irregularities have been reported. Care should be taken with

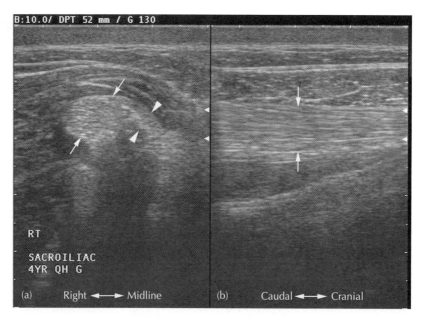

Figure 11.5   Ultrasonograms to show the appearance of the short dorsal sacroiliac ligament (DSIL) from the midligament region. (a) Transverse and (b) longitudinal ultrasonographic images of the right DSIL. The caudal extension of the thoracolumbar fascia (arrowheads) is visible medial to the right short DSIL (arrows). Image obtained with 10 MHz linear transducer, scanning depth = 5 cm.

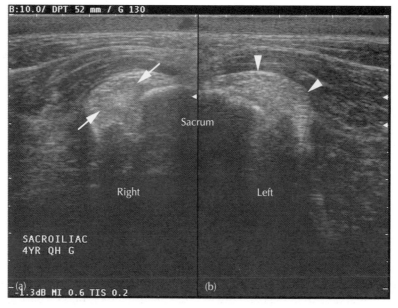

Figure 11.6   Transverse ultrasonograms to show the insertion of the (a) right and (b) left short dorsal sacroiliac ligaments (DSIL) onto the sacrum. (b) The left insertion is normal (arrowheads); however, a central core lesion (arrows) is present within the right DSIL (a). Image obtained with 10 MHz linear transducer, scanning depth = 5 cm.

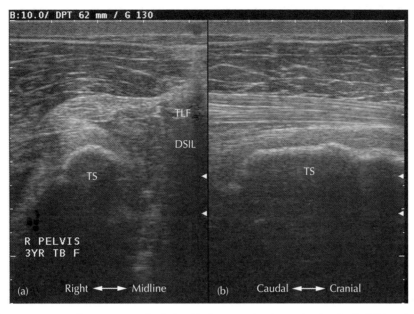

B:10.0/ DPT 62 mm / G 130

TLF

DSIL

TS

TS

R PELVIS
3YR TB F

(a)   Right ◄──► Midline   (b)   Caudal ◄──► Cranial

Figure 11.7   Ultrasonograms to show an unusual relationship between the thoracolumbar fascia (TLF) and short dorsal sacroiliac ligament (DSIL) at the level of the tuber sacrale (TS). (a) Transverse ultrasonogram and (b) longitudinal ultrasonogram. The TLF is located dorsal to the DSIL at the level of the TS. This anatomical variation is considered within normal limits, but is less commonly seen than a medial insertion of the TLF onto the short DSIL, shown in Figure 11.5. Image obtained with 10 MHz linear transducer, scanning depth = 6.2 cm.

interpretation of distance measurements from the skin to the bony surfaces of each tuber sacrale. Measurements can vary significantly depending on limb position as well as transducer placement/pressure on the skin surface. Care should also be taken when evaluating foals and juvenile horses, due to the fact that a large portion of each tuber sacrale is cartilaginous. Normal fetal cartilage is hypoechoic with a slightly speckled appearance. The underlying subchondral bone of the *tuber sacrale* will therefore have an altered shape compared with adults (Figure 11.8a). Varying degrees of ossification of the cartilage caps will be present in juveniles aged up to 2 years (Figure 11.8b). Such findings are typically bilaterally symmetrical and comparison can be helpful to differentiate bony pathology such as fractures or osteomyelitis from normal ossification.

Transcutaneous evaluation of the lateral surfaces of the sacrum should be attempted in all horses suspicious for sacral fracture. The transducer is positioned perpendicular to the long axis of the spine to the right and left of midline, caudal

to the tuber sacrale and iliac wings (Figure 11.9a). Bony surfaces should be smooth and slightly concave (Figure 11.9b). Transcutaneous visibility of the sacrum is highly variable, even with a low-frequency curvilinear transducer. Diagnostic images are frequently not obtained and close transrectal inspection should be performed. The long component of the DSIL can also be imaged using this technique. The long DSIL has an echogenic linear appearance that extends obliquely to the right and left of the sacrum (Figure 11.9b).

Transrectal evaluation

Transrectal ultrasonography is an important aspect of the lumbosacral study and includes evaluation of the sacrum, sacroiliac joints and lumbosacral junction (Figure 11.10a). All structures are located in close proximity to the rectal mucosa, and therefore a musculoskeletal or small parts program should be selected with a shallow depth

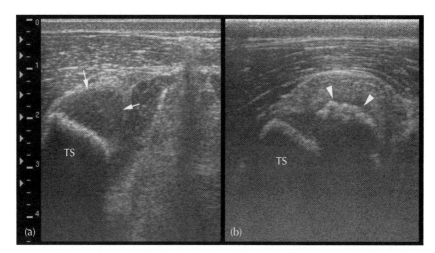

Figure 11.8 Ultrasonograms to show the transverse ultrasonographic images of the tuber sacrale (TS) in a 2-month-old foal (a) and a 2-year-old colt (b). Note the hypoechoic cartilage cap (arrows) overlying the ossified portion of the TS in the young foal (a) and the irregularly shaped area of ossification (arrowheads) within the TS cartilage of the juvenile horse (b). Varying degrees of ossification will be present in younger horses and are within normal limits. Image obtained with 10 MHz transducer, scanning depth = 4.5 cm.

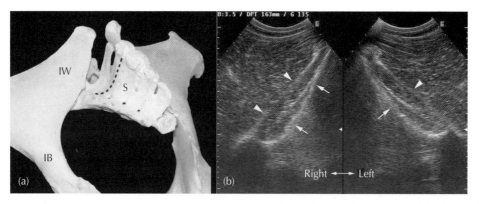

Figure 11.9 The ultrasonographic appearance of the sacrum: (a) a caudolateral view of an anatomical specimen of the pelvis and the sacrum (S) illustrating the sloping bony contour of the sacrum (dashed line) visible on transcutaneous ultrasonography. To perform transcutaneous ultrasonography the transducer is positioned caudal to the iliac wing (IW). Each side is evaluated independently by scanning to the left and right of the dorsal sacral processes. IB = iliac body (shaft). (b) A composite transverse ultrasonogram to show the ultrasonographic image of the sacrum (arrows) obtained using the technique shown in (a). The long (or lateral) portion of the right and left dorsal sacroiliac ligaments (arrowheads) is also visible and has an echogenic linear appearance that parallels the lateral aspect of the sacrum.

setting of 3–4 cm. The transducer (rectal or micro-convex) is directed dorsally along midline first to locate the disc space of L6–S1 at approximately mid-forearm to elbow's length (Figure 11.10b). The bony surfaces of the vertebral body of L6 and sacrum should be smooth. The disc space will appear somewhat triangular with a homogeneously hypoechoic appearance. To visualise the disc spaces of L5–6 and L4–5, the transducer is advanced further cranially along midline. These disc spaces will appear smaller than the lumbosacral junction. To view the right and left sacroiliac

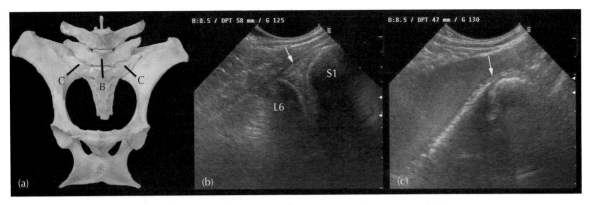

Figure 11.10   The ultrasonographic appearance of the lumbosacral region and sacroiliac joints: (a) a ventral view of an anatomical specimen of the ventral pelvis, sacrum, and sacroiliac and lumbosacral regions. Lines B and C indicate transducer placement to obtain transrectal images of the lumbosacral junction and sacroiliac joints, respectively. (b) A transrectal ultrasonogram to show the ultrasonographic image of the normal lumbosacral junction using transducer placement B on the anatomy specimen (a). The vertebral bodies of L6 and S1 have smooth bony surfaces. The intervertebral disc (arrow) has a somewhat triangular shape and a homogeneously hypoechoic appearance. (c) A transrectal ultrasonogram to show the ultrasonographic image of the normal sacroiliac joint (arrow), showing its tight articulation and smooth bony surfaces of the sacrum and iliac wing. Images obtained with 8.5 MHz microconvex transducer, scanning depth = 5–6 cm.

joints, the transducer is positioned slightly caudally from the lumbosacral junction and then to the right and left of midline, respectively. The normal joint should appear tightly articulated with relatively smooth bony surfaces (Figure 11.10c). Evaluation of the ventral aspect of the sacrum can also be performed to assist in the diagnosis of sacral fracture. Visible step defects and bony fragmentation are consistent with fracture; however, care should be taken not to misinterpret neural foramina as fractures.

Ultrasonographic evaluation of the pelvis

The primary indication for ultrasonographic evaluation of the equine pelvis is to rule out fracture; however, ultrasonography can also assist in the diagnosis of other coxofemoral joint disorders such as effusion/synovitis, osteoarthritis and luxation/subluxation. In contrast to small animal patients, fractures are usually unilateral in horses and therefore comparison to the contralateral hemipelvis can be useful when findings are questionable. Ultrasonography has many advantages compared with nuclear scintigraphy and radiography for the diagnosis of pelvic fractures. It is relatively inexpensive and can be performed in the

ambulatory setting without the risks and costs associated with transportation to a referral hospital. There are no exposure risks to personnel and general anaesthesia is not necessary. Although ultrasonography frequently provides a rapid diagnosis in horses with pelvic fractures, nuclear scintigraphy and/or radiography should be considered in highly suspect cases when ultrasonographic examination is negative.

Many horses can be evaluated using alcohol saturation of the hair coat, but images will generally be of better quality by clipping the hair, washing the skin with soap and water, and applying ultrasound gel. Evaluation of the tubera sacrale, coxae and ischii is performed with a high- or midrange-frequency transducer, because these structures are relatively superficially located, but evaluation of the bony surfaces of the iliac wing, iliac body and coxofemoral joint must be performed with a low-frequency (2–5 MHz), curvilinear or sector transducer. Transrectal ultrasonography should be performed in all cases, regardless of rectal palpation findings. It is not uncommon to identify a fracture via transrectal ultrasonography in horses that were unremarkable on rectal palpation. In addition, fractures of the ischium and pubis are rarely visible on transcutaneous examination.

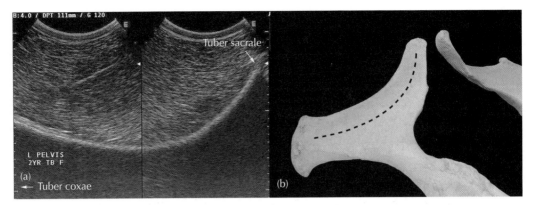

Figure 11.11   The ultrasonography appearance of the iliac wing as it extends from the tuber sacrale to the tuber coxae: (a) a composite longitudinal ultrasonographic image of the iliac wing; (b) a lateromedial view of an anatomical specimen of the iliac wing showing the site from which the ultrasonogram (a) was obtained (dotted line on anatomy specimen). The normal iliac wing has smooth convex bony surface. Image obtained with 4.0 MHz curvilinear transducer, scanning depth = 11 cm.

Deep structures of the pelvis

The iliac wing is most easily evaluated on longitudinal views by following a line drawn between the ipsilateral *tuber sacrale* and *tuber coxae*. Scanning depth should be set at 10–15 cm. Multiple slices through the iliac wing should be performed with special attention paid to the caudal border of the iliac wing in thoroughbred racehorses due to their propensity for stress fractures in this location. The normal iliac wing has a smooth concave surface (Figure 11.11). The examiner should be careful not to misinterpret "edge" artefacts caused by refraction of sound waves from fascial planes of overlying muscle bellies. This creates an artefactual gap in the bony surface at the mid-to-lateral portion of the iliac wing that may be confused with fracture (Figure 11.12).

The iliac body is evaluated by following its cortical surface from the *tuber coxae* towards the coxofemoral joint region. The iliac body demonstrates a smooth sloping bony surface on longitudinal views that becomes deeper relative to the skin surface as it nears the coxofemoral joint (Figure 11.13). An increased scanning depth of 15–20 cm is therefore required to visualise the entire bony surface. Similar to the iliac wing, longitudinal views are most useful to visualise step defects created by fractures, but transverse views may also be useful.

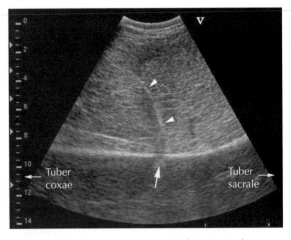

Figure 11.12   A normal longitudinal ultrasonographic image of the normal iliac wing with an artefactual defect (arrow) in its bony surface created from refraction of sound waves by the overlying fascial planes (arrowheads). This appearance should not be mistaken for a fracture. Image obtained with 4.0 MHz curvilinear transducer, scanning depth = 14 cm.

Evaluation of the coxofemoral joint is performed by sliding the transducer slightly caudally from a longitudinal image of the iliac body (Figure 11.14a). This produces a transverse image of the acetacular rim and femoral head at the cranial aspect of the coxofemoral joint (Figure 11.14b). Scanning depth is similar to that used for the iliac body (15–20 cm). The joint should appear tightly articulated, and all bony surfaces should be smooth and free of step defects. Visible joint effusion is not a common finding in normal horses. Examination of the craniodorsal and dorsal aspects of the coxofemoral joint is performed by sliding the transducer slightly dorsal and caudal from the cranial view and then rotating the transducer 70–90° in a clockwise direction when evaluating the left hemipelvis, or in a counter-clockwise direction when evaluating the right hemipelvis (Figure 11.14a). The transducer must also be directed somewhat ventrally at these locations to avoid obstruction of view by the greater trochanter of the femur. The caudal and ventral aspects of the joint cannot be visualised ultrasonographically.

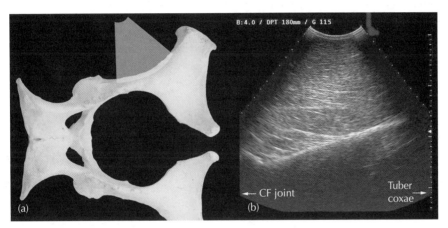

Figure 11.13 Ultrasonographic examination of the iliac body (shaft): (a) dorsoventral view of an anatomical specimen of the pelvis showing transducer orientation (grey segment) to obtain longitudinal views of the iliac body. (b) A normal longitudinal ultrasonogram to show the ultrasonographic appearance of the normal iliac body as it extends from the tuber coxae to the coxofemoral (CF) joint region. Image obtained with 4.0 MHz curvilinear transducer, scanning depth = 18 cm.

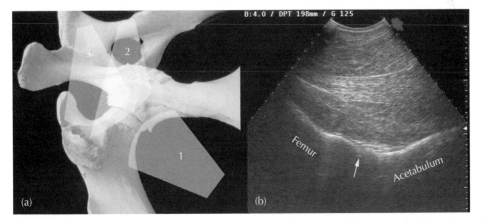

Figure 11.14 Ultrasonographic examination of the coxofemoral joint: (a) lateral view of an anatomical specimen of the coxofemoral joint showing transducer orientation (grey segments) to obtain transverse views of the cranial (1), craniodorsal (2) and dorsal (3) surfaces of the joint. (b) A normal transverse ultrasonogram to show the ultrasonographic image of the coxofemoral joint (arrow) with transducer orientation no. 2 (craniodorsal view) shown in (a). The articulation between the acetabulum and femoral head can be easily seen in most horses. All bony surfaces should be smooth. Image obtained with 4.0 MHz curvilinear transducer, scanning depth = 20 cm.

Superficial structures of the pelvis

The appearance of the *tuber sacrale* was described earlier in the chapter together with evaluation of the short DSILs. Evaluation of the *tuber coxae* is performed by placing the transducer directly on the point of the hip. The *tuber coxae* is located close to the skin surface and requires a shallow depth setting of 4–6 cm. The normal *tubera coxae* have a relatively smooth cortical surface, although some surface irregularities are within normal limits (Figure 11.15). Comparison with the contralateral side can be used in horses that are suspicious for fracture. Evaluation of the musculature ventral to the *tuber coxae* is important, because fracture fragments are typically displaced ventrally due to distraction by muscle attachments. Lastly, evaluation of the *tuber ischii* is performed by placing the transducer in the region of its palpable bony prominence approximately 20–30 cm ventral to the base of the tail. Compared with the *tuber sacrale* and *tuber coxae*, the *tuber ischii* requires an increased scanning depth of 6–12 cm. The normal *tuber ischii* has a smooth sloping appearance (Figure 11.16). Similar to tuber coxae fractures, tuber ischii fractures are often readily apparent due to ventral distraction by *semimembranosus* and *semitendinosus*. Similar to the *tuber sacrale* described earlier in this chapter, care should be taken when evaluating pelvic tuberosities in foals and juvenile horses caused by their cartilaginous centres of ossification. As ossification progresses, hyperechoic areas that appear within the cartilage can be mistaken for fractures. Comparison with the contralateral side can be useful in suspect cases.

Although not part of the pelvis, evaluation of the third trochanter of the femur should also be performed. Horses with third trochanter fractures often have a similar history and clinical findings as horses with back or pelvic injury. The third trochanter is located on the caudolateral aspect of the proximal third of the femur. Transducer orientation and its normal ultrasonographic appearance are shown in Figure 11.17. Evaluation is straightforward and fractures are easily recognisable in most cases.

Transrectal evaluation

Either a standard rectal transducer or a midrange-frequency microconvex transducer can be used. As all pelvic bony surfaces are located close to the rectal mucosa, a shallow scanning depth of 4–8 cm and a musculoskeletal or small parts program should be used. The bony surface of the ischium is readily evaluated by directing the transducer

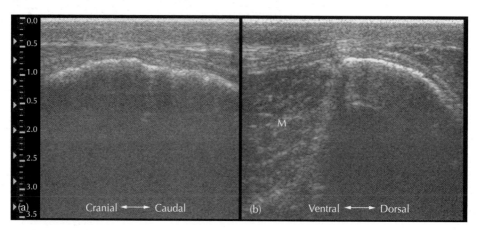

Figure 11.15 Ultrasonographic examination of the tuber coxae: (a) a normal transverse ultrasonogram and (b) a normal longitudinal ultrasonogram. The tuber coxae is seen to have a normal bony surface and ventral muscle attachments (M). Note the close proximity of the tuber coxae to the skin surface (within 1–2 cm). Image obtained with 10 MHz linear transducer, scanning depth = 3.5 cm.

ventrally upon entry into the rectum and then sweeping from left to right. The ischium should be smooth, although mild roughening will be seen along its symphysis on midline (Figure 11.18a, b). To visualise the pubis, the transducer is intro-duced further into the rectum, past the obturator foramen until the bony surface of the pubis is seen (Figure 11.18a, c). The transducer should again be swept from left to right to visualise the entire extent of the pubis. The axial surface of the acetab-

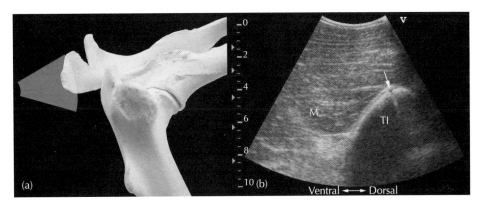

Figure 11.16 Ultrasonographic examination of the tuber ischii: (a) lateral view of an anatomical specimen of the proximal femur and its articulation with the ischium. The grey segment shows the transducer orientation required to view the tuber ischii and its ventral muscle attachments. (b) A normal ultrasonogram to show the appearance of the tuber ischii. The tuber ischii (TI) is seen to have a sloping bony contour and normal ventral muscle attachments (M). A physeal remnant (arrow) is evident in this 8-month-old colt. Image obtained with 5 MHz curvilinear transducer, scanning depth = 10 cm.

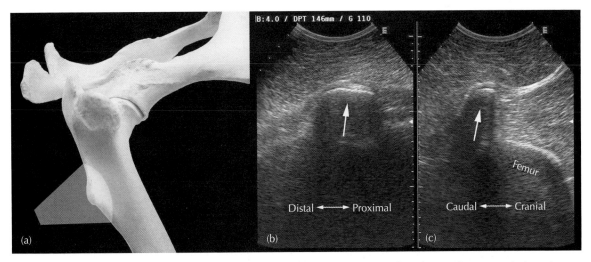

Figure 11.17 Ultrasonographic examination of the third trochanter of the femur: (a) lateral view of an anatomical specimen of the proximal femur and its articulation with the ischium. The grey segment shows the transducer orientation to obtain longitudinal views of the third trochanter. (b) A normal longitudinal ultrasonogram to show the ultrasonographic appearance of the third trochanter (arrow). The third trochanter is seen to have a smooth surface. (c) A normal transverse ultrasonogram, obtained by rotating the transducer 90° from that shown in (a). The third trochanter (arrow) has a slightly convex surface and is superficially located compared with the main portion of the femur.

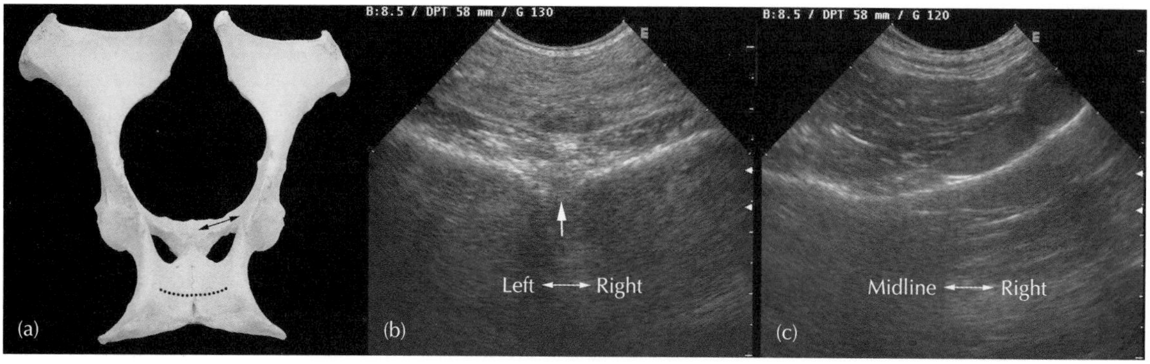

Figure 11.18   The transrectal ultrasonographic examination of the ischium and pelvis: (a) dorsal view of an anatomical specimen of the dorsal pelvis showing transducer placement to obtain transrectal images of the ischium (dotted line) and pubis (double arrow). (b) A transrectal ultrasonogram to show the ultrasonographic appearance of the normal ischium. The ischium is seen as a smooth bony surface with the exception of gap in the midline created by the ischial portion of the pubic symphysis (arrow). (c) A transrectal ultrasonogram to show the ultrasonographic appearance of the normal transrectal image of the right pubis. The pubis is seen as a smooth sloping bony surface. Both ultrasonographic images obtained with 8.5 MHz microconvex transducer, scanning depth = 5.8 cm.

ulum and iliac body can also be seen with transrectal ultrasonography and should demonstrate a smooth bony surface.

Further reading

1. Almanza, A. and Whitcombe, M.B. Ultrasonographic diagnosis of pelvic fractures in 28 horses. In: *Proceedings of the American Association of Equine Practitioners*. Lexington: AAEP, 2003: 34–41.
2. Denoix, J.M. Ultrasonographic evaluation of back lesions. *Veterinary Clinics of North America Equine Practice* 1999;**15**:131–139.
3. Gillis, C., Spinal ligament pathology. *Veterinary Clinics of North America Equine Practice* 1999;**15**:97–101.
4. Goodrich, L.R., Werpy, N.M. and Armentrout, A. How to ultrasound the normal pelvis for aiding diagnosis of pelvic fractures using rectal and transcutaneous ultrasound examination. In: *Annual Convention of the American Association of Equine Practitioners*. New Orleans: American Association of Equine Practitioners, 2006.
5. Haussler, K.K., Stover, S.M. and Willits, N.H. Developmental variation in lumbosacropelvic anatomy of Thoroughbred racehorses. *American Journal of Veterinary Research* 1997;**58**:1083–1087.
6. Henson, F.M.D., Lamas, L., Knezevic, S. and Jeffcott, L.B. Ultrasonographic evaluation of the supraspinous ligament in a series of ridden and unridden horses and horses with unrelated back pathology. *BMC Veterinary Research* 2007;**3**:3.
7. Shepherd, M.C. and Pilsworth, R.C. The use of ultrasound in the diagnosis of pelvic fractures. *Equine Veterinary Education* 1994;**6**:23–27.
8. Tomlinson, J.E., Sage, A.M. and Turner, T.A. Ultrasonographic abnormalities detected in the sacroiliac area in twenty cases of upper hindlimb lameness. *Equine Veterinary Journal* 2003;**35**:48–54.
9. Tomlinson, J.E., Sage, A.M. and Turner, T.A. Ultrasonographic examination of the normal and diseased equine pelvis. In: *Annual Convention of American Association of Equine Practitioners*. San Antonio: American Association of Equine Practitioners, 2000: 375–378.
10. Tomlinson, J.E., Sage, A.M., Turner, T.A. and Feeney, D.A. Detailed ultrasonographic mapping of the pelvis in clinically normal horses and ponies. *American Journal of Veterinary Research* 2001;**62**:1768–1775.

12 Thermography

Tracy A. Turner

Introduction

Back problems are considered a major cause of altered gait or performance in horses. Unfortunately the characterisation, localisation and identification of the painful area can be problematic. The incidence of back problems in general practice has been reported as 0.9% [1] and has been estimated as 2.2% of lameness cases [2]. The equine back covers a large area; it includes the axial skeleton from the withers to the sacroiliac joint and sacrum, and is covered with thick muscles, fascial tissues and the numerous ligaments. It is the complex nature of this large structure that makes diagnosis so difficult. Clinical signs are highly variable and imaging, using radiography, requires special equipment. Specific treatment for back pain can be performed only after identification of the site of pain and nature of the injury. It is these problems that make thermography a valuable tool in the identification of back problems. The objectives of clinical examination of the horse's back are to determine if back pain is present, the site or sites of pain, and the potential lesions for the pain. A number of confusing factors can make the diagnosis more difficult, specifically the effect of tack (saddles) and rider on the horse. Thermography aids each of these areas [3]. However, before any clinical discussion can be made, an understanding of the instrumentation and how it works, the principles of use and the physiology studied must be reviewed.

Instrumentation

Thermographic instrumentation, in the past, has been divided into contacting and non-contacting.

Contacting thermography

Contacting thermography uses liquid crystals in a deformable base [4, 5]. The crystals change shape according to the temperature that contacts them, and as they do they reflect a different colour of light. Therefore, the colour of a crystal represents a specific temperature. To use this technology for medical purposes, the liquid crystals are embedded into a flexible and durable latex sheet. This method has fallen out of favour because of numerous inherent problems in applying the technology. As a result of this, non-contacting thermography is the method of choice.

Non-contacting thermography

Two different technologies exist: cooled and uncooled. Cooled technology uses a detector of infrared radiation to measure temperature [6–8]. In addition, a series of focusing and scanning mirrors are used to systematically measure an entire field of view. The camera/detector is usually coupled to a cathode-ray tube and the intensity of the detected radiation is converted to an electrical signal. This signal is displayed on the cathode-ray tube as a black-and-white (grey scale) image of the object. The radiation intensity is directly proportional to the grey scale. Through the use of microchips, the black-and-white image can be made into a coloured image of the thermal picture (thermogram), hence a classic thermogram. As a result of the heat generated by the camera, the detector must be cooled to prevent interference from the machine heat. The complexity of the camera and the need to connect the camera to a computer makes this technology inconveniently portable.

The other technology available is uncooled technology. This technology employs a type of focal plane array, which, simply put, means that the infrared radiation is focused and measured on a series of detectors. These cameras have no moving parts and are contained in instruments the size of a handheld flashlight.

There are several factors to consider before purchasing a thermographic camera. Among the most important factors is the spectral range. For medical use, the range of 8–14 μm is ideal because this is the peak emissivity of skin. From a practical standpoint, there is also less environmental artefact at this range. The author prefers real-time thermography versus still thermography because real time eliminates any problems with motion; it also makes thermographic assessment more dynamic in that the operator can immediately observe change, and real time allows for faster imaging. Sensitivity refers to the amount of temperature difference that can be detected. Cooled units can differentiate within 0.01°C whereas most uncooled units can differentiate 0.08°C; although cooled is more sensitive, it is not applicable to veterinary thermography where 0.3°C is as sensitive as we need.

The final factor is portability and durability. In equine medicine, an instrument needs to withstand the rigors of daily use and it must be easy to carry. Relative to cooled units portability usually means increased cost. Also because of the detectors these units are usually more fragile. Uncooled cameras, using the focal array technology, are very portable and durable because there are no moving parts.

Principles of use

Heat is perpetually generated by the body, and dissipated through the skin by radiation, convection, conduction or evaporation [8]. As a result of this, skin temperature is generally 5°C (9°F) cooler than body core temperature (37°C). Skin derives its heat from the local circulation and tissue metabolism [9]. Tissue metabolism is generally constant, so variation in skin temperature is usually due to changes in local tissue perfusion. Normally, veins are warmer than arteries because they are draining metabolically active areas. Superficial veins will heat the skin more than superficial arteries, and venous drainage from tissues or organs with a high metabolic rate will be warmer than venous drainage from normal tissues.

The circulatory pattern and the relative blood flow dictate the thermal pattern, which is the basis for thermographic interpretation [8]. The normal thermal pattern of any area can be predicted on the basis of its vascularity and surface contour. Skin overlying muscle is also subject to temperature increase during muscle activity. Based on these findings, some generalisations can be made about the thermal patterns of a horse: the midline will generally be warmer [6, 8]; this includes the back, the chest, between the rear legs and along the ventral midline. Heat over the legs tends to follow the routes of the major vessels: the cephalic vein in front and the saphenous vein in the rear.

The thermal pattern of the back is warmest down the midline from the withers to the tail. There is a corresponding warm area from tuber coxae to tuber coxae. There will be isothermic bands of decreasing temperature on either side of the midline. In the lumbar area the isothermic bands are colder than they are over the thoracic area. The croup has a "T" pattern with a warm isothermic band from across the tuber coxae and down the midline. The areas over the gluteal are isothermic cold zones.

Injured or diseased tissues will invariably have an altered circulation [8]. One of the cardinal signs of inflammation is heat that results from increased circulation. Thermographically, the "hot spot" associated with the localised inflammation will generally be seen in the skin directly overlying the injury [4, 10]. However, diseased tissues may in fact have a reduced blood supply due to swelling, thrombosis of vessels or infarction of tissues [5, 11, 12]. With such lesions the area of decreased heat is usually surrounded by increased thermal emissions, probably due to shunting of blood.

Use in veterinary medicine

To produce reliable thermographic images the following factors need to be controlled: motion, extraneous radiant energy, ambient temperature and artefacts.

Motion

Motion can be controlled by immobilising the horse in stocks or using a qualified handler. The use of real-time thermography decreases the need for complete immobilisation. Chemical restraining agents to keep the horse from moving should be avoided because these drugs affect the peripheral circulation and cardiovascular systems, which could cause false thermal patterns to be produced; however, the author has not encountered this.

Extraneous radiant energy

To reduce the effects of extraneous radiant energy, thermography should be performed under cover shielded from the sun [8]. Preferably, thermography should be done in darkness or low-level lighting. Ideally, ambient temperature should be in the range of 20°C (68°F), but any temperature as long as the horse is not sweating is acceptable. Heat loss from sweating does not occur below 30°C (86°F), because radiation and convection are responsible for heat loss below that temperature. Very cold environmental temperatures may cause vasoconstriction of the lower legs and interfere with imaging. In these cases, low-level exercise to stimulate vasodilatation is necessary. The thermographic area ideally should have a steady, uniform airflow so that erroneous cooling does not occur. Practically, the horse should be kept from drafts. Likewise, the horse should be allowed time to acclimatise to the environment or room where thermography is performed. Typically, 10–15 minutes is adequate when going from a warm temperature to a cool one. However, up to 2 hours may be necessary when going from a cool environment to a warm one. In these cases, the acclimatisation can be sped up with low level exercise.

Artefacts

Artefacts are extraneous sources on the skin that can cause irregular images. Among these are debris, scar tissue, hair length, liniments, leg wraps, blankets and other equipment [8]. To avoid artefacts, make sure that all subjects are groomed and free of leg wraps, blankets or sheets for 2 hours whenever possible. Hair insulates the leg and blocks the emission of infrared radiation. But, as long as the hair is short and of uniform length, the thermal image produced is accurate. The skin should always be evaluated for changes in hair length that may cause false "hot spots" in the thermogram.

Multiple thermographic images of a suspect area should be made [13, 14]. The area in question should be evaluated from at least two directions approximately 90° apart, to determine if a "hot spot" is consistently present. The horse's extremities should be examined from four directions (circumferentially) [8]. Significant areas of inflammation will appear over the same spot on each replicate thermogram.

There are at least three ways in which thermography can be utilised in equine veterinary practice [11].

A diagnostic tool

In these cases, thermography is a physiological imaging method where a 1°C difference between two anatomically symmetrical regions indicates a region of inflammation and a decrease in temperature is as important as an increase in temperature. The image will identify an area of interest to pursue with an anatomical imaging method such as ultrasonography and/or radiography. The author finds that temperature differences as little as 0.3°C are significant.

To enhance the physical examination

In this case, thermography is used to identify changes in heat and therefore locate "areas of suspicion". Thermographic cameras are easily 10 times more sensitive than the hand in determining temperature differences. This method simply helps identify asymmetry and then the practitioner must use the information to determine the actual cause and significance of the temperature difference.

In a wellness programme

In this method, horses in training are followed on a routine basis, once weekly. Thermographic changes will occur 2 weeks before clinical changes. In these cases, thermography can be used to identify subclinical problems, and then training alterations can be made so that injury may be avoided altogether.

Thermography of the back

Thermography has been used to identify six different back injuries: overriding dorsal spinous processes (ORDSPs, kissing spines), dorsal spinous ligament injuries, muscle pain, withers injuries, sacroiliac problems and saddle fit problems [2]. To obtain a readable thermogram of the back, one must get high enough behind the horse to get a full view of the back. To be 90° to the back is ideal but not always positive, but less than 60° is not high enough to produce a good thermogram of the back. An alternative is to stand the horse under a reflective mirror and capture the back image through the horse's reflection.

The author uses two different thermal images to assess the back: one a thoracolumbar view and the second a croup view (Plate 25). The thoracolumbar view shows the withers and the sacrum and is especially good for looking at the mid-back. The croup view is best for evaluating the sacroiliac region. The thermal pattern is the most important aspect of assessing the thermogram of the back. It must be remembered that thermography establishes the location of a possible problem; it does not characterise the lesion. However, we will show that there are certain patterns that have been seen consistently with particular back problems.

The normal back pattern is: the warmest areas are down the midline, cooling slightly in the lumbar region and a warm cross from *tuber coxae* to *tuber coxae* and over the *tuber sacrale*, then same warmth down the middle of the croup (Plate 25). The warm area has symmetrical isothermic bands on either side. Any variation of this pattern

is due to either an artefact (thin hair, rubbed area) or a pathological process. If the lesion occurs along the midline of the thoracolumbar area, radiographs of the thoracolumbar spine are indicated. If the lesion occurs off the midline or in the croup region, we usually image the area with ultrasonography.

ORDSPs have been associated with any one of three different thermal patterns (T.A. Turner, personal communication, 2008):

1. Pattern 1: horses showed a "hot streak" perpendicular to the thoracic spine (Figure 12.1a).
2. Pattern 2: horses showed a "cold streak" perpendicular to the thoracic spine (Figure 12.1b).
3. Pattern 3: (the most common): horses showed a combination "hot spot"–"cold streak" pattern over the back (Figure 12.1c).

Our practice has evaluated 95 cases of ORDSPs over 3 years. In these cases the sensitivity of thermography for overriding spinous processes was 99%; however, the specificity was only 75%. This results in a positive predictive value of 94%. Compared with the positive predictive value of palpable pain in the thoracolumbar area for kissing spines, which is 74%, thermography performs well.

In contrast injuries to the supraspinous ligament or dorsal sacroiliac ligament injuries have not presented with this type of identifiable pattern [2]. Thermography changes associated with these injuries have been abnormal thoracolumbar thermal images. The specific changes may be increased heat, decreased heat or simply an abnormal back thermogram. After the identification of an abnormal thermogram, ultrasonography is used to identify the lesion (see Chapter 17).

Muscle injuries of the thoracolumbar region likewise do not have characteristic thermograms [2]. Typically, however, the thermal patterns will show either "hot spots" or "cold spots" off the midline (Figure 12.2). It is in these regions that we have concentrated ultrasonography to determine if muscle lesions can be seen. Withers injuries have all shown "hot spots" in the area of the withers, but nothing more characteristic than that. The croup muscles will show some specific changes [12].

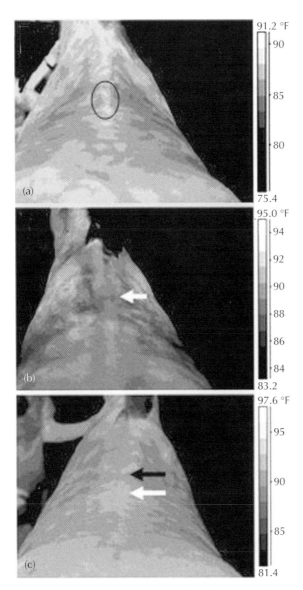

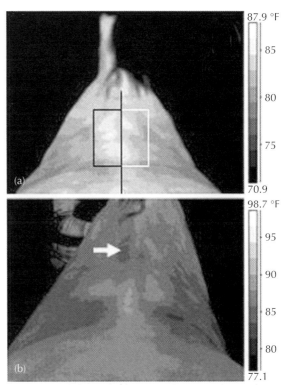

Figure 12.2   Two thermograms to show the pattern of distribution of body surface temperature in horses with suspected muscle pathology: (a) a horse with increased heat over muscle. The black line signifies midline, the black box is the region of "heat" on the left side and the white box is the corresponding "cooler" area on the right. (b) A horse with a "cold area" over the epaxial muscle just left of the midline (white arrow).

Figure 12.1   Three thermograms to show the pattern of distribution of body surface temperature in horses with overriding dorsal spinous processes (ORDSPs): (a) A horse with ORDSPs showing "hot spot" (circle). (b) A horse with ORDSPs showing the "cold streak" (white arrow). (c) A horse with ORDSPs showing the "hot" (black arrow) "cold" (white arrow) pattern.

Sacroiliac region thermography has shown several different patterns [2]. The most common pattern is a cold area centred over the region of the *tuber sacrale* (see Figure 10.4 in Chapter 10).

This finding of cold is hypothesised to be due to lack of normal movement in the sacroiliac region. This lack of movement can either result from primary pathology or be secondary to other causes of the horse not moving normally through the pelvic region. This has been corroborated by our clinical findings as well. Specifically, we find that only about half the horses exhibiting this thermal pattern actually show pain in the sacroiliac area. In addition, ultrasonographic evaluation reveals pathology in only about half the cases and this pathology usually looks chronic in nature.

We have seen either thinning of the cross-sectional diameter of the dorsal sacroiliac ligaments or, in a few cases, thickening of the ligaments. In these cases with the cold area, generally, if there is pain in the area we ultrasonographically examine the sacroiliac region. On the other hand, if there is no pain or the horse moves normally through the pelvis, we look for other causes of loss of back mobility. Pathology is seen much more commonly if the area over the tuber sacrale is hot or there is a hot spot centred over one *tuber sacrale* or the other (Figure 12.3). The pathology varies from hypoechoic areas within the dorsal sacral ligaments to generalised oedema in the region. This thermographic pattern is almost always associated with either pain or marked stiffness in the sacroiliac region.

Saddle fit thermography is very interesting (see Chapter 24) and requires multiple examinations

[3]. Thermography is an imaging modality that offers objective insight into saddle fit but has multiple other veterinary applications. In evaluating the dynamic interaction between the saddle and the horse's back, thermography will show not only the heat generated in contact areas on the saddle (Figure 12.4a), but also the physiological effects of the saddle on the horse's back (Figure 12.4b). A consistent technique provides the most useful information. Our protocol is to perform a baseline thermographic examination of the horse's back. Then the horse is saddled over a simple cotton pad with the girth as tight as it would be for riding, and the horse lunged for at least 20 minutes. The horse should be exercised at its normal gaits (walk, trot, canter) paying attention to dividing the lunging time equally in both direc-

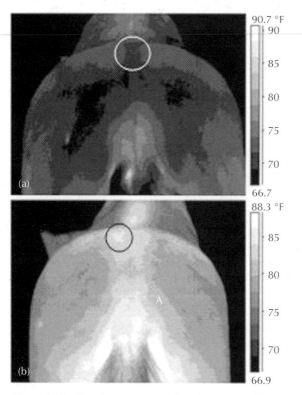

Figure 12.3 Two thermograms to show the pattern of distribution of body surface temperature in horses with suspected sacroiliac pathology: (a) a horse showing the "cold spot" (white circle) over the tuber sacrale indicating possible sacroiliac disease. (b) A horse showing a "hot spot" (black circle) over the left tuber sacrale indicating possible sacroiliac disease.

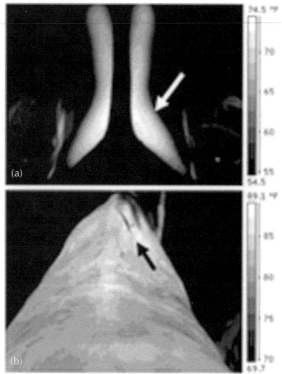

Figure 12.4 Two thermograms to show the pattern of distribution of body surface temperature in horses associated with the saddle: (a) a thermogram of the panels of a saddle; the right side of the saddle shows more heat (white arrow). (b) A thermogram of the horse where the saddle had been. The black arrow shows increased heat, correlating with the same region as the saddle in (b).

tions. The saddle is then removed and the panels of the saddle are assessed thermographically. The most important criterion is thermal symmetry. After the saddle is replaced, the back is reassessed. Again thermal symmetry is important. Most commonly because of the heat generated by the saddle, the horse's midline is now colder than the other structures under the saddle. In addition, the examiner is looking for focal hot spots, particularly along the spine, or hot or cold spots over the musculature. These abnormalities indicate problems caused by the saddle. The assessment is then repeated after a similar exercise session with the rider mounted. This evaluation allows consideration of the effect of the rider on the horse's back.

Conclusions

As our technological capabilities for equine practice increase and improvements are made in imaging the biological organism, our ability to make accurate diagnoses continues to improve. It is important to understand that no imaging techniques can replace or be used instead of the physical examination. Rather, all imaging techniques enhance only the database established by the physical examination, and each imaging modality offers unique specific information. Similarly, each imaging modality correspondingly has its own limitations.

Thermography is a physiological imaging modality [11]. It provides information about tissue physiology: specifically it gives insight into the circulation. It also provides information as to the location of injury or disease, as well as viability of the tissue, but it does not provide information as to the specific nature of the problem. This must be reserved for an anatomical imaging modality that identifies the structure of the tissues in question.

Radiography generally evaluates changes in bone. Identifications of these changes are used to determine injuries to bone. Unfortunately, except for fractures, most radiographic changes in bone often take 10–14 days to become evident [11, 15]. Furthermore, many of the bone changes are often permanent, so it can be difficult to determine if a change, especially a chronic change, is the cause of pain and lameness.

Thermography essentially images inflammation that usually implies pain [6, 8]. In this respect, thermography can directly help determine if a radiographic change is associated with inflammation, and therefore the possible cause of lameness.

Thermography and ultrasonography are complementary. Whereas thermography may be used to locate an injury, ultrasonography evaluates the injured structure's morphology and the size and shape of the injury. Ultrasonography can be used to follow the healing, but thermography evaluates "when" the inflammatory process is resolved [5, 11].

Thermography is a practical aid in the clinical evaluation of the horse. It is of particular help in the assessment of the horse's back. This modality specifically increases the accuracy of diagnosis. Thermography is an excellent adjunct to clinical examination, as well as being complementary to other imaging techniques such as radiology, ultrasonography and scintigraphy.

References

1. British Equine Veterinary Association. Survey of equine disease. *Veterinary Record* 1965;**77**:528–538.
2. Turner, T.A. Back problems in horses. In: *Annual Convention of the American Association of Equine Practitioners*. New Orleans: American Association of Equine Practitioners, 2003.
3. Turner, T.A. How to assess saddle fit in horses. In: *Annual Convention of the American Association of Equine Practitioners*. Denver: American Association of Equine Practitioners, 2004.
4. Hall, J., Bramlage, L.R., Kantrowitz, B.M., Page, L. and Simpson, B. Correlation between contact thermography and ultrasonography in the evaluation of experimentally-induced superficial flexor tendinitis. In: *Annual Meeting of the American Association of Equine Practitioners*. New Orleans: American Association of Equine Practitioners, 1987.
5. Townsend, H.G.G., Leach, D.H., Doige, C.E. and Kirkaldy-Willis, W.H. Relationship between spinal biomechanics and pathological changes in the equine thoracolumbar spine. *Equine Veterinary Journal* 1986;**18**:107–112.
6. Purohit, R.C. and McCoy, M.D. Thermography in the diagnosis of inflammatory processes in the horse. *American Journal of Veterinary Research* 1980;**41**: 1167–1174.

7. Purohit, R.C., McCoy, M.D. and Bergfeld, W.A. Thermographic diagnosis of Horner's syndrome in the horse. *American Journal of Veterinary Research* 1980;**41**:1180–1182.

8. Turner, T.A., Purohit, R.C. and Fessler, J.F. Thermography: A review in equine medicine. *Compendium of Continuing Education* 1986;**8**:855–861.

9. Love, T.J. Thermography as an indicator of blood perfusion. *Annals of the New York Academy of Sciences* 1980;**335**:429–437.

10. Bowman, K.F., Purohit, R.C., Ganjam, U.K., Pechman, R.D.J. and Vaughan, J.T. Thermographic evaluation of corticosteroids efficacy in amphotericin B induced arthritis in ponies. *American Journal of Veterinary Research.*1983;**44**:51–66.

11. Turner, T.A., Diagnostic thermography. In: Kraft, S.L. and Roberts, G.D. (eds), *Veterinary Clinics of North America Equine Practice.* Philadelphia: Saunders, 2001: 95–114.

12. Turner, T.A. Hindlimb muscle strain as a cause of lameness in horses. In: *Proceedings of the 35th Annual Convention of the American Association of Equine Practitioners.* Boston, MA: AAEP, 1989: 281.

13. Weinstein, S.A. and Weinstein, G. A clinical comparison of cervical thermography with EMG, CT scanning, myelography and surgical procedures in 500 patients. *Proceedings of the Academy of Neuromuscular Thermography* 1985;**2**:44–47.

14. Weinstein, S.A. and Weinstein, G. A review of 500 patients with low back complaints; comparison of five clinically-accepted diagnostic modalities. *Proceedings of the Academy of Neuromuscular Thermography* 1985;**2**:40–43.

15. Stromberg, B. The use of thermography in equine orthopedics. *Journal of Veterinary Radiology* 1974; **15**:94.

Section 3

The Diagnosis and Treatment of Specific Conditions

13 Traumatic Damage to the Back and Pelvis

Adam Driver and Rob Pilsworth

General principles

In many cases of pathological change in the skeleton of the equine athlete, predictable patterns of the site and nature of the pathology have been documented [1]. This is because many of the conditions that we encounter in our equine athletes are stress injuries produced by a focal accumulation of microdamage as a result of cyclical loading or overloading at specific sites. These sites are predetermined by the anatomy of the horse and the discipline that the horse is used for, which subjects certain areas to an increased likelihood of damage. In contrast, in traumatic damage to the spine and pelvis, these rules do not apply. The combination of the weight of the horse and the speed at which it was travelling, together with whatever inciting cause produces the traumatic damage, can lead to a bewilderingly complex array of injuries that can occur alone or in combination, e.g. after a fall a horse can sustain fractures to one, or several, elements of the pelvis, depending on how the horse falls and on to what it falls. Distinct clinical entities are therefore often merged and can be a diagnostic challenge.

Fracture of the dorsal spinous processes of the thoracic vertebrae (fractured withers)

Presentation and clinical signs

This injury almost always follows the horse rearing up over backwards and landing on the withers. There is usually a reluctance to walk, with the horse planting all four feet, similar to the presentation of a horse with quadrilateral acute laminitis. Great pain is usually exhibited initially with sweating and boarding of the entire musculature associated with the thoracolumbar spine. The head is usually held in hyperextension and the neck held rigid, in the horse's attempt to avoid movement of the nuchal ligament. Almost always several dorsal spinous processes (DSPs) fracture together and the entire segment of "freed" thoracic spines, along with the muscular insertions, is pulled to one side or the other of the midline. This normally results in a deviation of the line of the spine when viewed from the rear. This is sometimes more easily appreciated by palpation, by running the finger tips gently along the tips of the DSPs, than by visualisation, because the initial associated soft tissue swelling may obscure the spinal deviation.

The displacement of the fractured wither to one side also allows the proximal scapula on the contralateral side to protrude dorsally more than is normal. This should not be confused with a specific injury to the scapula, and is merely the result of displacement of the fractured segment of spine.

Diagnostic imaging

A radiographic examination of the withers region is recommended to confirm the diagnosis. The radiographs will show fracture and displacement of the DSPs and are usually diagnostic (Figure 13.1). In most cases of fractured DSPs, nuclear scintigraphy is probably not indicated. As stated elsewhere (see Chapter 8), care should be taken not to overinterpret the normal separate centres of ossification seen in the DSPs of all horses.

Treatment and prognosis

The treatment of fractured DSPs consists of administration of analgesics and non-steroidal anti-

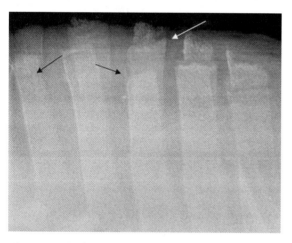

Figure 13.1   A lateromedial radiograph of the withers region (T5–9) showing fracture and displacement of the thoracic dorsal spinous processes (four fractures are apparent in this radiograph) .The normal separate centres of ossification (white arrow) should not be mistaken for fractures of the tip of the process (black arrow). This case shows the considerable overriding of the fracture, which results in "sinking" of the contour of the wither.

inflammatory drugs (NSAIDs) in the initial shock-like state. The horse should then be confined to the stable for at least 4 weeks to allow the fractured segment of the spine to stabilise in its new position. In the initial period, the horse will be unwilling to lower the head. Feed, hay and water should therefore be provided in elevated mangers. The temperature of the horse should be monitored daily, but, as the concurrent use of NSAIDs can artificially suppress pyrexia, occasional blood samples should be taken to guard against the possible development of pleuropneumonia. The risk factors for pleuropneumonia have been documented to increase as a result of impaired drainage of bronchial secretions, which follows continued elevation of the head and neck [2].

The prognosis for return to full function is usually good, but the horse will require care with saddling because of possible traumatic impingement between the front of the saddle and the new position of the withers. The apparent asymmetry often becomes less marked with time as the acute swelling subsides. In rare instances, the parent bone of one or more of the fractured DSPs can erode its way through the intervening tissues and ulcerate the skin. Should this occur, surgical treatment for removal of this spiculated sharp piece of bone will be necessary to avoid the development of chronic discharging fistula and infection of the associated site.

Fractures of the thoracolumbar vertebral column

Fractures of the vertebral column include fractures of the articular facet joints and fractures of the vertebral body and laminae. Each of these are considered in turn.

Fractures of the articular facet joints.

Presentation and clinical signs

Clinically horses present with localised marked muscle spasm, guarding, reluctance to flex the back and severe pain when the back is manipulated. A mild scoliosis towards the affected side may be present when the horse is observed from behind.

Diagnosis

The diagnosis of articular facet joint fractures has, historically, been a difficult challenge. However, with the advent of nuclear scintigraphy, the fractures can be readily seen within the spine. The fractures result in focal moderate-to-marked, increased radiopharmaceutical uptake at the site of the articular facet joint. This is in the dorsal region of the vertebral body, similar to the position where vertebral laminar stress fractures are seen in racehorses (see Chapters 15 and 22). Once a lesion is suspected, radiography can be targeted at the site of the lesion (see Chapter 8). Specialist dorsomedial–ventrolateral oblique (DMVLO) projections, highlighting the facet joints, can also be beneficial in demonstrating fractures (see Chapter 8). Ultrasonography may be helpful in some cases. In the acute phase, ultrasonography may visualise incongruity of the bone surface at the fracture site when performed diligently. In the chronic phase callus formation will be visible around the joint.

Treatment and prognosis

The treatment of a fractured articular facet is conservative. This conservative therapy comprises box rest for a period of 4–6 weeks, together with the administration of NSAIDs at least for the first 2 weeks. If the fracture is diagnosed in the chronic phase, with arthropathy or ankylosis of the facet joint, periarticular injection with corticosteroids may be beneficial, along with supportive therapy for epaxial muscular spasm and altered exercise. Overall, however, the prognosis for return to exercise is guarded at best.

Fractures of the vertebral body and laminae

Presentation and clinical signs

The horse presenting with vertebral body fractures will have clinical signs dependent on the degree of spinal cord compression and neurological compromise. Vertebral body fractures can cause a range of presentations, including cases in which no neurological changes are seen and the horse demonstrates severe back pain, to cases in which minor nervous damage is caused, leading to neurogenic atrophy of the epaxial musculature. In severe cases spinal cord damage leads to complete recumbency or "dog sitting" (hindlimb paralysis with functional forelimbs), with paralysis and loss of deep pain response in the hind limbs. It must also be noted that the clinical signs can change with time depending on the ongoing swelling or haemorrhage around and in the spinal cord. Vertebral fractures are often a result of high-speed falls or impact with static objects, leading to the initial examination often being performed in difficult surroundings.

Diagnosis

A thorough clinical and neurological examination is essential to determine the severity and prognosis of the trauma. It should be remembered that, in any traumatic incident, the neurological signs seen could be associated with cranial trauma, so the entire nervous system should be evaluated, including the cranial nerves. The examinations should aim to determine the site of the lesion and the severity. By evaluating the presenting upper motor neuron (UMN) and lower motor neuron (LMN) signs the location of the lesion can be identified. UMN signs include mild weakness and ataxia, spastic bladder paralysis and hypermetria, and hyperreflexia. LMN signs include marked weakness or paresis, flaccid paralysis of the bladder, hyporeflexia and, over a short period of time, marked neurogenic muscle atrophy. The spine can be divided into regions producing characteristic signs (summarised in Table 13.1).

Table 13.1 A summary of the clinical signs of traumatic damage at different sites of the spinal column

Site of damage	Clinical signs of damage
C6–T2	Front legs – LMN signs Hind legs – UMN signs Spastic urinary incontinence
T3–L3	Front legs – normal Hind legs – UMN signs Spastic bladder incontinence
L4–S2	Front legs – normal Hind legs – LMN Flaccid bladder paralysis, loss of anal sphincter tone and reflex and tail tone

LMN, lower motor neuron; UMN, upper motor neuron.

Lesions between C6 and T2 produce LMN signs in the front limbs and UMN signs in the hindlimbs, with spastic urinary incontinence. Lesions between T3 and L3 produce UMN signs in the hind limbs, spastic bladder incontinence, normal front limbs, and with time possible neurogenic atrophy of the muscles of the back in that region. Lesions between L4 and S2 produce LMN signs in the hindlimbs, flaccid bladder paralysis, loss of anal sphincter tone and reflex and tail tone, and normal front limbs. The proprioceptive system should also be evaluated during the neurological examination, to help determine the severity of the lesion. Mild compression will produce placement deficits and ataxia, the same as UMN signs. Moderate compression can result in paresis or paralysis of voluntary movements and reflexes, and a loss of skin sensation. Severe compression or transection will lead to a loss of deep pain sensation.

Once the lesion has been localised, and if the horse retains enough motor neuron and proprioceptive control to be moved, radiography is the imaging modality of choice to determine the fracture configuration and help determine the prognosis and treatment plan. Sometimes, however, although a vertebral fracture is suspected the diagnosis will only be made *post mortem*.

In cases of severe fracture dislocation of the spine, e.g. after collision with a motor vehicle or a very severe fall in competition, the veterinarian is often presented with a recumbent horse, in a difficult situation. The full neurological examination is difficult in these circumstances. A pragmatic approach has to take into account the welfare of the horse and the needs of the situation, if, for example, on a public road or in a competition arena. Any horse that, after a known fall or collision, is fully conscious, but remains recumbent and has made no attempt to rise for more than an hour, with associated hemi- or tetraplegia, can be considered a justifiable case for euthanasia, even in the absence of a definitive diagnosis [3].

Treatment and prognosis

Treatment is aimed at aggressive anti-inflammatory and antioxidant therapy (summarised in Table 13.2). This will include corticosteroid and NSAIDs such as dexamethasone (up to 0.2 mg/kg i.v.) or methylprednisolone sodium succinate

Table 13.2   Drugs that may be used in the treatment of vertebral fractures and their recommended dosages

Drug	Recommended dosage
Dexamethasone	Up to 0.2 mg/kg i.v.
Methylprednisolone sodium succinate	2–4 mg/kg
Flunixin meglumine	1 mg/kg i.v.
Mannitol	1 g/kg (20% solution over 20 min)
Dimethylsulphoxide	1 g/kg (10% solution twice a day)

(Solu-Cortef) (2–4 mg/kg i.v.) and flunixin meglumine (1 mg/kg i.v.). Mannitol use has also been proposed to reduce vasogenic oedema (1 g/kg maximum dose given as a 20% solution over 20 minutes). Antioxidative therapy includes dimethylsulphoxide (DMSO) (1 g/kg as a 10% solution twice a day) and vitamins E and C supplementation. Strict box rest and maintaining the horse in a quiet environment are essential. In most cases traumatic fracture of the back holds a poor-to-hopeless prognosis, however, with most fractures proving fatal.

Pelvic factures

Fractures of the tuber coxae

Presentation and clinical signs

Fractured *tubera coxae* often follow a history of impact with an inanimate object, usually a door frame, or after a fall on to a hard surface [4]. In the racehorse these can present as an acute fracture after hard work, but probably as the end-stage of stress pathology at the site rather than after trauma [5].

Complete fractures of the *tuber coxae* present with marked asymmetry of the bony prominences of the pelvis, with the fractured *tuber coxae* normally displaced ventrally and cranially into the sublumbar fossa. This displacement is due to the continued, unopposed contraction of the muscles that originate on the *tuber coxae*: the external abdominal oblique, superficial gluteal and *tensor fasciae latae*. This cranioventral displacement gives the condition its colloquial name of "knocked-down hip".

Clinically, a fractured *tuber coxae* causes a moderate-to-marked lameness, with gross asymmetry of the *tuber coxae*, as noted previously, giving a pathognomonic presentation. Crepitus and swelling may also be present at the site of the fracture, along with a moderate-to-marked pain response to palpation.

Diagnosis

Further diagnostic tests are not often required to diagnose the fracture, but the remainder of the pelvic girdle should be fully assessed, particularly if the inciting incident is unknown, or if the incident consisted of a high-speed fall, because further fractures may also be present. Ultrasound examination is the modality of choice to assess the integrity of the remainder of the pelvic girdle, and can also be used to confirm the primary diagnosis (Figure 13.2).

Treatment and prognosis

Treatment for a fractured *tuber coxae* consists of box rest for 8–12 weeks to allow for stabilisation of the fracture pieces in their new positions. The main complications that can occur include progression to a compound fracture if the sharp bone margins from the fracture bed penetrate the skin,

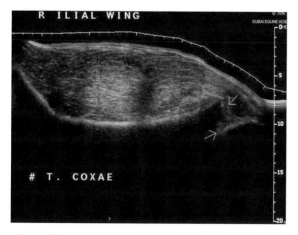

Figure 13.2 An ultrasound scan of a displaced fracture of the tuber coxae. Note the clear gap (white arrows) between the iliac surface and the displaced bone fragment.

leading to infection and potential sequestration of the fracture fragment if the blood supply is compromised. In these cases surgical débridement of infected or necrotic bone may be required, along with antibiotic therapy and management of the discharging lesion.

The prognosis for return to exercise is guarded, with an expected mechanical restriction of the stride length due to the occurrence of altered pelvis conformation. However, despite this expected impairment, many racehorses with this injury return to full competitive athletic function in that discipline after healing, so the prognosis depends to some extent on the expected and acceptable level of gait impairment after recovery.

Fractures of the ilial wing and shaft

Presentation and clinical signs

Ilial wing fractures are most common in the racehorse because this is a predilection site for stress fracture, but can also result from a fall at high speed. Due to the traumatic nature of the latter fractures, they can occur in any configuration. Fractures are most commonly unilateral but can be bilateral. Horses present with marked or non-weight-bearing lameness on the affected side, and will show signs of marked pain, including spasm of and sweating over the gluteal musculature, a hunched-up appearance, and a reluctance to move or bear weight. There is frequently asymmetry of the *tuber sacrale*, with the affected side displacing ventrally if the fracture is complete and at its base. If the fracture is at the base of the shaft or extends from the wing into the shaft, there is particularly high risk for laceration of the internal iliac artery, leading to the horse presenting in hypovolaemic shock, often with swelling of the upper thigh region as the blood is forced through the fascial planes. In these cases the horse will sometimes exsanguinate rapidly.

Ilial shaft fractures can occur in isolation or as part of a complex fracture of the pelvis. In the authors' experience these fractures hold a greater risk for laceration of an internal iliac artery and exsanguination of the horse than the ilial wing fracture described above. The horse will present with marked lameness or be non-weight bearing, with spasm of the gluteal muscles, similar to an ilial wing fracture. If the fracture is complete, the ipsilateral *tuber coxae* may appear ventrally displaced compared with the contralateral side. Frequently there is also crepitus or distinct "clicking" as the horse shifts weight with complete fractures. A rectal examination may allow the clinician to palpate the fracture site and associated haemorrhage on the axial margin of the shaft.

Diagnosis

Ultrasonography is the imaging modality of choice for confirmation of diagnosis [6, 7]. The normal ilial wing has a continuous, smooth, hyperechoic, curving bone margin when scanned through the gluteal muscle mass. A fracture will present as a discontinuity or "step" in the hyperechoic bone margin (Figure 13.3), frequently with an area of anechoic/hypoechoic haemorrhage around the site, with disruption of the overlying, normal, hypoechoic/echogenic, striated muscular pattern. The wing should be scanned in both a longitudinal and a transverse plane, paying particularly close attention to the caudal margin, which is often the

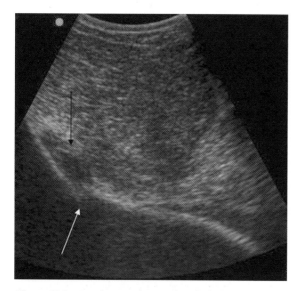

Figure 13.3   An ultrasound scan of an ilial wing fracture. Displaced fractures such as these show an easily demonstrated abrupt "step" in the surface of the ilium (white arrow), often associated with an area of hypoechogenicity resulting from haemorrhage within the muscle (black arrow).

only site that will present with an incongruity in incomplete fractures. Caution should be observed when interpreting acoustic shadowing caused by focal neurovascular bundles or fascial plane intersections that will extend to the wing margin and cause a focal anechoic spot, creating a false-positive finding. Linear, curvilinear or microconvex probes with frequency range from 3 MHz to 5 MHz are all suitable for examining the ilial wing.

Ultrasonography of the shaft can be technically more difficult to perform than examination of the ilial wing and a thorough knowledge of the structural anatomy of the pelvis is required. It is essential that the probe be aligned parallel to the shaft, otherwise obliquity can create false "steps" in the shaft, which may be misdiagnosed as fractures. The shaft should be examined over its entire length, from the base at the ilial wing to the raised cup of the acetabulum at the coxofemoral joint. Similar to the shaft, the fracture site will present as a disruption or "step" in the normal, smooth, sharply defined, hyperechoic bone margin, with hypoechoic/anechoic haemorrhage in the surrounding soft tissues. Ultrasound examinations can often give a false-negative result in the acute phase, when the fracture is incomplete. At *postmortem* examination a common configuration of these fractures is such that the cranial exit point of the fracture is on the ventral aspect of the shaft, at the junction with the iliac wing, and the fracture line extends along the shaft, similar to the splitting of a log along its length. It will be appreciated that, as only the dorsal aspect of the shaft can be evaluated with ultrasonography, the fracture cannot be identified until complete collapse or displacement occurs.

Nuclear scintigraphy may be useful in confirming a diagnosis of a fractured ilial wing or shaft, particularly in some shaft fractures when ultrasonographic evaluation is inconclusive, but it should not be performed until 5–7 days after the inciting incident to minimise the risk of false-negative results (see Chapter 9). These false-negative results (i.e. failure to diagnose the fractures) are probably a result of attenuation of the gamma radiation due to the overlying muscle mass, or disruption of the blood supply to the fracture site limiting supply of radiopharmaceutical to the bone after the acute fracture. Depending on the severity of lameness and stability at the fracture site, it may not be possible to transport a horse to a scintigraphy facility safely.

Prognosis and treatment

Treatment, as with all pelvic fractures, is conservative, with box rest for a minimum of 8–12 weeks. Many authors also recommend cross-tying of the horse during the first 3- to 4-week period, until the fracture site is stable, to prevent laceration of the internal iliac artery. Managing the cross-tied horse is essential to a successful outcome. The horse should be untied at least four times a day to feed from the ground. The rectal temperature should be monitored twice daily or, if NSAIDs are being administered, routine haematology testing performed every 48 hours, to ensure early detection of any developing pleuropneumonia. The contralateral limb should be closely monitored for signs of laminitis if the horse is non-weight bearing or severely lame on the fractured side, and appropriate support therapy including deep bedding or bedding on sand, aspirin (20 mg/kg p.o. twice daily) and acepromazine (0.02–0.04 mg/kg i.m. or p.o. twice daily). Frog support such as Styrofoam pad or sole support material should also be applied, but this is frequently not possible in the acute phase of the fracture. Pain relief for the horse must be balanced between allowing the horse to remain comfortable and minimising morbidity, while maintaining the inherent protective mechanisms of pain. All four limbs will require careful bandaging to minimise the degree of distal limb oedema, and these bandages should be changed twice daily. The horse should be placed in as quiet a stable as possible and should be able to see what is happening in its surrounding environment so that it is not startled or surprised. There should always be a piece of twine between the headcollar and each shank connecting the horse to the overhead rope or wall rings, to prevent the horse from throttling itself if it decides to lie down.

The prognosis for uncomplicated ilial wing fractures is good for a return to racing. Fractures of the ilial shaft hold a guarded-to-poor prognosis for a return to racing, not only due to the increased risk of exsanguination, but also because the increased pain associated with these fractures increases the risk of contralateral laminitis and other complications such as contracture of *biceps femoris*, *semimembranous* and *semitendinous*, and upward fixation of the patella.

Fractures of the ischium and *tuber ischii*

Presentation and clinical signs

These fractures occur predominantly from falling over backwards or reversing into inanimate objects at speed. The horse has a marked-to-severe unilateral lameness, with pain and progressive swelling over the affected *tuber ischii*. Fractures within the ischium itself are rarer and often present with minimal external clinical signs, so presenting a greater diagnostic challenge. Occasionally, in displaced fractures there may be laceration of the internal pudendal or obturator blood vessels, which can lead to haemorrhage and progressive swelling of the caudal thigh and ultimately death, but this is less common than in ilial shaft or wing fractures. Clinically there is pain to palpation of the affected tuber ischii and, if the fracture is complete, asymmetry between the *tubera ischii*. There is frequently a marked reduction in the cranial phase of the stride of the limb on the affected side.

Diagnosis

Diagnostic techniques that are useful in the diagnosis of these fractures include ultrasonography, nuclear scintigraphy and radiography. Ultrasonography of the ischium is a greater technical challenge than that of the ilial wing (Figure 13.4). False-negative findings often occur due to the fracture being incomplete or non-displaced. Nuclear scintigraphy can be a useful technique to demonstrate a fracture not visible using ultrasonography (Figure 13.5), but again can produce false-negative results for up to 2 weeks after the inciting incident. Radiography requires a high-power generator to produce the exposure factors required to obtain a diagnostic image. However, it can be a valuable tool to confirm the diagnosis (Figure 13.6) and determine the prognosis, especially if the fracture is within the body of the ischium and may involve the caudal aspect of the coxofemoral joint.

Treatment and prognosis

Treatment is based on box rest for 4 weeks followed by gradually increasing daily hand walking for a further 4 weeks. These cases are normally left loose in the stable, and not tied up. The prognosis for return to competition is fair for simple fractures of the tuber ischii, although, if there has been displacement of the fracture fragment, there may be long-term mechanical restriction of the stride length. The prognosis for complete fractures of the ischium are dependent on the involvement of the coxofemoral joint, and generally hold a guarded

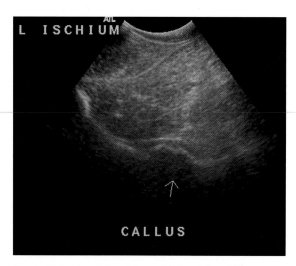

Figure 13.4   An ultrasound scan of the surface of the ischium. The irregular contour is the result of callus (white arrow) over the site of a healing, non-displaced, ischial fracture.

prognosis, with those extending into the joint having a grave prognosis.

Pubic fractures

Presentation and clinical signs

Fracture of the pubis in isolation is an infrequent occurrence but normally follows a fall or the horse slipping and spread-eagling the hind legs. Horses affected with pubic fractures tend to stand in a "hunched-up" manner and often have the tail raised. They may walk with a very short protraction indicative of severe pain and bilateral hindlimb lameness. This can mimic the signs of severe exercise-induced rhabdomyolysis. There may be associated swelling of the vulva and perineal region in the female. There is usually an unwillingness to move after a standstill.

Diagnosis

In these cases radiography is impractical because only radiography under general anaesthesia will produce diagnostic images of the region, and the risks of fracture displacement involved with general anaesthesia are usually considered too great to proceed. Nuclear scintigraphy can be useful if the appropriate images are acquired. Nuclear scintigrams obtained in the usual dorsoventral manner rarely identify the fracture because of the screening effect of the overlying spine and musculature, and the small bone mass of the pubis (and hence origin of signal) causes significant

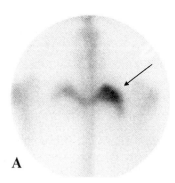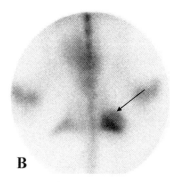

Figure 13.5   Nuclear scintigrams of an ischial fracture: (a) caudocranial view of the caudal pelvis; (b) dorsoventral view of the caudal pelvis. The black arrows show an area of increased radionuclide uptake in the tuber ischii on both views. This fracture was not visible after ultrasonographic examination in the acute stage, as is often the case with traumatic impaction fracture in this site. The horse reared and fell in the stable 2 weeks previously, and was lame subsequently.

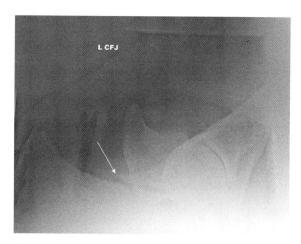

Figure 13.6 A radiograph demonstrating a fracture of the tuber ischii. This radiograph is obtained by using a standing oblique radiographic projection. Here a fracture of the ischium (white arrow) is seen extending into the coxofemoral joint.

attenuation of the signal. However, a caudal view, obtained with the camera face parallel to the posterior surface of the thighs, with the tail gently pulled to one side, gives excellent visualisation of fractures of the pubis, which appear as an intense area of increased radiopharmaceutical uptake in the midline between the femora. Rectal examination can also be rewarding. The symphysis pubis should be palpated with the horse standing fully weight bearing, and then the horse rocked gently from side to side by an assistant while the hand remains over the pubic symphysis. Motion of one hemi-pelvis in relation to the other is often appreciated in conjunction with crepitus at the site.

Fractures and dislocation of the coxofemoral joint

Presentation and clinical signs

Fractures of the coxofemoral joint are often a result of the horse slipping and falling on a hard surface or "doing the splits". The horse will present with a non-weight-bearing lameness for both fracture and dislocation. In the dislocated joint the femoral head is usually displaced dorsally and cranially, and as a result the leg may appear shortened, the stifle rotated outwards more than the contralateral

limb and the greater trochanters may not be symmetrical, although these changes can be difficult to assess. These horses may also have upward fixation of the patella due to the altered position of the femur to the quadriceps muscle mass. In horses that have landed on their side and fractured the acetabular cup by punching the femoral head inwards, there can be few signs except severe pain. A rectal examination may identify swelling or sharp bone edges around the dorsal axial surface of the acetabulum, but often it is the ventral portion of the cup that is fractured, which cannot be palpated. If the horse is able to move then crepitus may be appreciated either externally or during the rectal examination. As with all pelvic fractures there is marked-to-severe muscle spasm and guarding with marked pain, which may be mistaken for severe exertional rhabdomyolysis.

Diagnosis

Diagnostic imaging techniques that may be used in these cases include ultrasonography, nuclear scintigraphy and radiography. Ultrasonography can be disappointing as many of the fracture configurations are not accessible for scanning. However, most commonly with dislocated coxofemoral joints or comminuted fractures, there will be a loss of the normal relationship between the femoral head and dorsal acetabular rim, or it may not be possible to identify the joint at all due to shadowing from the greater trochanter. If the joint is intact distension of the joint may be identifiable. Rectal ultrasonography may also be beneficial in identifying callus or incontinuities on the axial margin of the acetabulm. Nuclear scintigraphy can also be disappointing in these cases, particularly if performed close to the inciting incident, as discussed above. Generally there should be a minimum delay of 5–7 days and preferably 14 days before performing the scan. The most common positive finding is a localised moderate-to-marked increased radiopharmaceutical uptake around the joint. Oblique, dorsal and caudal views may be required to definitively determine that the uptake is actually associated with the joint. Radiography, as with fractures of the *tuber ischii*, requires a high-power generator, but can be very useful in identifying fractures. The use of an oblique lateral view in the standing horse has proved useful [8] (see Figure 13.6) in identifying traumatic injury to the coxofemoral joint. The main limitation of radiography and scintigraphy is the necessity to move the horse, which is often not possible, due to a persistent non-weight-bearing lameness.

Treatment and prognosis

The prognosis for dislocation or fracture of the coxofemoral joint in the adult horse is grave in most cases. General anaesthesia and reduction of the dislocation have been described, but in most cases reduction is not achieved or is unstable, and dislocation recurs on recovery or shortly afterwards. Fractures of the coxofemoral joint, even if stable and non-displaced, will ultimately lead to significant osteoarthritis of the joint and permanent lameness.

Multiple, complex, comminuted fractures of the pelvis

Presentation and clinical signs

Obviously any combination of fractures of the pelvis can occur if sufficient trauma is imparted to the horse. Severe fractures involving the acetabulum and iliac shaft after a fall may result in the horse remaining recumbent and apparently being unable to rise. This is presumably because of the severe pain, in addition to instability of the coxofemoral joint on the affected side. These fractures will often be associated with intense haemorrhage and a shock-like state may ensue. The horse may attempt and attain the "dog-sit" position only to fall back down to the ground. The signs can mimic those of a spinal fracture with partial or total transection of the spinal cord, but careful examination of tone in the limbs and tail may show the normal spinal reflexes to be intact, although in "shocked" horses this is sometimes not the case. Rectal examination in a recumbent horse in distress is dangerous and should not be attempted, and it is sometimes impossible to make an antemortem diagnosis. If severe unilateral fracture is present, the horse may well be able to rise if rolled over onto the other side and this should be attempted, with care, before consideration of euthanasia [3].

Where the horse is able to rise, it will show a severe unilateral or bilateral hindlimb lameness, and unwillingness to move. Combinations of one or more of the clinical signs described in the previous section may be present, which will aid in the assessment of viability of treatment.

Diagnosis

The diagnosis of a complicated fracture is made using a combination of clinical signs, radiography, nuclear scintigraphy and ultrasonography.

Treatment and prognosis

The basic principles of treatment of pelvic fracture have been described in detail [5] and in an earlier section in this chapter. Essentially, the treatment is almost always conservative, with box rest for a minimum of 8–12 weeks, with a recommended period of 3–4 weeks cross-tying of the horse. As previously stated, careful thought should be given to the likely end-result of treatment in cases of severe or multiple pelvic fracture at the outset.

Sacral fractures

Presentation and clinical signs

These can occur either alone or in combination with fractures to one or both iliac wings. As a result of the important nerves that exit from the spine in this region, the sacral fracture can be accompanied by a variable set of neurological symptoms (see Chapter 4). Fractures situated cranially in the sacrum may cause nerve root injuries of the entire cauda equina which may have symptoms in the pelvic limbs, as well as the normal cauda equina complex of urinary incontinence, flaccid paralysis of the anal ring and paralysis of the tail. Fractures situated more caudally often involve only symptoms involving urination, defecation and loss of skin tone around the perineum, in association with flaccid paralysis of the tail. In the mare the flaccid paralysis of the vulva can cause abrupt and marked pneumovagina, which can be distressing to the horse and produce an excitable fear-response behaviour. Urinary dribbling will be noted and rectal examination often reveals faecal accumulation within the rectum.

Diagnosis

Horses affected with complete displaced fracture of the sacrum have a characteristic appearance with an abrupt angle change visible just caudal to the tuber sacrale (Plate 26) and apparent hollowing of the caudal pelvis and coccygeal region. Radiographic confirmation of sacral fracture is difficult and not without significant radiation hazard. More specific information can be obtained from a nuclear scintigraphic examination of this site where images taken from the lateral, dorsal and caudal perspectives will give complete information for the site and severity of the injury. Rectal examination, both manual and together with ultrasonography using a rectal probe, can also be used to assess a sacral fracture, but great care should be taken as the rectum often "balloons" and becomes atonic as a result of the neurogenic damage incurred. Ultrasound examination of the sacrum has been described [9]. Localised hyperaesthesia or pruritus has been reported following non-displaced fractures of the sacrum, which have healed and in which subsequent callus formation has presumably exerted pressure on nerves [10]. The formation of callus and scar tissue after a fracture may lead to the development of cauda equina syndrome some time after the original inciting incident. Damage to the nerve roots innervating skeletal muscle also results in very rapid, often very focal, neurogenic muscle atrophy, which will result in marked depressions in the contour of the quarters adjacent to the sacrum.

Treatment and prognosis

Horses affected with the cauda equina syndrome must have supportive care. If the bladder is paralysed it will need to be emptied three times daily by catheter or an in-dwelling catheter left in situ. If the rectum is ballooned and atonic, as is often the case, manual evacuation of faeces will be required. This in itself is not without risk given the lack of tone in the rectal wall. Antibiotic cover with trimethoprim sulphonamide combinations is advisable given the urine stasis that will be present in the bladder. The urine soaking of the hind limbs will lead to scalding of the skin if barrier creams and meticulous hygiene are not used. The tail can become very excoriated because of constant soaking with urine and faeces, and may require

subsequent amputation. However, this is often best left until it is obvious whether the horse will recover some degree of function and not require permanent nursing care.

The medical treatment of sacral fractures has been well summarised [11]. Initially this consists of treatment to diminish inflammatory changes around the nerves such as intravenous DMSO drips, the use of corticosteroids and NSAIDs can be helpful from the acute injury to approximately 14 days after injury. At this stage, it is considered that the inflammatory effect on the nerves will have diminished and, if neurological symptoms persist after this time, they are likely to be the result of partial or complete transection of the nerves rather than neuropraxia. In this situation axon re-growth is reported to occur at approximately 1 mm/day and the practicality of salvaging the horse depends on the length of the nerve that has to re-grow. It has been suggested that, if there is no improvement in the condition after 2 months from the date of the original injury, nerve damage may be permanent requiring long-term intensive care [11]. Surgical decompression of the sacrum has been described as a treatment for a chronic sacral fracture that led to permanent pruritus on the croup. In this description the tail was also amputated and the horse made a complete recovery [10].

The prognosis is obviously dependent on the site and severity of the sacral fracture, in conjunction with the willingness of the connections of the horse to undertake prolonged intensive and expensive medical care to allow recovery.

Coccygeal fractures

Presentation and clinical signs

These fractures can follow the horse rearing up and landing on the posterior aspect of the coccyx and can occur together with ischial fractures. Usually there is some degree of flaccid paralysis of the tail and an area of hyperaesthesia immediately proximal to the fracture site where the horse is extremely resistant to manual palpation. In the filly the tail may become soaked in urine because of the horse's inability to raise the tail during urination, and remedial steps have to be taken to avoid scalding in this situation. The horse may appear agitated and ill at ease and may mimic the signs of exercise-induced rhabdomyolysis or colic. Fractures can occur at any site but the most common is Cy1–2.

Diagnosis

Radiography of the coccyx is relatively easily carried out. The tail hairs can be used to extend the coccygeal vertebrae horizontally so that they can be imaged in the standing lateral position. Nuclear scintigraphy may be helpful and indicated in cases of suspected incomplete fracture if there is a specific pain response to palpation.

The innervation of the coccygeal muscles is derived from the coccygeal nerves. There are normally five pairs of these, the dorsal and ventral branches of which anastomose to run as nerve trunks immediately adjacent to the vertebrae on either side of the tail. Obviously the specific site and severity of injury will determine the degree of atonia and lack of sensation in the tail. The apparent flaccid paralysis may resolve fairly speedily if there is no involvement of the sacrum, and is often the result of neuropraxia after acute swelling rather than complete transection of the nerves.

Treatment and prognosis

As long as there has not been complete severance of the nerves the horse normally regains control of the tail within a period of 2–6 weeks once the swelling and pressure changes subside. If the nerves are severed, full function may take much longer to return, and some degree of dysfunction become permanent. Healing is often accompanied with a subsequent mal-angulation of the coccygeal vertebrae, but this does not appear to interfere with the horse's athletic function in many cases and the prognosis is usually favourable.

References

1. Stover, S.M., Johnson, B.J., Daft, B.M. et al. An association between complete and incomplete stress fractures of the humerus in racehorses. *Equine Veterinary Journal* 1992;**24**:260–263.
2. Raidal, S.L., Love, D. and Bailey, G.D. Inflammation and increased numbers of bacteria in the lower respiratory tract of horses within 6–12 hours of confinement with the head elevated *Australian Veterinary Journal* 1995;**72**:45–47.
3. Williams, J. and Dyson, S.J. Management of a recumbent horse. In: *A Guide to the Management of Emergencies at Equine Competitions*. Newmarket, Suffolk: EVJ Ltd, 1996: 58–63.
4. Dyson, S.J. Pelvic injuries in the non-racehorse. In: Ross, M.W. and Dyson, S.J. (eds), *Diagnosis and Management of Lameness in the Horse*. St Louis: Saunders, 2003: 491–501.
5. Pilsworth, R.C., Diagnosis and management of pelvic fractures in the thoroughbred racehorse. In: Ross, M.W. and Dyson, S.J. (eds), *Diagnosis and Management of Lameness in the Horse*. St Louis: Saunders, 2003: 484–490.
6. Reef, V.B., ed. Musculoskeletal ultrasonography. In: *Equine Diagnostic Ultrasound*. Philadelphia: W.B. Saunders Co., 1998: 149–150.
7. Shepherd, M.C. and Pilsworth, R.C. The use of ultrasound in the diagnosis of pelvic fractures. *Equine Veterinary Education* 1994;**6**:23–27.
8. Barrett, E.L., Talbot, A.M., Driver, A.J., Barr, F.J. and Barr, A.R.S. A technique for pelvic radiography in the standing horse. *Equine Veterinary Journal* 2006;**38**:266–270.
9. Almanza, A. and Whitcombe, M.B. Ultrasonographic diagnosis of pelvic fractures in 28 horses. In: *Proceedings of the 49th American Association of Equine Practitioners*. New Orleans, LO: AAEP, 2003: 50–54.
10. Collatos, C., Allen, D., Chamber, J. and Henry, M. Surgical treatment of sacral fracture in a horse. *Journal of the American Veterinary Medicine Association* 1991;**198**:877–879.
11. MacKay, R.J. The cauda equina syndrome. In: Robinson, N.E. (ed.), *Current Therapy in Equine Medicine 4*. Philadelphia: W.B. Saunders, 1997: 311–314.

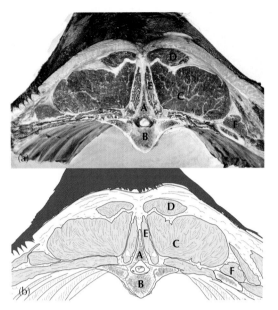

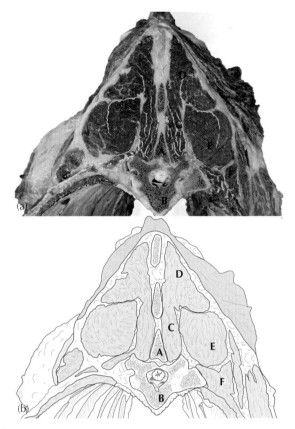

Plate 1 The cross-sectional anatomy of thoracic vertebra 1: (a) postmortem section; (b) line diagram. A, dorsal spinous process; B, vertebral body; C, longissimus dorsi; D, longissimus dorsi (spinalis); E, multifidus; F, iliocostalis.

Plate 2 The cross-sectional anatomy of thoracic vertebra 7: (a) postmortem section; (b) line diagram. A, dorsal spinous process; B, vertebral body; C, multifidus; D, longissimus dorsi (spinalis); E, longissimus dorsi; F, iliocostalis.

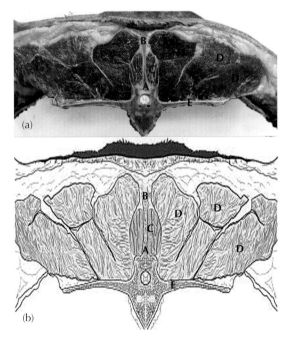

Plate 3 The cross-sectional anatomy of lumbar vertebra 2: (a) postmortem section; (b) line diagram. A, dorsal spinous process; B, supraspinous ligament; C, multifidus; D, longissimus dorsi; E, transverse process.

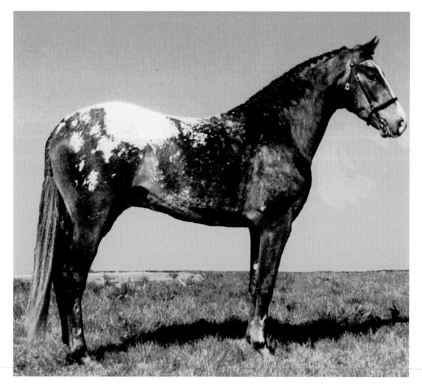

Plate 4 A photograph of a normal horse. The horse is stood "four square" on a flat surface outside to allow general appraisal of the conformation of its back and fore- and hindlimbs, as well as assessing its general condition and muscling.

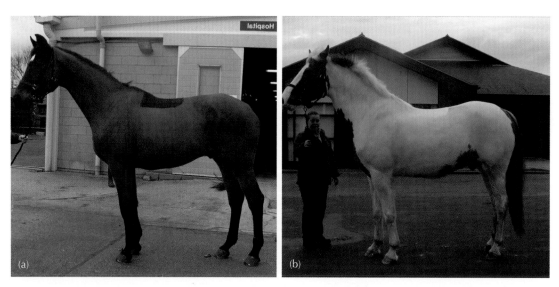

Plate 5 Photographs of horses with different conformation: (a) a "short-backed" horse; (b) a "long-backed" horse. This refers to the distance between the withers and the tuber sacrale relative to the other dimensions of the horse.

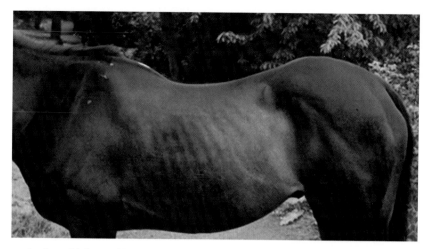

Plate 6 A photograph of an old thoroughbred horse. This horse does not have any clinical signs of back pain but has age-related lordosis (dipping).

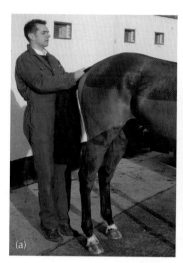

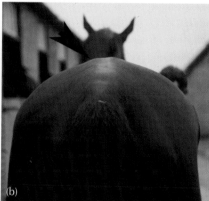

Plate 7 Two photographs to demonstrate the assessment of the back from behind. (a) It is important to view the dorsal midline of the back of the horse from behind the horse. The horse is stood straight and aligned through its neck, back and quarters. This is a very effective way of assessing the back and pelvis conformation and muscling. (b) There is a lowered tuber sacrale and gluteal muscle wastage on one side of the horse. These clinical signs may suggest chronic sacroiliac disease, although it may be incidental as a cause of back or pelvic pain.

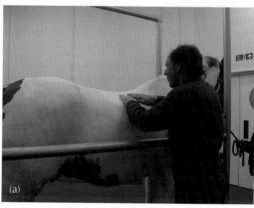
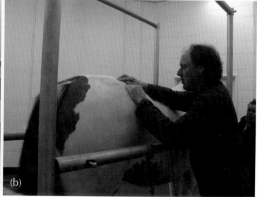

Plate 8 Two photographs to demonstrate palpation of the back: (a) the thoracolumbar spine and (b) the area around the tuber sacrale. Examination of the tuber sacrale should be carried out and the area lateral to it should be carefully palpated for any evidence of pain, fibrosis or thickening.

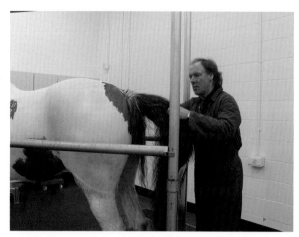

Plate 9 A photograph to demonstrate the assessment of flaccidity of the tail and croup region, asymmetry of the tail, and for any evidence of cauda equina neuritis.

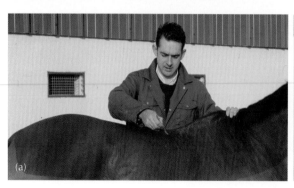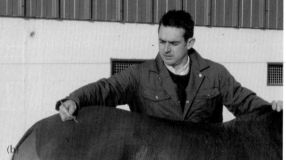

(a)

(b)

Plate 10 A photograph to demonstrate the application of pressure: (a) thoracic region; (b) gluteal region. In the normal horse pressure on to the caudal thoracic area leads to dorsiflexion (dip).

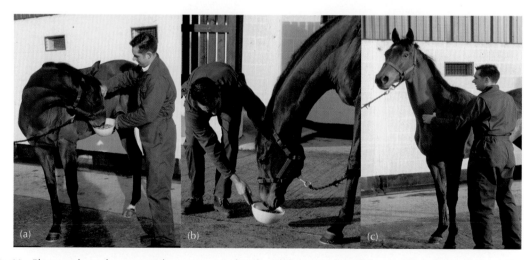

(a)

(b)

(c)

Plate 11 Photographs to demonstrate the assessment of neck mobility using a small bowl of feed. The neck should be palpated on both sides and assessed for symmetry, swelling, muscle spasm and sites of pain. In (a) the ability of the horse to flex laterally to left and right is assessed. In (b) and (c) the ability of the horse to (b) lower and (c) raise its head and neck is assessed.

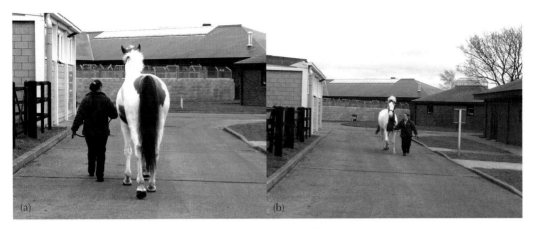

Plate 12 Photographs to demonstrate the horse being viewed: (a) at walk; (b) at trot.

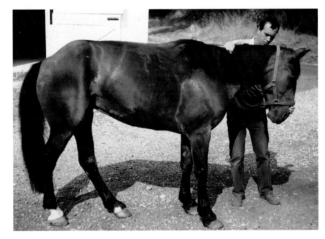

Plate 13 A photograph to demonstrate the re-examination of a horse that had severe back pain. The horse is being asked to move backwards by the handler. Note how it is resisting this by the positioning of its legs and body.

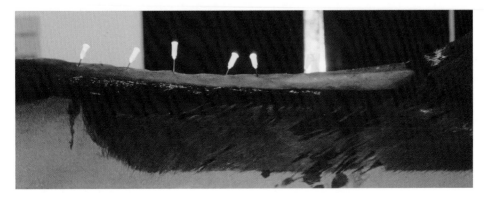

Plate 14 A photograph to show the placement of needles for the injection of local anaesthetic between dorsal spinous processes. This horse had back pain and its performance was assessed before and after injection of a small amount of local anaesthetic into specific sites of dorsal overlapping spinous processes under ultrasonographic guidance.

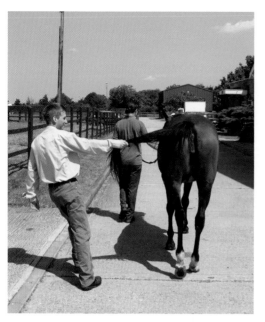

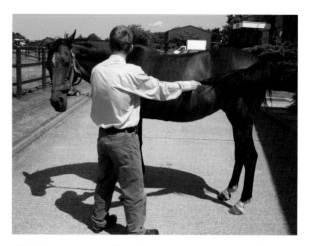

Plate 16 A photograph to show a horse being tested for subtle signs of weakness in the pelvis and thoracic limbs. Such weakness may be exacerbated by pulling on the tail and head collar at the same time while circling the horse.

Plate 15 A photograph to show a horse being tested for extensor weakness. This test is performed by pulling the tail. Extensor weakness may be evident if the horse is easily pulled to the side when walking.

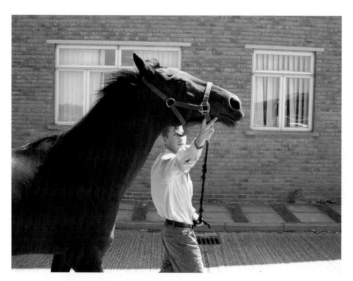

Plate 17 A photograph to demonstrate the raising up of the head while walking. By raising the head, subtle signs of ataxia may be made more evident.

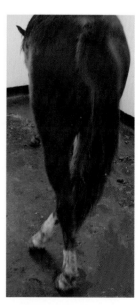

Plate 18 A photograph to show abnormal limb placement of the hindlegs. This limb placement would imply that the horse has proprioceptive deficits.

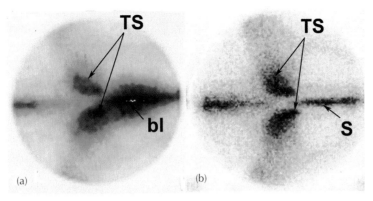

Plate 19 Nuclear scintigrams to show the effects of repeat scanning of the pelvis after urination. Dorsoventral views of the caudal pelvis. (a) Scintigram shows a large "hot spot" associated with the bladder (bl). The paired *tubera sacrale* (TSs) are not readily distinguishable from the bladder shadow. (b) After urination the *tuber sacrale* are clearly seen and the sacrum (S) is now visible.

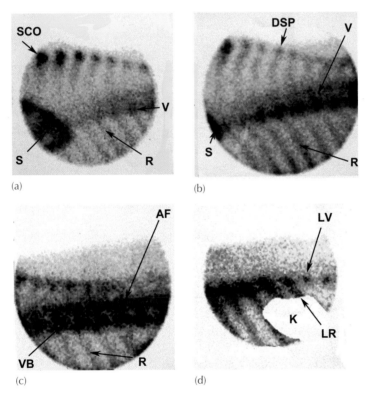

Plate 20 Nuclear scintigrams to show the normal scintigraphic appearance of the thoracolumbar spine in the most frequently acquired views. (a) Lateromedial scintigram of cranial thoracic region. Note the increased uptake on the caudal border of the scapula (S) and associated with the secondary centres of ossification (SCO) of the cranial thoracic vertebrae. The vertebral bodies (V) and ribs (R) have poor uptake. (b) Lateromedial scintigram of mid-thoracic region. There is still an increased uptake on the caudal border of the scapula. The dorsal spinous processes (DSPs) of the mid-thoracic vertebrae and the ribs have poor uptake. The vertebral bodies have moderate uptake. (c) DLVMO oblique scintigram of mid-thoracic region. The uptake in the vertebra is separated into dorsal and ventral parts. High uptake of radionuclide is seen dorsally in the articular facets (AF) and ventrally in the vertebral bodies (VB). The ribs have poor uptake. (d) Lateromedial scintigram of the caudal thoracic region with the kidney region (K) masked out. The cranial vertebral bodies have moderate uptake, whereas the first two lumbar vertebrae (LV) have less. The last thoracic vertebra is located by identifying the last rib (LR).

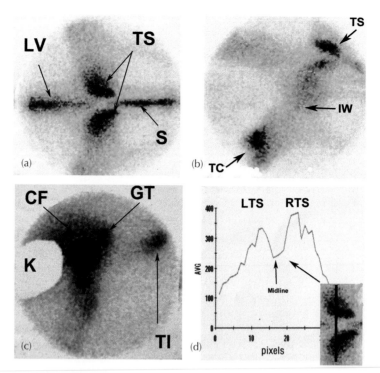

Plate 21 Nuclear scintigrams to show the normal scintigraphic appearance of the pelvis in the most frequently acquired views. (a) Dorsoventral scintigram of the cranial pelvis. The paired *tuber sacrale* (TS) are seen to be comma shaped either side of the midline. The lumbar vertebrae (LV) are seen cranial to the *tuber sacrale* and the sacrum (S) is caudal to the *tuber sacrale*. (b) Dorsolateral–ventromedial oblique (DLVMO) scintigram of cranial pelvic region. Moderate uptake is seen associated with the *tuber coxae* (TC) and *tuber sacrale*, with mild uptake in the ilial wing (IW). (c) Lateromedial scintigram of the caudal pelvis. The bladder region (B) has been masked out. Moderate uptake is seen associated with the coxofemoral joint (CF). The greater trochanter (GT) of the femur is visible. There is mild uptake also associated with the *tuber ischii* (TI). (d) An example of profile analysis of the sacroiliac region in a normal horse. The scintigram insert shows the paired *tuber sacrale* with the profile line drawn on. The radionuclide counts under this line are calculated and a graphic profile produced (main picture). The profile shows two peaks associated with the left and right *tubera sacralae* (LTS and RTS), with a dip between them indicating the midline of the horse. AVG, average.

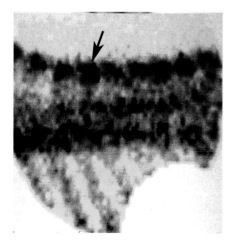

Plate 22 Lateromedial nuclear scintigram of the caudal thoracic region to show the appearance of radionuclide uptake in the region of the dorsal spinous processes (DSPs). There are a number of DSPs showing focal marked increase in uptake (black arrow highlights the most focal uptake).

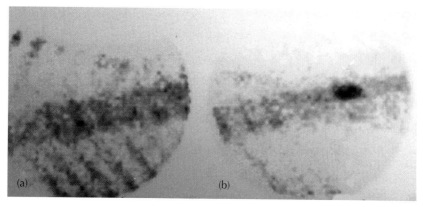

Plate 23 DLVMO nuclear scintigrams to show the appearance of a vertebral lamina stress fracture. (a) Mid-thoracic region – no abnormal increase in radionuclide uptake. (b) Caudal thoracic region – a marked increase in radionuclide uptake is seen associated with the articular facet, consistent with the diagnosis of a stress fracture.

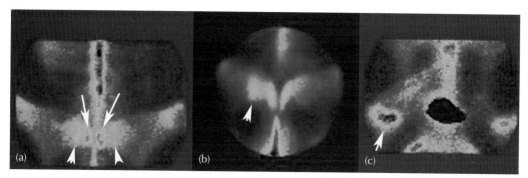

Plate 24 Pelvic scintigrams: (a) dorsoventral view: bilateral moderate increase in uptake in the region of the sacroiliac joint (arrowheads) either side of the tuber sacrale (white arrows); 10-year-old showjumper. (b) Dorsoventral view: marked focal increase in uptake at the junction of the medial and middle third of the left ilium consistent with a stress fracture (arrowhead); 2-year-old thoroughbred. (c) Caudal view: bladder masked. Marked increase in uptake within the soft tissues and greater trochanter of the left hip (white arrow); 4-year-old national hunt horse.

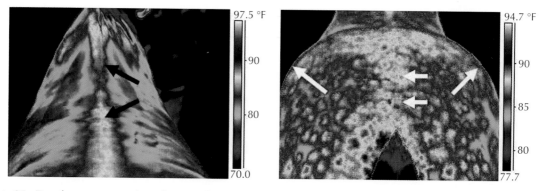

Plate 25 Two thermograms to show the normal pattern of distribution of body surface temperature: (a) thermogram of the thoracolumbar region of the back of a normal horse; the midline is the warmest (yellow stripe; black arrows). (b) Thermogram of the lumbosacral and gluteal regions of the back of a normal horse, the warmest area (yellow) is along the midline and from tuber coxae to tuber coxae (white arrows).

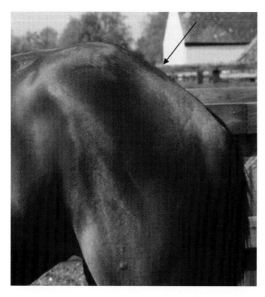

Plate 26 A photograph of a horse showing the pathognomonic clinical appearance of sacral fracture, i.e. the abrupt abnormal angle change caudal to the tubera sacrale.

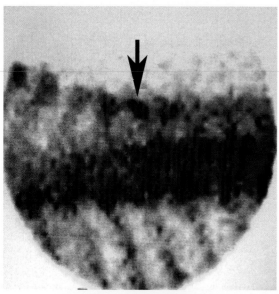

Plate 27 Lateromedial nuclear scintigram of the mid-thoracic region to show the scintigraphic appearance of overriding dorsal spinous processes (DSPs). This is seen as a focal area of markedly increased radionuclide uptake (arrow).

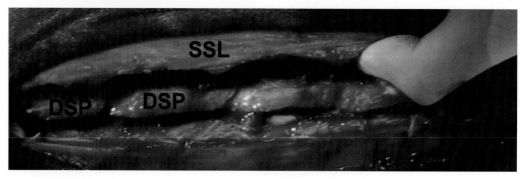

Plate 28 An intraoperative photograph during surgery to resect overriding dorsal spinous processes (DSPs). A midline incision has been made, the supraspinous ligament (SSL) transected longitudinally and the summits of the DSPs exposed (DSP).

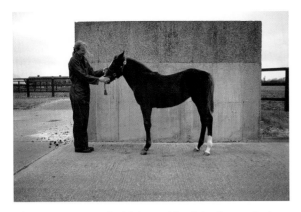

Plate 29 A 6-month-old thoroughbred that has marked lordosis (a dipped-back appearance).

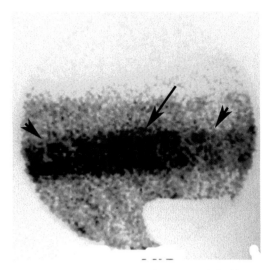

Plate 30 A DLVMO (dorsolateral–ventromedial–oblique) scintigram of the caudal thoracic region. This horse has osteoarthritis of the articular facets in the caudal thoracic region (arrow). Normal radionuclide uptake is seen cranial and caudal to the osteoarthritis (arrowheads). The radionuclide uptake in the region of the osteoarthritis is mild.

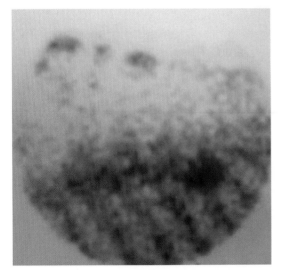

Plate 31 A lateromedial scintigram of the mid-thoracic region to show the appearance of vertebral spondylosis. There is an increase in radionuclide uptake associated with the ventral aspect of the vertebral bodies.

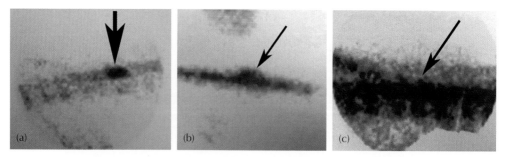

Plate 32 Scintigrams showing the appearance of a vertebral lamina stress fracture at presentation and 6 months later after rest. (a) Lateromedial view: presentation. The stress fracture is seen as a marked focal increase in radionuclide uptake (arrow). (b) Dorsoventral view: presentation. The stress fracture is seen to be unilateral – the increase in radionuclide uptake is one side of the spine (arrow). (c) Lateromedial view: obtained 6 months after (a). The stress fracture is no longer detectable (arrow shows original position).

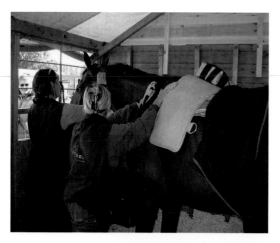

Plate 33 Combined treatment with physical therapy, ultrasound and massage machine for a 3-day event horse during a competition.

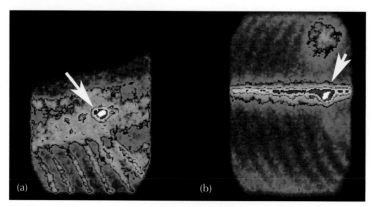

Plate 34 Nuclear scintigrams to show the scintigraphic appearance of a typical racehorse injury, the stress fracture of the lumbar lamina. A lateromedial (a) and a dorsoventral (b) view are shown. There is a focal area of increased radionuclide uptake in the articular facets (arrows), which is seen to be mainly on the left-hand side on the dorsoventral scintigram.

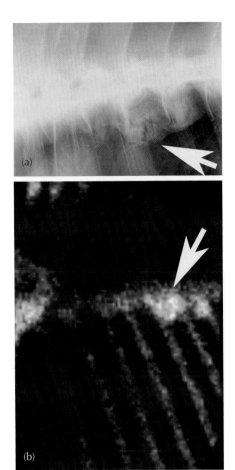

Plate 35 (a) A lateromedial radiograph and (b) a lateromedial nuclear scintigram showing ventral spondylosis (arrows) of the caudal thoracic region in a racing thoroughbred.

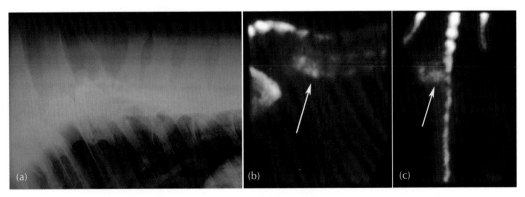

Plate 36 (a) A lateromedial radiograph, (b) a lateromedial nuclear scintigram and (c) a dorsoventral scintigram to show the appearance of a congenital deformity, scoliosis (arrows), in the spine of a young thoroughbred racehorse.

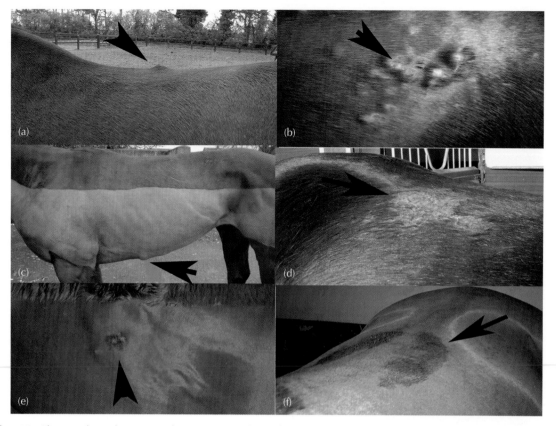

Plate 37 Photographs to demonstrate the appearance of superficial skin lesions caused by poor management. (a) Haematoma under the saddle region; (b) nodular collagen necrosis; (c) girth gall on the ventral chest; (d) photograph showing the effect of sand trapped between the saddle and skin – an outbreak of these occurred simultaneously in one yard; (e) folliculitis affecting the side of a thoroughbred – note the 'runners' radiating from the lesion; (f) patchy sweating under the saddle area caused by local trauma.

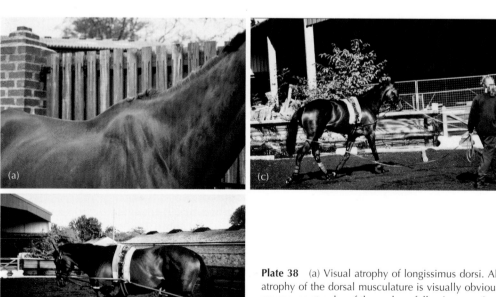

Plate 38 (a) Visual atrophy of longissimus dorsi. Although the atrophy of the dorsal musculature is visually obvious the primary cause was atrophy of the scalene following a racing fall, when the horse landed on its head. (b) A horse learning to work in long reins. The rehabilitation therapist is preventing the hindquarters from tracking out; the horse is leaning on the side reins. (c) The horse is in self-balance and ready to start a rehabilitation programme.

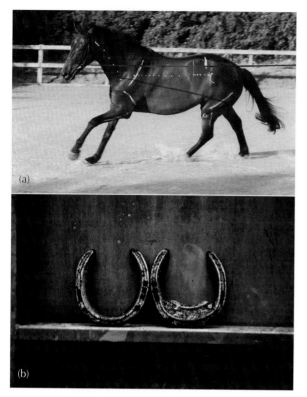

Plate 39 (a) Horse on a lunge, falling in, on a circle. The areas marked in white suggest areas of skeletal stress. (b) The shoe on the right has had one-third of a normal second shoe welded to its inner border at the toe. This has increased the weight by 75 g. A weighted shoe is used when a horse has reached the stage of ridden rehabilitation.

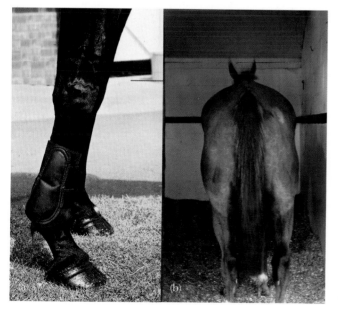

Plate 40 (a) Boot weighing 220 g applied to the right front. This type of loading can be used during exercise on a horse walker, or with care when a horse is worked in long reins or led out in hand. (b) This horse developed back pain secondary to the disparity between the hindquarter masses and was referred to the author because the rider had a good feel left diagonal, poor right diagonal. The horse first became uncomfortable in the T18–L1 area and was classed as "cold backed". The second area of discomfort, T6–8, was not apparent for 6 months when the horse refused to be girthed.

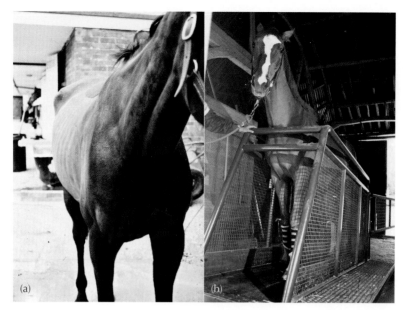

Plate 41 (a) Case referred as unrideable. The picture shows a loss of the left pectoral muscle and right gluteal muscles. This horse has developed a dipped back. (b) The type of treadmill found in many rehabilitation units. Useful for the restoration of balanced stride length.

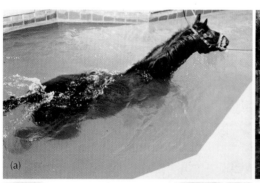

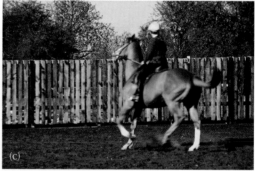

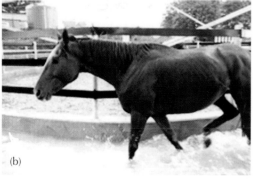

Plate 42 (a) Horse swimming in a balanced, and therefore useful, manner. (b) A horse in the sea walker. In this case the water depth has been adjusted to ensure that the hindlimb action uses the loin musculature. It is hypothesised, considering the principle of agonist/antagonistic muscle activity, that iliopsoas must also be activated. (c) Ridden work introduced too early in the programme.

14 Overriding Dorsal Spinous Processes

Frances M.D. Henson and Jessica A. Kidd

Anatomy of the dorsal spinous processes

As discussed in Chapter 1, a typical thoracic vertebra is made up of a vertebral body, a vertebral arch and vertebral processes (see Figures 1.3 and 1.4 in Chapter 1). The vertebral body provides the surface against which the intervertebral disc sits, whereas the vertebral arch provides a gap in the osseous structure through which the spinal cord runs. The vertebral processes are the sites of attachment for various ligaments and muscles and are named the dorsal spinous processes (DSPs), the transverse processes (TPs) and the articular processes (APs). The DSPs project dorsally from the vertebra into the surrounding musculature. These elongated bony prominences are believed to serve an important function as levers for the soft tissue attachments of the vertebral column.

The DSPs vary in their length, shape and angulation in different regions (Figure 14.1). The DSP of T1 is small, but the DSPs in the cranial thoracic vertebral region are markedly elongated in the region of T2–8 to form the withers. The apex of the withers is formed by the DSPs of T4–7. From an apex at T6 or T7 the length of the DSP decreases sharply down to approximately T12; the height of the DSPs decreases slightly down to the anticlinal (approximately T15–16) vertebrae and then increases to the last lumbar vertebra.

Both the shape and the angulation of the DSPs depend on the anatomical site from which they arise. DSPs from vertebrae T1–10 are narrow and tend to be quite straight (Figure 14.1). At T11–16 they have a marked beak-shaped outline and are wider at their base than at their apex. Dorsally they form the cranially pointing 'beak' with a rounded caudal aspect at their summits. From T1 to T14 the DSPs are angled dorsocaudally (i.e. towards the tail). At the anticlinal vertebra, the DSP is upright and then from T17 to L6 the DSPs are angled dorsocranially (towards the head) (see Figure 1.2 in Chapter 1).

Each DSP arises from a separate vertebra and therefore each has its own theoretical space above the vertebra. Therefore, it is considered that, in the normal horse, there is a gap between each DSP, visible on lateromedial radiography. The size of the 'normal' gap is more than 5–7 mm. However, in many cases the DSPs do not have separate space in the back, but make contact with adjacent vertebra – impinging or overriding dorsal spinous processes (ORDSPs) (Figure 14.2). In severe cases of overcrowding the DSPs are even seen to overlap. It must be noted that, when two DSPs are sufficiently close together, given time a false joint will actually form between the two bones in order to stabilise the interface (Fig 14.3).

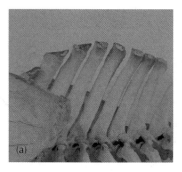 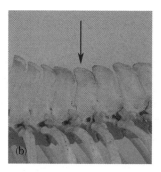 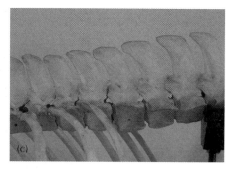

Figure 14.1 A postmortem specimen of the back of a horse, showing the different shapes of the dorsal spinous processes (DSPs) at different regions of the spine. Note that the cranial DSPs incline caudally and the caudal DSPs incline cranially. The anticlinal vertebra (see Chapter 1) is indicated in (b) with a black arrow.

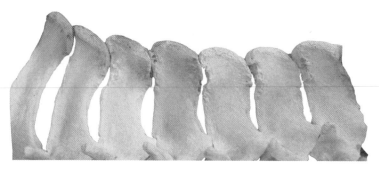

Figure 14.2 A postmortem specimen of the dorsal spinous processes (DSPs) of thoracic vertebrae T11–16. There are overriding DSPs in all the bones. Note the marked remodelling at the sites of overriding T12–16.

Incidence

DSP impingement has affected animals of the equine species for many, many years with the condition even being found in the extinct *Equus occidentalis* [1]. In more recent times Jeffcott reported that impingement of the DSPs was the most common cause of back pain in horses [2], and this is certainly the authors' clinical impression. However, it must be emphasised that the demonstration of an anatomical abnormality does not necessarily mean that this is the cause of back pain in an individual and ORDSPs can be found in many athletic and performance horses with no clinical signs of back pain. Indeed the question "Where is the source of pain in cases of ORDSPs?" is frequently posed. Some horses have ORDSPs throughout their athletic careers, with no obvious clinical signs of back pain. Indeed, in many cases the ORDSPs simply form painless false joints at

the sites of impingement. Clearly not enough is known at the current time about the pathogenesis of the pain in this condition.

The formation of false joints between some affected DSPs is, presumably, a response by the bones to their unexpected proximity. These false joints involve the remodelling of both cranial and caudal DSPs, often in a very marked fashion. This remodelling usually takes the form of a flattening and widening of the opposing bony edges of the DSPs (see Figure 14.4). Histologically, the false joints are cartilaginous.

Although the true incidence of pain arising from ORDSPs in the horse population is not known, the anatomical abnormality itself is extremely common. The anatomical incidence of ORDSPs has been described radiographically and *post mortem*. Postmortem studies have reported an incidence of between 86% and 92% [3, 4], whereas radiographic surveys have reported the incidence

Fig 14.3 A close-up of postmortem specimens of the dorsal spinous processes (DSPs) of thoracic vertebrae T14–17. Note the flattening and widening of the areas of bone in contact; these changes are indicative of false joint formation.

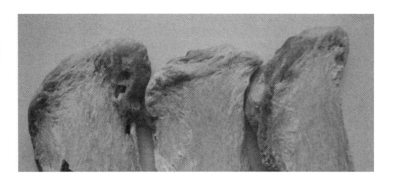

of ORDSPs as 34% (normal horses) and 33% (horses with a history of thoracolumbar pain) [2, 5]. There is a difference in incidence of ORDSPs in different breeds; the thoroughbred has a higher incidence of ORDSPs, possibly due to the shape of the summits of the DSPs (thoroughbreds have a markedly beak-shaped summit to the DSPs) and in horses undertaking different athletic endeavours. Jumping horses and dressage horses are reported to have the highest incidence of lesions.

Pathogenesis

ORDSPs may arise by a number of different mechanisms. In the simplest case the horse simply has a thoracolumbar spine that has the DSPs closer together than another individual, e.g. horses that are 'short backed' (see Chapter 6) have to fit the same number of vertebrae and their DSPs into a smaller length than a 'long-backed' horse, and the ORDSPs will occur due to a crowding of the DSPs into the space provided. In other cases, the horse will have an apparently normal length of back, but the DSPs themselves are more markedly 'beak shaped', meaning that there is increased chance of a DSP contacting the DSP immediately adjacent to it.

ORDSPs can also theoretically arise when the back undergoes excessive dorsiflexion (e.g. as potentially occurs in jumping horses) or spinal manoeuvres (e.g. as occurs in high-quality dressage horses). However, biomechanical studies have shown no evidence for increased movement in the T13–18 region compared with other parts of the thoracolumbar spine, and so this explanation may not be correct. Another hypothesis is that the weight of a saddle and rider causes a downward force on the T13–18 area, consequently forcing the DSPs in this region to become close together. However, given that ORDSPs have been described in unbroken/unridden horses and horses that compete in athletic but non-ridden disciplines (driving, trotting races), this too seems unlikely.

Site of pathology

Although all thoracic and lumbar vertebrae have DSPs, ORDSPs do not occur with similar frequency in the different areas of the thoracolumbar spine. They are almost unknown in the cranial withers region and are most commonly seen between T13 and T18 [5, 6]. In 1979 Jeffcott [5] reported that soft tissue pathology in the back tended to occur in the cranial and caudal parts of the spine, whereas ORDSPs were centred around the mid-point of the back. The reason for this distribution is not known. It may merely be a function of the anatomy of the horse, in that this is the site that has less space per DSP in all horses. As stated above, this does not seem to be a site of increased movement that may cause the DSPs to move closer together, nor is it likely that rider weight has an effect.

History

Horses can present with ORDSPs at any age. In non-racing competition horses, there seem to be three categories of presentation: young animals (3–4 years) that exhibit clinical signs of back pain when broken in and first ridden, young competition animals (6–9 years) that fail to train on as expected and are found to be suffering from

ORDSPs, and older horses (10+ years) that have been competing satisfactorily and then begin to suffer back pain, apparently from ORDSPs. Any breed and sex can be affected, although thorough-bred geldings have been reported to be overrepresented in some case series [5].

Horses subsequently found to be suffering from ORDSPs present with a number of owners' complaints, ranging from reluctance to being saddled/mounted to a subtle loss of performance. The clinical signs reported include resistance to being saddled or girthed (even the development of "phobic" behaviour when approached with a saddle), vague signs of back discomfort and back stiffness, poor performance, poor jumping, bucking and general reluctance to work. In extreme cases the horse is dangerous and unrideable.

Clinical examination

The clinical signs of ORDSPs, in the authors' opinion, cover the entire spectrum of signs of back pain in the horse. In some horses there are apparently no clinical signs at the time of the examination (even though ORDSPs are clearly demonstrable using diagnostic imaging), whereas in other horses extreme reactions are demonstrated. For the purposes of this chapter the authors are assuming that a basic examination will take place, as described in Chapter 6. The aim of the following section is to highlight any particular aspects of the clinical examination of horses with ORDSPs that are of importance.

A visual inspection of the horse is performed first. Assessment should be made as to whether the horse has a 'short-backed' appearance, indicating that a crowding of DSPs may be occurring. The musculature of the thoracolumbar spine should be visually assessed for evidence of atrophy or swelling. In cases of chronic back pathology and pain, atrophy of *longissimus dorsi* is often noted, leading to the summits of the DSPs becoming almost visually apparent in some animals.

Once the horse has been visually examined, palpation of the dorsal midline of the back should be performed to identify the presence of any heat, pain and swelling, and to assess the flexibility of the spine. A discussed in Chapter 6, this is ideally performed in stocks, in which the horse cannot evade the movements required during the examination.

During the clinical examination for ORDSPs particular attention must be paid to the presence of any obvious areas of pathology in the midline region. As regards dynamic tests of back soundness, one of the most consistent clinical signs of ORDSPs is a reluctance towards/resistance to dorsiflexion of the spine (dipping). In some cases a marked response to this test will be seen, with the horse sinking to the floor. Often this reluctance to dorsiflex the back is accompanied by marked spasm of *longissimus dorsi* and/or a show of anxiety or bad behaviour from the horse. However, in some cases, particularly when the back pain is severe, the horse may not move the back at all in response to thoracic pressure, i.e. the dorsiflexion response will be absent. This gives the clinical impression of "guarding" the painful site. The horse will often, however, appear anxious and unsettled during the application of the pressure.

Following an examination at rest the horse should be assessed in-hand at walk, trot and canter in straight lines and on the lunge. Ideally the horse should also be seen ridden with its normal jockey or another suitably experienced rider. Caution must be exercised before asking anyone to ride a horse that is known, by the veterinary surgeon, to be a danger to the rider or people on the ground.

Diagnosis

Once back pain is established the clinical diagnosis of ORDSPs should be made in two stages. First, any anatomical evidence of ORDSPs must be demonstrated and, second, the functional evidence of pain arising from ORDSPs must be demonstrated. As a large number of horses will have anatomical evidence of ORDSPs as discussed above [7], with no signs of pain, the proof of functional pain is the most important diagnostic step.

Diagnosis of anatomical abnormalities

The anatomical abnormality of ORDSPs can be demonstrated by radiography, nuclear scintigraphy and ultrasonography.

The use of radiography in the diagnosis of ORDSPs

The ease with which ORDSPs can be identified on lateromedial radiographs is both a diagnostic blessing and curse! It is a blessing because it means that lesions can be easily seen and clearly demonstrated. Conversely, it is a curse because this is often the only site that is investigated diagnostically by some practitioners, who wrongly interpret changes at this site as indicative of clinical pathology and do not go on to look for any other cause of pain. This leads to an incorrect diagnosis and, worse, in some cases, a needless and unsuccessful surgical procedure.

On radiography, DSPs are usually seen to be separate from their neighbours, with no evidence of remodelling or sclerosis on their cranial and caudal borders (Figure 14.4). When ORDSPs occur a number of radiographic abnormalities can be seen. These include DSPs that are simply touching, DSPs that have sclerosis of their cranial and caudal borders and DSPs that have radiolucencies on their cranial and/or caudal borders (Figure 14.5. In severe cases, marked remodelling is seen (Figure 14.6). These radiographic changes have been described by a number of authors and grading systems introduced (see Chapter 8); however, there is no evidence that the grade of the changes correlates with clinical pain.

In addition to the radiographic grading scores described in Chapter 8, a grading score that describes the situation along the whole back, rather than an individual DSP, has been described by Petersson et al. [8] (Table 14.1).

The use of nuclear scintigraphy in the diagnosis of ORDSPs

As described in Chapter 9, a nuclear scintigraphic examination can be very useful in the identification of active ORDSPs. Nuclear scintigraphy works on the principle that the radiolabel will bind to areas of remodelling bone. Therefore, physiological or pathological sites of osteoclast/osteoblast activity will be identified. Nuclear scintigraphy is, therefore, a sensitive indicator of active bone remodelling in the DSPs. However, it must be appreciated that active bone remodelling is *not synonymous with pain* [9]. Some horses with demonstrable pain arising from ORDSPs may have minimal increase in radionuclide uptake on a nuclear scintigraphic examination of this site, whereas other horses with focal areas of increased radionuclide uptake in the DSPs may show no signs of back pain (see Chapter 9).

On nuclear scintigraphy ORDSPs are detected by the presence of a focal increase in radionuclide uptake in the summits of the DSPs. In some cases

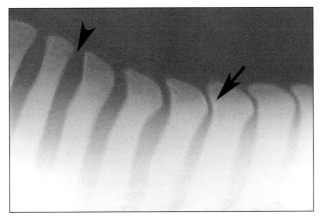

Figure 14.4   Lateromedial radiograph of the mid-thoracic region to show the distances between adjacent dorsal spinous processes (DSPs). There is a clear gap between DSPs in the cranial region of the radiograph (arrowhead). More caudally there is mild sclerosis of the cranial and caudal borders of the DSPs (arrow) and they are positioned more closely together.

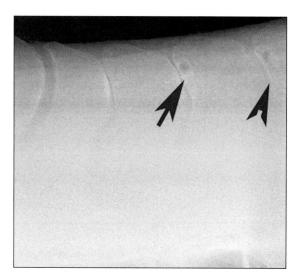

Figure 14.5   Lateromedial radiograph of the mid-thoracic region to show contact between adjacent dorsal spinous processes (DSPs) and area of radiolucency at these points of contact (arrow). In one part there is some radiographic evidence of false joint formation (arrowhead).

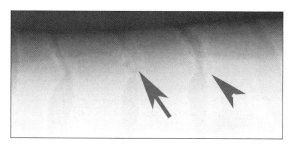

Figure 14.6   Lateromedial radiograph of the mid-thoracic region to show contact between adjacent dorsal spinous processes (DSPs) and marked areas of remodelling at these points of contact (arrow). In the caudal space there is evidence of marked lysis of bone (arrowhead).

Table 14.1   A grading score for the classification of overriding dorsal spinous processes in the thoracolumbar spine [8]

Grade	Description
I	Narrowing of two or more interspinous spaces with sclerosis and/or rarefaction
II	Impingement between two or more spinous processes with sclerotic and/or radiolucent areas
III	Impingement and overriding with sclerotic and/or radiolucent areas between two or more spinous processes

treatment aspect, e.g. surgical treatment of ORDSPs is not recommended in the presence of other concurrent back pathology [6].

The use of ultrasonography in the diagnosis of ORDSPs

As discussed in Chapter 10 ultrasonography can be useful in the diagnosis of ORDSPs. It can be used to identify the summits of the DSPs on longitudinal section and to ascertain the distance between the DSPs (see Figure 10.3 in Chapter 10). It can identify the presence of remodelling at the summits between the bones and can provide evidence of overlapping DSPs. The technique of ultrasonography of this site is detailed in Chapter 10. Ultrasonography can also be very useful in the diagnosis of active ORDSPs because it can be used to identify the spaces between the DSPs for placement of diagnostic analgesia.

Diagnostic local analgesic

Although the techniques described above can provide information about the presence of ORDSPs they do not provide proof that the ORDSPs are causing the clinical signs of back pain. To prove this, diagnostic analgesia of the affected ORDSPs is performed. Before placement of the local analgesia the clinical signs exhibited by the horse must be established. Thus, the horse must be examined in a reproducible manner, often including ridden exercise. The horse is then injected with local anaesthetic and the horse re-examined exactly as it was before the injection at 10 and at 30

only one DSP is affected (Plate 27); in others several DSPs are affected (see Plate 22).

Nuclear scintigraphy is also very useful to the veterinarian because it provides information on the presence of bone remodelling at sites other than the DSPs within the back and pelvis, e.g. the scintigraphic examination may reveal focal areas of increased radionuclide uptake in the DSPs but it may also reveal increased radionuclide uptake in, for example, the articular facets of the thoracic vertebrae [7, 10]. This is important not only from the diagnostic aspect of the case, but also from the minutes post-injection. The clinician and rider/handler, where appropriate, must then decide if there has been a positive response to the analgesia.

Anaesthesia of the DSPs can be achieved in a number of ways. Ideally, in order to avoid false-positive results due to diffusion of the local anaesthetic away from the DSPS, a small volume should be accurately placed between the affected DSPs. However, by virtue of the fact that these bones are overriding, it follows that the gap that should be the target of the anaesthetic is not present, so it is not possible, in such cases, to inject into the interspinous space. An infiltration of the soft tissues around the interspinous space is all that can be reasonably achieved.

The exact site can be identified radiographically and radio-opaque markers placed on the skin to provide landmarks for subsequent injection. Alternatively ultrasound can identify the areas of ORDSPs. Once the anatomical site(s) has been chosen the local anaesthetic infiltration should be performed by injecting 5–10 ml mepivacaine either side of the suspected lesion to a depth of approximately 5 cm. It is usual to provide analgesia to all of the affected DSP spaces at the same time for diagnostic purposes, rather than try to isolate any particular lesion (Plate 14).

Theoretically this infiltration technique could de-sensitise other structures in the region. The supraspinous ligament (see Chapter 10) may well be anaesthetised, but a detailed ultrasound examination of the ligament can identify and rule out lesions of supraspinous ligament desmitis (see Chapter 17). Epaxial muscle analgesia may also occur, but it is considered that such focal analgesia would be unlikely to significantly affect injuries to such large structures. Similarly, placement of the local anaesthetic too deep may lead to inadvertent analgesia of the articular facets of the vertebrae. Pathology at this site should, however, be ruled out on radiographic and nuclear scintigraphic examination (see Chapters 8 and 9).

Treatment

Once a diagnosis of ORDSPs has been made, treatment should be instituted. A number of different treatment options are available including conservative/medical and surgery. Few detailed comparisons between treatment modalities have been reported; however, one comparison between medical and surgical treatment of ORDSPs was made by Petersson et al. [8]. These authors showed that surgical treatment was associated with a better outcome (72% return to former function compared with 22% for those undergoing non-surgical treatment).

Conservative and medical treatment

Conservative treatment of ORDSPs includes rest, physiotherapy and anti-inflammatory medication. Case selection for conservative treatment is relatively straightforward. It is usual to treat most cases of proven ORDSPs conservatively/medically in the first instance, unless there are specific indicators to the contrary. It is also advisable to be patient with conservative/medical therapy in those older horses who have clearly had anatomical ORDSPs for some considerable time, but who are only now showing acute signs of back pain. In these animals it is reasonable to assume that they have exacerbated a usually quiescent region and the aim of therapy here is to reduce inflammation and allow the horse to return to its non-painful state.

The aim of rest in the management of ORDSPs is to reduce the inflammation associated with the bone contact, bone remodelling and soft tissue damage. As we know that, given time, ORDSPs form a non-painful false joint, theoretically many horses should have the capability to progress to this state. However, not all horses/owners/trainers have the time and/or inclination to undertake prolonged rest. Rest to reduce inflammation alone should be of sufficient length to be beneficial (between 3 and 9 months rest may be necessary). It is recommended that this rest be combined with oral, systemic, non-steroidal anti-inflammatory drugs (NSAIDs) in order to reduce inflammation at the sites of contact. Physiotherapy and rehabilitation therapy can also be helpful in these cases with exercises such as repeated ventroflexion exercises aimed at "opening up" the back (see Chapters 23–25).

More direct medical treatment of ORDSPs is also widely used, particularly in competition horses that are required to continue performing. Intralesional medication may be anti-inflammatory (e.g. corticosteroids) or analgesic (e.g. Sarapin injection). Corticosteroids are a potent anti-inflammatory and can be injected between DSPs or adjacent to ORDSPs if the interspinous space is no longer present. The dose of corticosteroid used depends on the number of DSPs affected and the drug used. A number of different drug doses have been reported including 10 mg triamcinolone or 40–60 mg methylprednisolone acetate or 0.5–1.0 mg flumethasone or 1.5–2.5 mg dexamethasone per space [6, 9]. In competition horses the rules of the organisation under which the horse competes must be observed regarding drug withdrawal times.

An alternative to corticosteroid treatment is the use of intralesional Sarapin, a sterile aqueous solution of soluble salts of the volatile bases from *Sarraceniaceae* species (pitcher plant). Sarapin is believed to exert its action by blocking pain from the affected site by an, as yet, unknown mechanism. It is administered in a similar fashion to the corticosteroids described above. It is reported to provide long-term analgesia in some horses, but is not, however, licensed for such use.

In addition to these intralesional medications other treatment techniques have been described. The use of mesotherapy to treat back pain is well established in Europe. Mesotherapy relies on the principle of inhibition of nerves carrying painful information from the deep structures within a spinal segment by the stimulation of nerves from more superficial structures. Mesotherapy is performed by administering multiple intradermal injections of saline/corticosteroid/local anaesthetic at the level of the lesion and caudal to it [9]. This therapy is reported to be very beneficial in some patients.

Extracorporeal shock wave therapy (SWT) may also be beneficial in treating cases of ORDSPs. SWT uses high-energy ultrasonic acoustic radiation to impart energy into tissues under treatment. In horses it is used particularly in the treatment of ligamentous insertion pathology, e.g. proximal suspensory desmitis. However, it is believed to have analgesic properties and may help to provide analgesia to sites of pain. The exact mechanism by which SWT works is not known; however, a number of theories have been discussed, including the idea that microtrauma caused by repeated shock waves in the affected area induces neovascularisation and promotes an environment more conducive for healing. In the treatment of ORDSPs it is recommended that the horse repeat three treatments with SWT, 7–10 days apart on three occasions before being re-assessed for an improvement.

Surgical treatment

Surgical treatment of ORDSPs is based on the removal of DSPs that have been identified to be causing a clinical problem using the diagnostic procedures described above. This procedure was first described by Roberts [11], and later by a number of other authors. *Case selection is extremely important to the success of this surgery.* It is vital to be certain that the back pain is arising from those DSPs to be resected and that there is no evidence of concurrent pathology. The presence of, for example, articular facet disease is a contraindication for surgery.

The indications for surgery are cases in which conservative/medical therapy has not worked and cases that would be considered to benefit from immediate surgical relief. There is no evidence in the literature that the prognosis after surgery is affected by the chronicity of the disease process.

Surgical technique

The original method of surgical removal of ORDSPs described removal of the affected bony portions by an open approach under general anaesthesia. However, an open standing technique and an endoscopic technique of DSP removal have also been described. At the current time the open, general anaesthetic surgical technique is most widely used.

Open method under general anaesthetic

Before anaesthesia the DSPs that are to be resected are marked using radio-opaque skin markers under radiographic guidance. The aim of the surgery is to remove as few DSPs as possible; thus if there are two or three DSPs in close apposition only one is removed; if there are four DSPs in apposition only two are removed.

The horse is anaesthetised and placed in lateral recumbency. Care must be taken in positioning the horse because it is extremely important to ensure that the spine is straight and free from rotation, and that the skin surface of the dorsum is on the edge of the operating table. This positioning facilitates access to the soft tissues ventral to the DSP in surgery. The skin is clipped and prepared for aseptic surgery. Two approaches to the DSPs can be used. The authors prefer a midline incision made through the skin, subcutis and supraspinous ligament, although an incision just lateral to the DSPs has also been described [6]. (A slight modification to these techniques is the use of localised small incisions directly over the affected DSP, through which it is removed.)

Whichever technique is used the incision should be long enough to include one DSP cranial and one DSP caudal to the DSPs to be resected. The soft tissue attachments to the DSPs (supraspinous and interspinous ligaments and multifidus muscles primarily) are blunt dissected away from the bone to a depth of 5–8 cm (Plate 28). The surrounding musculature is then held back from the surgical site using large retractors (hand-held or self-retaining depending on surgeon preference). The DSPs to be removed are then resected using a hand-held oscillating saw. It is important to ensure that not just the easily accessible summits are resected – palpation of the surgical site will allow identification of the areas of overriding and remodelling, and the surgeon should aim to ensure a minimum gap of 5 mm between the remaining bodies of each DSP [6]. Before closure it is recommended that the top 5–10 mm of the adjacent, remaining DSPs be removed with the oscillating saw in order to prevent a large, step-like change in the contour of the back after surgery. The surgical incision is closed in routine fashion, including closure of the supraspinous ligament. It is recommended that the wound be protected in the initial postoperative period by a stent bandage sewn in place.

Endoscopic method under general anaesthesia

Endoscopic resection of the DSPs has been described by Desbrosse et al. [12]. This surgery is performed under a general anaesthetic with the horse in lateral recumbency. The affected portion of the ORDSP is identified endoscopically and removed with rongeurs and burrs. This surgical procedure has the advantage of being minimally invasive and may well prove to be the method of choice for resection in the future.

Ostectomy in the standing, sedated horse

Subtotal ostectomy of dorsal spinous processes in sedated horses has also been described [13]. This procedure is performed in the standing horse. Analgesia of the region is provided by local infiltration of local anaesthetic solution (40–60 ml per site) around the affected DSPs and surrounding soft tissues to a depth of approximately 10 cm. The affected portion of the ORDSP is identified and removed with an oscillating saw. This surgical procedure has the advantage of avoiding a general anaesthetic and its inherent risks and expenses, and is reported to reduce haemorrhage at the surgical site.

Surgical complications and bone reactions after resection of ORDSPs

There are few significant complications of surgical resection of ORDSPs. The most common complications are wound infection with/without wound breakdown (reported as between 3.5% and 20% [6, 14]. Swelling and seroma formation at the surgical site are also reported. In the authors' experience wound infection, although not common, can be persistent and require long courses of antibiotics to treat it.

Longer-term consequences of surgical resection of ORDSPs are remodelling of the remaining, adjacent vertebrae, although this is considered to be reduced if the summits are removed as described above ("bevelling"). In addition, there is new bone formation at the surgical site, although this is not of clinical consequence. The superficial cosmetic outcome can be excellent, with horses capable of return to a showing career if required.

Surgical outcome

Surgical treatment for ORDSPs has a favourable outcome. In one large series of 215 horses 72% of horses were reported to return to full use, with the treatment being curative [6]. In the authors' experience this operation is extremely successful if performed on genuine cases of ORDSPs. However, given the limitations of the diagnostic techniques available to equine clinicians when compared with other species (no MRI or CT scanners for use on the backs of horses), there must be many cases that have concurrent pathology, which we just cannot locate at the current time. It is these individuals that will not respond well to surgical treatment.

Conclusion

ORDSPs are the most common anatomical abnormality reported in the horse with back pain; however, it must be remembered that a diagnosis of ORDSPs cannot be made on diagnostic imaging alone. Functional evidence of pain must be proven. ORDSPs can be successfully managed medically, but should this not prove successful an excellent surgical option for therapy can be offered.

References

1. Klide, A.M. Overriding dorsal spinous processes in the extinct horse *Equus occidentalis*. *American Journal of Veterinary Research* 1989;**50**:592–593.
2. Jeffcott, L.B. Disorders of the thoracolumbar spine of the horse – a survey of 443 cases. *Equine Veterinary Journal* 1980;**12**:197–210.
3. Haussler, K.K. Osseous spinal pathology. *Veterinary Clinics of North America: Equine Practice* 1999;**15.1**: 103–111.
4. Townsend, H.G.G., Leach, D.H., Doige, C.E. and Kirkaldy-Willis, W.H. Relationship between spinal biomechanics and pathological changes in the equine thoracolumbar spine. *Equine Veterinary Journal* 1986;**18**:107–112.
5. Jeffcott, L.B. Radiographic examination of the equine vertebral column. *Veterinary Radiology* 1979;**20**:135–139.
6. Walmsley, J.P., Pettersson, H., Winberg, F. and McEvoy, F. Impingement of the dorsal spinous processes in two hundred and fifteen horses: case selection, surgical technique and results. *Equine Veterinary Journal* 2002;**34**:23–28.
7. Erichsen, C., Eksell, P., Holm, K.R., Lord, P. and Johnston, C. Relationship between scintigraphic and radiographic evaluations of spinous processes in the thoracolumbar spine in riding horses without clinical signs of back problems. *Equine Veterinary Journal* 2004;**36**:458–465.
8. Pettersson, H., Stromberg, B. and Myrin, I. Das thorkolumbe, interspinale Syndrom (TLI) des Reitpferdes – Retriospektiver Vergleich konservativ und chirurgisch behandelter Falle. *Pferdeheilkunde* 1987;**3**:313–319.
9. Denoix, J-M. and Dyson, S.J. Thoracolumbar spine. In: Ross, M.W. and Dyson, S.J. (eds), *Diagnosis and Management of Lameness in the Horse*. Philadelphia: Saunders, 2003: 509–521.
10. Erichsen, C., Eksell, P., Widstrom, C. et al. Scintigraphy of the sacroiliac joint region in asymptomatic riding horses: scintigraphic appearance and evaluation of method. *Veterinary Radiology and Ultrasound* 2003;**44**:699–706.
11. Roberts, E.J. Resection of thoracic or lumbar spinous processes for the relief of pain responsible for lameness and some other locomotor disorders of horses. *Proceedings of the American Association of Equine Practitioners* 1968;**14**:13–30.
12. Desbrosse, F.G., Perrin, R., Launois, T., Vanderweerd, J-M.E. and Clegg, P.D. Endoscopic resection of dorsal spinous processes and interspinous ligaments in ten horses. *Veterinary Surgery* 2007;**36**: 149–155.
13. Perkins, J.D., Schumacher, J., Kelly, G., Pollock, P. and Harty, M. Subtotal ostectomy of dorsal spinous processes performed in nine standing horses. *Veterinary Surgery* 2005;**34**:625–629.
14. Lauk, H.D. and Kreling, I. Surgical treatment of kissing spines syndrome – 50 cases. II. Results. *Pferdeheilkunde* 1998;**14**:123–130.

15 Miscellaneous Osseous Conditions

Frances M.D. Henson

Introduction

In addition to the pathological conditions that are commonly reported in the back and pelvis, e.g. overriding dorsal spinous processes (ORDSPs) (see Chapter 14), suspraspinous ligament (SSL) desmitis (see Chapter 17) and sacroiliac dysfunction (SID, see Chapter 18), a number of other clinical entities are seen infrequently. These include:

- anatomical abnormalities
- degenerative conditions
- infectious conditions
- stress fractures
- neoplasia
- miscellaneous.

Anatomical abnormalities

From time to time the veterinarian will be presented with a horse that appears to have an anatomical abnormality of the back or pelvis. Often these will be foals or young horses that have congenital defects; in other cases the condition is apparently acquired. A number of different anatomical abnormalities of the equine back are recognised including lordosis, kyphosis, scoliosis and vertebral malformation [1]; abnormalities of the pelvis are rarely reported. The incidence of structural abnormalities is relatively low; Jeffcott [2] reported that these abnormalities accounted for 2.9% of a series of 443 horses that presented with thoracolumbar pathology.

Lordosis

Lordosis of the back is seen as a significant dipping of the back in the thoracolumbar region. The back of the horse follows a natural dip just after the withers but is then roughly horizontal, rising gently to the tuber sacrale. In cases of lordosis, however, this dip is exaggerated. Lordosis can be considered to be primary – when the horse is born with this condition or acquires it in early life – or secondary to some external factor. To some extent older horses all develop secondary lordosis with age, acquiring a dipped back conformation over time.

The diagnosis of lordosis is made on the clinical signs (Plate 29). Radiography of the thoracolumbar region may be useful to identify whether or not the abnormality is due to malformation of the vertebrae. There is no treatment for lordosis; some horses with mild lordosis can be useful riding animals, others cannot be fitted for saddles and/or are unable to weight bear comfortably.

Kyphosis

Kyphosis of the back is seen as a rising or upward arching of the back in the thoracolumbar region. As discussed above the back of the horse rises gently to the tuber sacrale. In cases of kyphosis, however, this rising is exaggerated into a definite upward arch. This is usually most apparent in the lumbar region.

As with lordosis, kyphosis may be considered a primary or a secondary condition. In the primary condition the kyphosis is present at birth or apparent in early life and can be considered congenital. It has also been reported to be associated with scoliosis (lateral deviation of the spine, see below) [3, 4]. In most of these congenital cases it is due to malformations in the vertebral column. Kyphosis has been reported to occur secondary to back trauma (e.g. fractured thoracic vertebrae [5]) and in some horses with bilateral hindlimb pain, particularly young horses – anecdotally, and in the author's experience, particularly those with stifle pain. This kyphosis disappears when the lameness has been treated.

The diagnosis of kyphosis is made on the clinical signs. Radiography of the thoracolumbar region may be useful to identify whether the abnormality is due to malformation of the vertebrae, vertebral fracture or other vertebral trauma. In addition, in cases of secondary kyphosis careful attention should be paid to whether or not hindlimb lameness is present. There is no treatment for primary kyphosis; most horses with mild-to-moderate kyphosis can be useful riding animals.

Scoliosis

Scoliosis of the back is seen as a deviation of the vertebral column from the midline when the horse is viewed from above. Primary scoliosis is reported in foals and young horses, often associated with vertebral body hypoplasia and hemivertebrae [6]. The diagnosis of scoliosis is made on clinical signs and radiography is very useful to determine whether or not the scoliosis is accompanied by vertebral body malformations, which are usually present (see Figure 8.4 in Chapter 8). There is no specific treatment for scoliosis in the horse, although therapeutic manipulation may be of benefit in mild acquired cases [7].

Degenerative conditions

Degenerative conditions are relatively common in the equine spine. These conditions include osteoarthritis of the articular facets of the thoracolumbar spine, ventral spondylosis and discospondylosis.

Osteoarthritis of the articular facets

Osteoarthritis (OA) occurs at a number of sites in the equine back. Of these sites, OA of the articular facets of the thoracic and lumbar spine is quite commonly identified as a possible source of back pain.

Articular facet disease is not straightforward. First, little is known about the normal ageing of the equine spine and how the articular facets in "normal" horses change over time. Jeffcott [8] states that OA at this site is common in older horses, but that it is probably not clinically significant. Indeed, in the few studies that have been reported, the incidence of articular facet joint changes is high, e.g. in one postmortem study of thoroughbred racehorses, Haussler et al. [9] reported that 97% of the horses examined had a degree of lumbar vertebrae articular facet degeneration. Although the incidence of articular facet changes is high, the clinical significance of OA at this site is not fully understood, so the veterinarian must be cautious about assuming that the presence of visible articular facet OA automatically means that this is the cause of the back pain in the horse. However, synovial intervertebral articulation lesions are more consistently associated with back pain than ORDSPs, in both the author's experience and the experiences of others [10].

Denoix [11] reports that articular facet pathology in the lumbar vertebrae and the thoracolumbar junction is one of the most common spinal conditions associated with back pain. In humans OA of the articular facets, ankylosing spondylitis and rheumatoid arthritis are all considered to be significant sources of back pain. At present it can be concluded that insufficient is published in the literature about this pathology and its clinical significance in the horse to be able to conclusively predict whether or not the presence or absence of articular facet degeneration is significant. However, clinically it is considered that evidence of articular facet degeneration is a significant finding in horses with back pain, especially when both radiographic evidence and scintigraphic evidence are available, indicating active remodelling at the site.

Diagnosis of articular facet OA

It is reasonable to assume that articular facet OA is more likely in the middle-aged to older horse as is true with all arthritic/degenerative disease in the horse. The clinical signs of articular facet OA are varied. Most cases will present with a history of mild-to-moderate chronic back pain and poor performance. It is rare, in the author's experience, for these horses to show marked and dramatic signs of back pain. In many individuals that animal will still be competing at the level at which it is expected to be, but with a reduction in results/placings/scorings. These signs are all typical of a low-grade, chronic back problem.

On clinical examination horses with articular facet OA show classic clinical signs of back pain (see Chapter 6), which will lead the clinician to suspect that there is genuine back pathology. OA of the facets is then diagnosed using nuclear scintigraphy, radiography and ultrasonography. However, although demonstration of pathological changes at the facets is straightforward, proving that they are the source of the pain remains virtually impossible.

A nuclear scintigraphic examination of the back is particularly useful in the diagnosis of articular facet OA because it will reveal the presence of increased radionuclide uptake over the affected articular process(es) and can provide valuable information on bone remodelling in both the thoracic spine and the lumbar spine. Uptake associated with OA at this site is usually mild to moderate in intensity (Plate 30), and may be difficult to detect above the background uptake at this site. This mild uptake is in marked contrast to the high uptake seen at this site in, for example, lamina stress fractures (Figure 15.1).

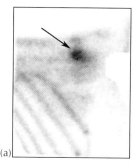 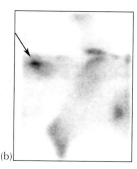

(a)   (b)

Figure 15.1   Scintigrams showing a ventral laminar stress fracture in the lumbar region. (a) DLVMO (dorsolateral–ventromedial–oblique) scintigram. The stress fracture is seen as a marked focal increase in radionuclide uptake (arrow). (b) Lesion-oriented view. The stress fracture is seen as a marked focal increase in radionuclide uptake (arrow). Compare the intensity of the radionuclide uptake in the stress fracture with that seen in osteoarthritis (Plate 30). (Courtesy of R. Pilsworth.)

A radiographic examination is essential for the diagnosis of articular facet OA. Dorsomedial–20° ventrolateral–oblique (DM20°VLO) views are recommended in order to visualise the articular facets (see Chapter 8).

As discussed in Chapter 8 normal articular facets are readily identified on the ventrolateral–dorsomedial–oblique (VLDMO) views (see Figure 8.8). In the thoracic region the facets are seen as "L"-shaped joints, described as having a cranial oblique branch and a caudal vertical branch [10]. In the thoracolumbar junction and the lumbar region the joint spaces become more linear and are seen to run at an angle of 40° to the horizontal.

Radiographic changes associated with OA in the articular facets include loss of the joint space, sclerosis around the joint and new bone formation associated with the joint (Figure 15.2 and see Figure 8.8). More detailed radiographic changes associated with facet OA have been well described by Denoix [11], who has developed a grading system. However it must be recognised that recognition of basic sclerosis around the articular facet and identification of new bone formation (see Figure 8.15) may be all that is possible in the standing horse with most X-ray machines in most clinics.

In addition to nuclear scintigraphy and radiography, ultrasonography can be very helpful in the

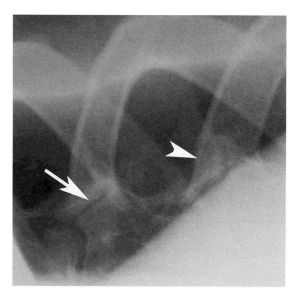

Figure 15.2   A dorsomedial–20° ventrolateral–oblique (DM20°VLO) radiograph showing osteoarthritis (OA) of the articular facets. A normal facet is seen (arrow) cranial to a facet affected by OA – marked new bone formation is seen (arrowhead).

diagnosis of articular facet OA. Transverse ultrasonography of the articular facets has been described using a 2.5- to 5-MHz probe (see Chapters 10 and 11, and in particular Figure 11.3) and can produce good images of the region. Although technically tricky, this ultrasonography may be useful in identifying dorsal new bone formation (Denoix categories 4 and 6 detailed above) at the site (see Figure 22.1 in Chapter 22), particularly in cases in which nuclear scintigraphy/radiography has identified a potential problem.

Although it is relatively straightforward to obtain diagnostic imaging evidence of OA in the articular facets, the interpretation of the findings can be difficult. Ideally, as at other sites of pain arising from OA in the horse, the response to local anaesthesia at the site should be ascertained before ascribing clinical significance to a lesion. However, there are a number of significant difficulties associated with injections of local analgesia into the articular facets of the thoracic and lumbar spine and, in practice, local analgesia is rarely employed to make a diagnosis. The difficulties of using local anaesthetic to diagnose OA of the facet joints include the technical difficulty of the injection, although use of ultrasonographic guidance (see

Chapter 10) can be very helpful. However, placement of the anaesthetic actually into the joint is at best an approximation in most cases and should be interpreted as such. Other difficulties with the technique include the risk of local anaesthetic diffusing from the site of the injection to the spinal cord or outflow nerves. Such diffusion carries with it the risk of temporary paresis of the patient. An ultrasound-guided technique of injection of the nerves proposed to innervate the articular facets has been described [12]. Thus targeted analgesia of the medial branch of the dorsal ramus of the spinal nerve can be attempted (see Chapter 10).

Treatment of articular facet OA

General treatment

Once a diagnosis of articular facet degeneration has been made treatment options must be considered. Unfortunately, there is no absolute specific treatment for this condition and it is often considered that management of the clinical signs is the most that can be achieved. To reduce the pain arising from the pathology, general therapies involve resting the horse to reduce the load and movement on the joint, or in extreme cases retirement of the horse from the activities that may be exacerbating the condition. The use of systemic non-steroidal anti-inflammatory drugs (NSAIDs) to reduce the inflammation around the joint is of merit in this condition, as it is in treating OA at other sites in the horse. Physiotherapy and extracorporeal shock wave therapy have also been suggested to be efficacious, although there are no published data available on the effect of these treatment modalities for articular facet OA.

Specific treatment

Specific therapies that have been described to treat articular facet OA include corticosteroids, Sarapin, tiludronate and mesotherapy.

Perilesional anti-inflammatory injections of corticosteroids, in a similar fashion to which OA would be treated elsewhere in the horse, have been described by a number of authors. Injection of the corticosteroids actually into the joints is very difficult, even under ultrasound guidance, although it can be done. Most clinicians inject into the multifidus muscle surrounding the articular facet, on either side of the horse, just 2 cm off the midline, preferably using ultrasound guidance. The injection should be performed under aseptic conditions and corticosteroids (to a total dose of 20 mg triamcinolone acetate or 140 mg methyl-prednisolone acetate per horse) administered. In competition horses, the rules of the governing council under which the horse is competing must be observed with regard to withdrawal times.

In addition to injecting corticosteroids, the use of perilesional injections of Sarapin, a sterile aqueous solution of soluble salts of the volatile bases from *Sarraceniaceae* (pitcher plant) is also common, based on the management of human lumbar facet joint pain in which it has been found that Sarapin can provide pain relief [13]. Sarapin does have an advantage over corticosteroids in having no reported side effects in the horse. However, some clinicians have suggested that as multifidus contains proprioreceptive nerve endings that are important for vertebral movements, injections at this site are not recommended, although Sarapin is reported to have specific noci-ceptor effects. These specific effects are possibly based on an ammonium ion antagonism action, although the exact mechanism of action of Sarapin has not yet been elucidated.

The use of intravenous tiludronate (Tildren) has been advocated by one clinical research group [14], which reported promising results. This method of treatment certainly does have some logic because tiludronate is licensed for use in the treatment of OA at other sites in the horse, and this treatment may prove to be extremely useful in the management of this difficult disease in the future.

Finally, the use of mesotherapy to treat articular facet disease is well established in Europe and relies on the principle of inhibition of nerves carrying painful information from the deep structures within a spinal segment by the stimulation of nerves from more superficial structures. Thus mesotherapy is based on administering multiple intradermal injections of saline/corticosteroid/local anaesthetic at the level of the lesion and caudal to it [11]. This therapy is reported to be very beneficial in some patients, with a substantial improvement expected in 7–14 days, lasting from 3 to 12 months.

Ventral spondylosis

New bone formation on the ventral aspect of the vertebrae in the thoracolumbar region is termed "vertebral spondylosis" (Figure 15.3). Although extremely common in humans and dogs, ventral spondylosis is considered to be relatively rare in the horse, although it may well be an ageing change. Little is currently known about the pathogenesis and significance of ventral spondylosis in the horse and the interpretation of the clinical significance of the condition in the horse is extremely difficult. Indeed, even among experienced veterinarians dealing with a high caseload of horses with back pathology, there is currently no consensus opinion over the significance of the lesions. Some consider ventral spondylosis the condition to be clinically insignificant, and some highly significant, particularly if the lesion can be demonstrated to be currently active (see below).

Diagnosis

Ventral spondylosis is diagnosed on radiography. It is a relatively rare finding and only occasionally seen on radiographs obtained during an examination of a horse with suspected back pathology. Radiographically, ventral spondylosis is seen as a spectrum of severity of new bone formation ventrally on the vertebral body, associated with the

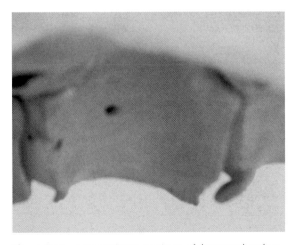

Figure 15.3 A postmortem specimen of the ventral surface of two intervertebral disc spaces showing new bone formation associated with ventral spondylosis. The bone is seen as spur formation either side of the disc space.

disc space (see Figure 8.14 in Chapter 8). In cases in which there is active new bone formation at the site, nuclear scintigraphy will show a focal area of increased radionuclide uptake associated with ventral aspect of the vertebral column (Plate 31).

Although the diagnosis of ventral spondylosis is easy, given access to sufficiently powerful radiographic equipment and nuclear scintigraphy, there is, as yet, no method available for proving that it is the source of the back pain exhibited by the patient. Local analgesic techniques for this site are not described, so obtaining proof of the significance of the lesion is difficult. It is not unreasonable, however, in cases in which there are clear radiographic signs of ventral spondylosis and focal increased radionuclide uptake at the site and, in the absence of other back pathology, to consider ventral spondylosis as clinically significant.

Treatment

There is no specific current treatment for ventral spondylosis in the horse. However, the general therapies that were discussed above for the management of articular facet OA are equally applicable. Rest, treatment with NSAIDs and physiotherapy should all be considered. Theoretically, on the basis that "active" lesions are painful, once the spondylosis has formed the clinical signs should abate.

Discospondylosis

Again, compared with humans and dogs the incidence of discospondylosis is extremely low in the horse. It is likely, however, given the difficulty in diagnosing the condition, that subclinical cases are more frequent than currently recognised. In the horse it is considered that degenerative disc disease is extremely rare, but that disc degeneration secondary to external trauma may well occur. It has been proposed that trauma to the discs and associated structures, through falls and repeated, strenuous exercise, lead to progressive spondylosis associated with the disc.

The clinical signs of discospondylosis in the thoracolumbar spine are similar to those reported for discospondylitis (see below) but do not include the signs reflecting the infectious organism. The

horse may show moderate-to-severe back pain and a variety of neurological signs. The diagnosis is achieved through radiography of the vertebral column, which should demonstrate the collapsed disc space and new bone formation depending on the anatomical site of the lesion. Nuclear scintigraphy is also useful in identifying any active bone remodelling associated with the pathology. However, the major diagnostic problem remains in the differentiation between infectious and non-infectious disc disease. There is no specific treatment for non-infectious discospondylosis in the horse at the current time.

Infections of the back and pelvis

Spondylitis/discospondylitis

Infection in the back can be divided into infection within either the vertebrae (spondylitis/vertebral osteomyelitis) or the vertebrae and the intervertebral disc (vertebral discospondylitis). Both these conditions are rare in the horse, but often devastating when they occur. Spondylitis and discospondylitis are usually caused by haematogenous spread of organisms, usually bacteria. Both conditions are more common in foals in which there has been a failure of passive transfer. A number of organisms have been reported as being associated with spinal infections in the horse, including streptococci, staphylococci, mycobacteria, and *Rhodococcus* and *Aspergillus* species. Infective osteitis is extremely rare in the pelvis, although there have been isolated case reports, including infection of the pubic symphysis with *Rhodococcus equi* [15].

Diagnosis

The diagnosis of spondylitis can be very difficult because the clinical signs of osteomyelitis and discospondylitis are initially vague and can be quite variable. The early clinical signs of spinal infections are acute localised spinal pain and signs of systemic infection, which may progress until other systems become involved, i.e. neurological signs are seen, due to either direct spinal cord involvement or meningitis. The horse can present with a range of clinical signs including pyrexia, lethargy, and back stiffness with or without signs of nerve compression. Haematology may well indicate a leukophilia, neutrophilia and hyperfibrinogenaemia. If the infection is located close to the spinal column it may erode into the spinal canal and cerebrospinal fluid collection, and analysis may provide further evidence of an infectious process.

Diagnostic imaging may be very useful in identifying a lesion; radiographic views of the thoracic and lumbar spine may reveal evidence of infection. Radiographically, vertebral endplate lysis with sclerosis surrounding is seen, often associated with some ventral new bone formation (ventral spondylosis) [16], and in some cases the infection can be associated with a prolapsed disc [17]. Where available, nuclear scintigraphy should be employed in suspected cases because it is a very sensitive indicator of the bone remodelling caused by the infection. Nuclear scintigraphy will identify bone infection as a marked focal increase in radionuclide uptake (Figure 15.4).

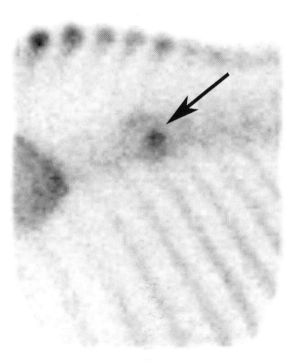

Figure 15.4 A lateromedial scintigram of the mid-thoracic region to show the appearance of vertebral infection. There is increased radionuclide uptake associated with the vertebral body. (Courtesy of R. Pilsworth.)

Treatment

Unfortunately the treatment of spondylitis can be difficult and often unrewarding, particularly in cases in which neurological signs have occurred before a diagnosis has been made. Treatment relies on the use of long-term, high-dose antibiotics, anti-inflammatory drugs and supportive therapy where required [18].

Fistulous withers

"Fistulous withers" is a rare condition that refers to chronic inflammation within the supraspinous bursa that runs over the summits of the DSPs in the withers region. Fistulous withers can be either primary or secondary. Primary cases are caused by inflammation, or parasitic or infectious diseases. In these cases initially the infection is within the bursa; however, over time the infected tissue ruptures and a draining fistula develops. In addition primary fistulous withers can, in severe, chronic cases, lead to osteomyelitis and periostitis of the DSPs.

Brucella abortus and *Actinomyces bovis* are most commonly isolated from cases of fistulous withers [19]; however, in cases when the withers have become damaged by trauma other opportunistic organisms may be isolated. In addition *Onchocerca* species have been associated with the development of the condition.

Fistulous withers can also be seen secondary to trauma to the withers region, e.g. after a fracture of the DSPs of the cranial thoracic vertebrae.

Clinical signs

The clinical signs of fistulous withers differ according to whether the lesion is open or closed. In earlier, closed cases the clinical signs are of a soft tissue swelling over the withers region that is usually associated with pain. In open cases there is an open, draining wound in the withers region, again usually with associated pain in the area. In some cases systemic illness is also present – depression, pyrexia and possible anorexia.

Diagnosis

The main diagnostic step to be taken is to ascertain whether the draining tract is due to a primary infection or whether there is some underlying condition leading to the formation of a draining tract, e.g. fractured withers. Aspiration of the fluid within the swelling is useful in closed lesions in order to identify the presence of an infectious agent. Radiography and nuclear scintigraphy (Figure 15.5) can be used to rule out primary or secondary bony involvement and ultrasonography is also useful to determine the extent of the lesion and whether there are any, for example, foreign bodies within the lesion that may be causing the problem. Ultrasonography is also useful in more chronic cases in which the supraspinous ligament can also become infected.

In addition to the diagnostic steps outlined above, it is advisable to test whether the horse is seropositive for *Brucella abortus* because this is a zoonosis and subject to control measures in some countries.

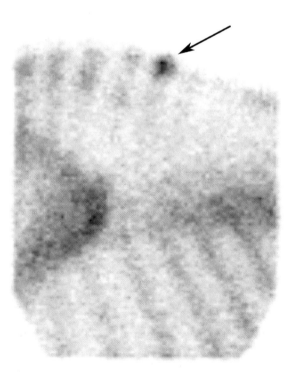

Figure 15.5 A lateromedial scintigram of the cranial thoracic region showing the appearance of dorsal spinous process (DSP) infection. There is infection in the DSP (arrow), seen as an increase in radionuclide uptake. (Courtesy of R. Pilsworth.)

Treatment

The treatment of fistulous withers can be very difficult and unrewarding. In simple cases medical therapy can be attempted. This usually consists of a long course of broad spectrum antibiotics, e.g. trimethoprim/sulphonamide combinations [20], together with the use of NSAIDs and local anti-inflammatory measures such as hydrotherapy, hot packing and topical administration of dimethyl sulphoxide (DMSO). In unresponsive and/or severe cases, and cases in which there is bony involvement, surgical treatment may be necessary, which involves resection of the damaged tissue and excision of the DSPs of affected vertebrae.

Stress fractures

Fractures of the back and pelvis are either traumatic (see Chapter 13) or stress fractures. Although traumatic fractures can occur in all types of horses, stress fractures are confined to those athletic horses undergoing strenuous and repetitive exercise. For stress fractures of the back and pelvis this means that racehorses are the animals affected. There is a high prevalence of stress fractures in racehorses. In the UK the incidence of stress fractures has been estimated as comprising 57% of the total fractures seen in racehorses [21]. Two sites of stress fracture of the back and pelvis are recognised: the vertebral lamina stress fracture and the pelvic stress fracture.

Stress fractures are characterised clinically by:

- being confined to predilection sites within the bone
- being incomplete fractures that may progress to complete fractures
- the presence of periosteal or endosteal callus.

Pathophysiology of stress fractures

Pelvis stress fracture (see also Chapter 13)

Pelvic stress fractures are usually seen to originate on the caudal border of the ilium directly over the region of the sacroiliac joint. The fracture lines then propagate either craniodorsally or craniolaterally towards the tuber sacrale or tuber coxae. These fractures are seen as focal increase in periosteal proliferation at the site of the fracture with or without a propagating fracture line.

Diagnosis of pelvic stress fractures

Pelvic stress fractures can be diagnosed on ultrasonography and/or nuclear scintigraphy. Nuclear scintigraphy reveals the stress fracture as a focal area of markedly increased radionuclide uptake originating on the caudal border of the iliac wing (see Plate 24b). Ultrasonography permits the identification of alterations in the bone surface [22]. On ultrasonography the classically described "step" or incongruency in the hyperechoic bone margin is seen (see Figure 13.3, Chapter 13).

Treatment

The treatment of the pelvic stress fracture is described in Chapter 13 but consists, essentially, of rest.

Vertebral lamina stress fracture

Vertebral lamina stress fractures (VLSFs) were first described by Hassler and Stover [23] in a postmortem survey of thoroughbred racehorses. VLSFs were reported to occur in the caudal part of the thoracic or lumbosacral spine and were seen in 50% of the horses examined. The site of the VLSFs is consistent between horses: they are found on the cranial aspect of the vertebra, near the junction of the articular process and the DSP, and they are continuous with the articular surface of the articular facet (Figure 15.6). These stress fractures usually continued onto the articular surface, leading to articular cartilage fissures and damage. VLSFs were found to be most common at L1, with a decrease in incidence either side of this segment [23].

Diagnosis

VLSFs can be diagnosed using nuclear scintigraphy, radiography and ultrasonography. A nuclear scintigraphic examination will reveal a very marked focal increase in radionuclide uptake at a very similar site to the articular facet, just dorsal

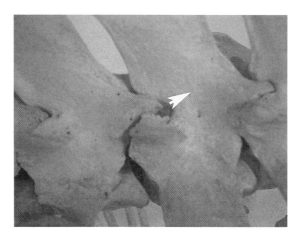

Figure 15.6 A postmortem specimen of the articular facet region of three vertebrae. The site of vertebral stress fractures is shown (arrow head). The stress fractures are reported to originate from the lamina on the edge of the articular facet.

to the vertebral bodies in the lumbar region (see Figure 15.1). OA of the articular facets will also cause a focal increase in radionuclide uptake in this region, but the amount of uptake is marked in the VLSF and mild to moderate in the articular facet disease as a general rule. Radiography can be useful when the VLSF affects those vertebrae that can be imaged successfully (the thoracic vertebrae) and when the VLSF is associated with new bone formation at this site. However, it may not be possible to differentiate new bone formation caused by the VLSF from new bone formation resulting from OA of the articular facets in some cases.

Ultrasonography can also be used to identify new bone formation associated with VLSFs; however, the subtle fracture lines of the VLSF are not appreciable with ultrasonography in most cases and, again, it may not be possible to differentiate the changes from those associated with OA of the articular facets. Although it is clear that diagnostic imaging techniques do not differentiate clearly between stress fractures and OA at this site, the history and signalment of the horse should be very helpful in making the diagnosis.

Treatment

The treatment of VLSFs is, as with most stress fractures, rest. The horse should be put onto a reduced plane of exercise and the high intensity exercise stopped. However, as noted above, the progress of the lesion can be monitored scintigraphically (Plate 32).

Neoplasia

The incidence of neoplasia affecting the back and pelvis is extremely low in the horse. Primary osseous tumours are rare at any site in the equine skeleton and the vertebral column is an extremely unlikely site to find tumours even in cases of skeletal neoplasia. Likewise the vertebral column and pelvis are unlikely sites to find secondary metastatic tumours. If a bone tumour is suspected, radiography and nuclear scintigraphy can be very useful to identify remodelling, new bone formation and bone lysis at the site of the tumour. At the current time the prognosis for neoplasia of the back and pelvis is very poor to hopeless, regardless of the tumour type.

Miscellaneous conditions of the vertebral bodies

In addition to the conditions described above there are occasional case reports in the literature of unusual findings in the back and pelvis. These include incidental findings of vertebral body deformations (usually hemivertebrae), disc enthesiopathy (due to deformity of adjacent vertebrae) and dorsal bony extension of the vertebral fossa found in the caudal thoracic area. Most of these conditions are incidental findings *post mortem* and are not proven causes of back pain.

References

1. Rooney, J.R. Congenital equine scoliosis and lordosis. *Clinical Orthopaedics and Related Research* 1969;**62**: 25–30.
2. Jeffcott, L.B. Disorders of the thoracolumbar spine of the horse – a survey of 443 cases. *Equine Veterinary Journal* 1980;**12**:197–210.
3. Kirberger, R.M. and Gottschalk, R.D. Developmental kyphoscoliosis in a foal. *Journal of the South African Veterinary Association* 1989;**60**:146–148.
4. Lerner, D.J. and Riley, G. Congenital kyphoscoliosis in a foal. *Journal of the American Veterinary Medical Association* 1978;**172**:274–276.
5. Kothstein, T., Rashmir-Raven, A.M., Thomas, M.W. and Brashier, M.K. Radiographic diagnosis: Thoracic spinal fracture resulting in kyphosis in a horse. *Veterinary Radiology and Ultrasound* 2000;**41**:44–45.
6. Wong, D., Miles, K. and Sponseller, B. Congenital scoliosis in a quarter horse filly. *Veterinary Radiology and Ultrasound* 2006;**47**:279–282.
7. Faber, M., Van Weeren, P.R., Scheepers, M. and Barneveld, A. Long-term follow-up of manipulative treatment in a horse with back problems. *Journal of Veterinary Medicine Series A* 2003;**50**:241–245.
8. Jeffcott, L.B. The horse's back – soft tissue and skeletal problems – their diagnosis and management. Presented at the Dubai International Equine Symposium, Dubai, 1996.
9. Haussler, K.K., Stover, S.M. and Willits, N.H. Pathology of the lumbosacral spine and pelvis in Thoroughbred racehorses. *American Journal of Veterinary Research* 1999;**60**:143–153.
10. Denoix, J.M. and Dyson, S.J. Thoracolumbar spine. In: Ross, M.W. and Dyson, S.J. (eds), *Diagnosis and Management of Lameness in the Horse*. Philadelphia: Saunders, 2003: 509–521.
11. Denoix, J.M. Lesions of the vertebral column in poor performance horses. Presented at the World Equine Veterinary Association Symposium, Paris, 1999.
12. Vandeweerd, J.M., Desbrosse, F., Clegg, P. et al. Innervation and nerve injections of the lumbar spine of the horse: a cadaveric study. *Equine Veterinary Journal* 2007;**39**:59–63.
13. Manchikanti, L., Pampati, V., Bakhit, C.E. et al. Effectiveness of lumbar facet joint nerve blocks in chronic low back pain: a randomised clinical trial. *Pain and the Physician* 2001;**4**:101–117.
14. Coudry, V., Thibaud, D. and Riccio, B. Efficacy of tiludronate in the treatment of horses with signs of pain associated with osteoarthritic lesions of the thoracolumbar vertebral column. *American Journal of Veterinary Research* 2007;**68**:329–337.
15. Clark-Price, S.C., Rush, B.R., Gaughan, E.M. and Cox, J.H. Osteomyelitis of the pelvis caused by *Rhodococcus equi* in a 2 year old horse. *Journal of the American Veterinary Medical Association* 2003;**222**:269–272.
16. Sweers, L. and Carsten, A., 2006, Imaging features of discospondylitis in two horses. *Veterinary Radiology and Ultrasound* **47**:159–64.
17. Furr, M.O., Anver, M. and Wise, M. Intervertebral disc prolapse and discospondylitis in a horse. *Journal of the American Veterinary Medical Association* 1991;**198**:2095–2096.
18. Hillyer, M.H., Innes, J.F., Patteson, M.W. et al. Discospondylitis in an adult horse. *Veterinary Record* 1996;**139**:519–521.

19. Gaughan, E.M., Fubrini, S.L. and Patterson, M.W. Fistulous withers in horses: 14 cases (1978–1987). *Journal of the American Veterinary Medical Association* 1988;**201**:121–124.

20. Cohen, N.D., Carter, G.K. and McMullan, W. Fistulous withers; the diagnosis and treatment of open and closed lesion. *Veterinary Medicine* 1991;**86**:416–418.

21. Verheyen, K.L.P. and Wood, J.L.N. Descriptive epidemiology of fractures occurring in British Thoroughbred racehorses in training. *Equine Veterinary Journal* 2004;**36**:167–173.

22. Pilsworth, R.C., Sheperd, M.C., Herinckx, B. and Holmes, M.A. Fracture of the wing of the ilium, adjacent to the sacroiliac joint, in Thoroughbred racehorses. *Equine Veterinary Journal* 1994;**26**:94–99.

23. Haussler, K.K. and Stover, S.M. Stress fractures of the vertebral lamina and pelvis in Thoroughbred racehorses. *Equine Veterinary Journal* 1998;**30**:374–381.

16 Muscular Disorders of the Equine Back

Richard J. Piercy and Renate Weller

Introduction

Muscle disorders that affect the equine back can be broadly divided into two categories, depending on whether the condition is generalised (e.g. an exertional myopathy) or localised (e.g. a muscle tear). The investigation of such cases will depend largely on the presenting clinical signs; however, often it may be difficult to determine whether the problem is localised to the back or whether, in fact, the signs are a manifestation of a more general problem.

Difficulty in discriminating between generalised and localised conditions partly reflects the underlying pathology. In particular, the response shown by skeletal muscle is somewhat limited despite varied underlying causes. Disruption of muscle fibre homoeostasis results in osmotic imbalance: normally the myoplasmic Ca^{2+} concentration is tightly regulated and maintained at a resting concentration that is 60–100 times lower than that of the extracellular fluid; however, damage or disease allows Ca^{2+} to enter the cytoplasm from the interstitial fluid or sarcoplasmic stores, thereby activating destructive cellular proteases and inhibiting mitochondrial respiration [1, 2]. Cell death by necrosis is often associated with inflammatory responses that result in the chemotaxis of circulating neutrophils and macrophages, the removal of damaged tissue and collagen deposition, which if extensive may result in fibrosis. However, in many circumstances, there is muscle disease without a marked inflammatory response [3].

The regenerative capacity of muscle is dependent on a population of normally quiescent 'stem cell'-like cells, known as satellite cells, which occupy a position beneath the fibre's basement membrane but outside the fibre's sarcolemma. Fibre damage results in satellite cell activation, division and transformation into myoblasts – cells that eventually fuse to form immature myotubes and subsequently new myofibres [4]. This process may take several months; in the intervening period, histopathology reveals immature fibres of variable sizes with internally located nuclei (Figure 16. 1) [5]. Regeneration is, however, limited by the extent to which reinnervation and revascularisation are possible when these modalities are compromised, and the degree of damage to the fibres' basement membranes [6]. It is generally assumed that when the basement membrane is compromised there is a greater propensity for fibrosis and scar formation [6].

Diagnostic procedures

Clinical examination

Clinical signs vary depending on the extent of the underlying disease. Localised tears or inflammation will manifest as guarding or avoidance

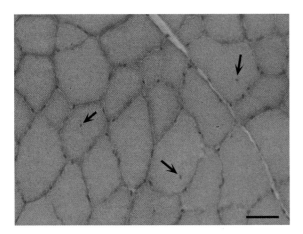

Figure 16.1 Semimembranosus muscle biopsy sample: 11-year-old thoroughbred mare with a history of repeated episodes of exertional rhabdomyolysis. Note the internalised nuclei (arrows). Haematoxylin and eosin stain. Bar = 50 μm.

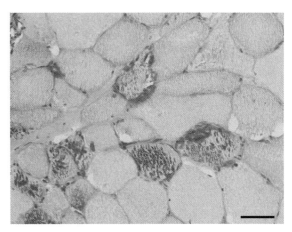

Figure 16.2 Semimembranosus muscle biopsy sample stained with periodic acid–Schiff (PAS) following diastase digestion: 8-year-old cob gelding with exertional rhabdomyolysis. Note the abundant pink-staining inclusions in multiple fibres, consistent with abnormal polysaccharide and a diagnosis of polysaccharide storage myopathy. Bar = 50 μm.

responses to deep palpation of the region, whereas horses with generalised myopathies may show more severe systemic signs. Mild-to-moderately affected animals are tachycardic, with firm hindlimb, epaxial and gluteal musculature that is painful when palpated and results in a stiff gait. Pigmenturia may be evident in more severely affected animals: furthermore, these animals will often have severe pain and be severely tachycardic and tachypnoeic. They may sweat profusely and be unwilling to move or become recumbent.

Biochemistry

Many muscle strains and tears may not be detectable through routine biochemical assessment; however, more generalised conditions (such as the exertional myopathies) or severe localised muscle damage are likely to be represented by elevations in the activities of the muscle-derived enzymes, creatine kinase (CK) and aspartate transaminase (AST; also called aspartate aminotransferase). CK remains the most convenient and specific marker of acute muscle damage, peaking at 4–6 hours after acute muscle damage [7]. AST activity usually peaks about 24 hours after an episode and may remain elevated for several days to weeks [8, 9]. In some horses, provocative exercise testing may

be informative: although individual clinicians vary in their methodology and interpretation of such testing, a positive response is often regarded when a horse has shown a 250% rise in CK activity 2–4 hours after 20–30 minutes of moderate lunged exercise [10]. Note, however, that not all horses with underlying myopathic conditions show a consistent positive response to such testing.

Biopsy

Muscle biopsy is indicated in an animal that is presented because of suspected back pain, where no other credible cause has been identified and, in particular, when there are persistent elevations in serum muscle enzyme activities or when a horse has shown a significant rise in muscle-derived enzymes after an exercise test. The site of the biopsy should be based on results of the physical examination; however, epaxial, gluteal and semimembranosus muscles are usually chosen [9, 10]. A semimembranosus muscle biopsy is likely to result in fewer complications and is generally indicated in suspected generalised myopathic conditions such as polysaccharide storage myopathy (Figure 16.2). Both open and needle biopsy techniques have been described and, ideally, both fresh and formalin-fixed samples should be submitted to a specialist laboratory.

Ultrasonography

Ultrasonography is widely used for the evaluation of soft tissue structures in the horse. Although it is mainly used for tendons, ligaments and joints, its use for the evaluation of equine muscle has been described [11, 12].

Technique

For accurate and repeatable assessment the skin over the area of interest has to be clipped and thoroughly cleansed. Soaking the skin for a few minutes usually improves image quality. An ultrasound machine used for the evaluation of the flexor tendons is suitable for the ultrasonographic examination of the epaxial muscles. The epaxial muscles vary in depth depending on the location and a 5–10 MHz transducer with a central frequency of 7.5 MHz will allow visualisation of the muscles iliocostalis, longissimus dorsi, spinalis and multifidus. Due to its heterogeneous architec-ture longissimus dorsi should be assessed at multiple locations along its length.

Muscle tissue appears less echogenic ultrasonographically than the connective tissue enveloping the muscle fascicles. This results in a speckled or marbled appearance of muscle on transverse scans (Figure 16.3), and multiple, parallel, linear lines on longitudinal scans (Figure 16.4). Aponeurotic sheets appear as hyperechogenic lines within muscles or separating muscle bellies (Figure 16.4). Each muscle has a characteristic ultrasonographic appearance that is dependent on its architecture and its contraction status: care should be taken to standardise the ultrasonographic examination by ensuring that the horse is positioned on a level surface, equally weight bearing on all four limbs, with the head and neck positioned in line with the back.

Indications for ultrasonography

Ultrasonography has been used to diagnose muscle tears, myositis, haemorrhage, foreign bodies and abscesses, although this has not been described for these lesions in equine back muscles. In some horses with suspected muscle strain based on a localised increase in uptake of radiopharma-

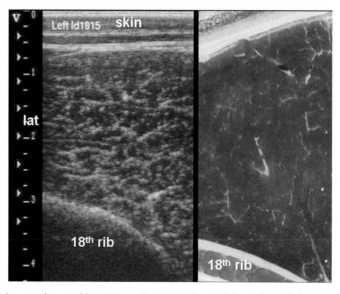

Figure 16.3   Transverse ultrasound scan of longissimus dorsi at the level of the eighteenth thoracic rib and the corresponding dissection. Muscle tissue appears less echogenic than the connective tissue enveloping the muscle fascicles, resulting in a speckled appearance.

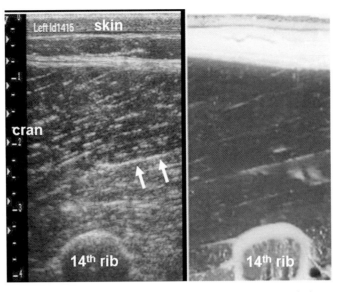

Figure 16.4   Longitudinal ultrasound scan of longissimus dorsi at the level of the fourteenth thoracic rib, 15 cm ventral to the midline, and the corresponding dissection. Muscle is less echogenic compared with the connective tissue, and the muscle fascicles appear as multiple, parallel, linear lines; aponeurotic sheets appear as distinct hyperechoic lines within muscles (arrows) and separating muscle bellies.

ceutical over the thoracolumbar region, an increase in echogenicity with changes in pennation angle have been found on ultrasonography.

Ultrasonography can also be used to evaluate muscle architecture as an indicator of muscle fitness, to monitor training and to assess horses with suspected back pain, with a view to determining efficacy of interventional treatments. Muscle architecture, including volume, fibre length and pennation angle, greatly influences muscle function [13]. These architectural parameters are used to calculate the physiological cross-sectional area of a muscle (which is proportional to the force potential of the muscle). The amount of fibrous tissue within a muscle also determines its passive force–length properties. Active and passive properties of the muscle are important in back function, because back muscles not only contribute to spinal movement, but are also crucial in spinal stabilisation [14, 15]. Muscle responds to its usage: atrophy or hypertrophy occurs with decreased and increased use (training), decrease or increase in muscle volume, and pennation

angle. The same effect has been observed in a cohort of six untrained ponies undergoing a 12-week low-intensity training programme (R. Weller and R.J. Piercy, 2008, unpublished data).

It is well documented in humans that back pain is associated with changes in the volume of back muscles [16]. Affected muscle groups undergo hypertrophy in the acute stage and atrophy with an increase of connective tissue in chronic cases. This seems to hold true for longissimus dorsi in the horse: preliminary data from horses with chronic back disorders show an increased fibrous: muscle tissue ratio, a decrease in muscle depth and a change in pennation angle in longissimus dorsi (R. Weller and R.J. Piercy, 2008, unpublished data). These measurements should be considered in the context of the overall muscular condition of the horse to differentiate between generally unfit animals and horses with impaired back muscle function. Note that pennation angle decreases from cranial to caudal and from dorsal to ventral, ranging from 30° to 45°, so standardisation of location is important.

Scintigraphy

Scintigraphic evaluation follows a standard procedure for musculoskeletal examination in the horse (see Chapter 9).

Generalised radiopharmaceutical uptake over the back muscles has been described in racehorses after an episode of exertional rhabdomyolysis. This has been reported 24 hours after treadmill exercise [17], but also up to 10 days after training [18]. These findings have been observed in the bone phase, rather than the soft tissue phase, of the scintigraphic examination. Not all horses with evidence of exertional rhabdomyolysis, however, show abnormal findings on scintigraphy. Figure 16.5 shows the scintigraphic findings in a horse with acute rhabdomyolysis. The image shows linear areas of increased radiopharmaceutical uptake 3 hours after injection of 1 GBq technetium-99 m-labelled methylene diphosphonate ([99mTc]MDP). Radiopharmaceutical uptake over specific portions of the epaxial muscle has also been identified in sport horses with concurrent ipsilateral hindlimb lameness, possibly due to muscle strains or tears [18]. This can be associated with an increase in echogenicity and changes in pennation angle on ultrasonography (see above).

Electromyography

An electromyographic (EMG) signal can be collected using surface or fine-wire needle electrodes, and provides information on the timing and amplitude of muscle activity and also clinical information regarding the state of innervation and pathology within the muscle.

Surface EMG

EMG using surface electrodes has been used to relate muscle activity to changes in gait characteristics in normal horses in different gaits and under different conditions [14, 15, 19]. It has also been used to assess the efficacy of physiotherapeutic intervention in horses and the effect of training aids (J.M. Wakeling, 2008, personal communication). The signal and its interpretation are very sensitive to the position and placement of the electrode over the muscle of interest and great vari-

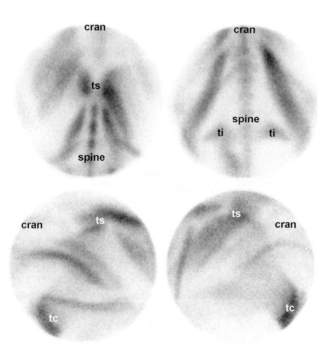

Figure 16.5 Scintigraphic images of a horse with acute rhabdomyolysis 3 hours after injection of [99mTc]methylene diphosphonate. The top two images show two dorsal views of the pelvis region, the two bottom images show a left lateral oblique and a right lateral oblique image (tc = tuber coxae, ts = tuber sacrale, ti = tuber ischii). Note the striped/linear increase in radiopharmaceutical uptake over the musculature typical for this condition.

ability can exist between signals collected from the same and between different animals. Electrodes are placed over the mid-belly region of the muscle of interest, so surface EMG is restricted to evaluation of superficial muscles.

To ensure a good quality signal, the area on which the electrode will be placed should be clipped and shaved. The skin should be wiped clean to remove any remaining dust and grease. The surface electrodes, which are usually self-adhesive, should then be placed onto the skin and held in place with suitable tape to help prevent movement and introduction of low-frequency noise artefact. The dimensions of the electrodes (size and interelectrode distance) should be known and reported, because these factors influence the signal components. Several manufacturers offer complete EMG systems with varying numbers of channels and sampling frequencies to suit different needs.

Needle EMG

A needle EMG requires specialist equipment and expertise and is indicated in cases where the clinician suspects neurogenic or primary myopathic disease. Unlike surface EMG, with needle EMG the clinician can evaluate very specific regions and the electrical activity of individual groups of muscle fibres. Normal muscle at rest is electrically inactive, so, after a brief period of activity caused by the placement of the needle disrupting muscle fibres (insertional activity), a resting muscle should quickly fall silent (unless the needle is close to a neuromuscular junction). Prolonged insertional activity is considered abnormal.

Electrical activity within the muscle after needle insertion can be either normal or pathological. Normal activity occurs when the muscle contracts, or is held contracted, making assessment in standing, conscious horses sometimes difficult to interpret (the latter is aided by a quiet environment, stocks and a sedated animal). Pathological findings include fibrillation potentials and positive sharp waves, which are often encountered with denervation. The reader is referred to additional sources for further information [20]. Generally, needle EMG is best interpreted in an anaesthetised horse, if practicalities allow.

Disorders: aetiopathogenesis and treatment

Muscle strains, bruises and tears

Although there may be a history of trauma, frequently muscle tears and strains at first go unnoticed because the condition may become painful only after several hours. Generally these injuries occur during exercise or while at pasture and, in some circumstances, injuries may result from inexperienced riding or poorly fitting saddles. Showjumpers and eventers are particularly prone to lumbar and gluteal strain, which may be reflected as unwillingness to jump or turn sharply; however, often, horses exhibit only mild-to-moderate lameness or stiffness. The propensity for muscle injury to result in chronic back pain, and in particular myofascial trigger points, is an active area of investigation. These points are regarded as the sites of painful nodules, located within taut bands of skeletal muscle [21, 22].

Adequate rest followed by a gradual return to exercise forms the mainstay of treatment in horses with these kinds of injuries. Non-steroidal anti-inflammatory drugs (NSAIDs, e.g. phenylbutazone 4.4 mg/kg i.v. or p.o. twice daily for 1 day followed by 2.2 mg/kg p.o. twice daily for several days, or flunixin meglumine 0.5–1.1 mg/kg i.v. or p.o. twice daily or once daily) provide analgesia and may help limit the fibrotic response. Various forms of physiotherapy, such as massage, electrical stimulation and swimming exercise may aid healing and speed recovery.

Exertional myopathies

Exertional myopathies have received considerable attention in recent years, as investigators have recognised that specific entities exist within this multifactorial syndrome. Horses with exertional myopathies usually have generalised disease, of which back stiffness, soreness and pelvic limb lameness may be part. There is convincing evidence that both acquired and genetic causes contribute to the clinical scenario: within the former group, overexertion, electrolyte imbalance, hormonal influence and infectious disease have all been proposed as potential causes [23]. Note, however, that many of these factors may be the precipitating cause of disease in a genetically susceptible animal.

Injury resulting from overexertion probably has several components and depends on the nature of the exercise, e.g. eccentric muscle contraction (contraction that occurs during muscle lengthening, as might occur as strain is taken in contracted back muscles on landing from a jump, is believed to result in more severe muscle damage than other types of contraction and, in particular, in sarcomeric disruption and damage to the excitation–contraction coupling mechanism and the sarcolemma [24]. The result is a local inflammatory response accompanied by oedema and the sensitisation of nociceptors [25].

Other factors that may contribute to overexertion-induced myopathy include metabolic exhaustion (e.g. in endurance animals) and antioxidant status. For the latter, evidence suggests that production of reactive oxygen species (such as free radicals) correlates with energy expenditure [26] and that oxidative stress occurs in horses, especially when ambient humidity and temperature are high. Causal links with myopathies and oxidative stress are hard to prove; however, although antioxidant supplementation does not attenuate exercise-induced elevations in muscle enzymes in horses [27], the link between vitamin E and/or selenium deficiency in foals with nutritional myodegeneration [28] suggests that antioxidants may play an important role. Animals with antioxidant deficiencies may be especially prone to damage or disease of other underlying cause.

There are two forms of exercise-related myopathy in horses with underlying genetic causes. These include a condition examined extensively in a group of thoroughbreds in the USA that has been termed "recurrent exertional rhabdomyolysis" (RER) [29] and another condition, termed "(equine) polysaccharide storage myopathy" (PSSM or EPSM) [30]. These conditions have clinical and clinicopathological similarities and are managed similarly, although they also have key differences and breed susceptibilities [31]. The word "recurrent" in thoroughbreds with exercise-related myopathy has been used variably to describe certain thoroughbreds with documented abnormalities in muscle calcium regulation [29], a wider group of thoroughbreds with an apparent inherited form of exertional rhabdomyolysis [32] and all thoroughbreds with a susceptibility to the syndrome. In humans there are many genetic causes of rhabdomyolysis (e.g. mutations in genes encoding enzymes involved in cellular metabolism or structural proteins); it is currently unknown how many different forms of rhabdomyolysis affect horses.

Recurrent exertional rhabdomyolysis

Estimates of prevalence or incidence of exercise-associated rhabdomyolysis in thoroughbreds suggests that 5–7% of thoroughbreds worldwide are affected [33, 34], although it remains unknown whether all these animals have the same disorder. Pedigree analysis of some lines of thoroughbreds in the USA supports autosomal dominant inheritance of the trait [35]. Given that acquired forms of rhabdomyolysis are common in humans and other species, it seems possible, or likely, that some thoroughbreds develop acquired forms of the syndrome as a result of triggering environmental or management factors. Despite this, a common underlying genetic predisposition within the breed remains a distinct possibility. Furthermore, it is possible that exertional myopathies in other breeds (such as standardbreds) may have an identical underlying cause.

The abnormality in muscle calcium regulation identified in some thoroughbreds shares certain experimental similarities to a condition recognised in humans and other species, known as malignant hyperthermia (MH). In particular, muscle from horses with RER and other species with MH is hypersensitive to agents (such as caffeine and halothane) that stimulate release of calcium from the muscle calcium store (sarcoplasmic reticulum) through a calcium release channel known as the ryanodine receptor (RYR1) [29]. However, although MH has been reported in some horses after halothane anaesthesia, and indeed, although an RYR1 receptor mutation has been identified in MH-susceptible quarter horses [36], thoroughbreds with abnormal calcium regulation do not share the same mutation, and there is evidence to suggest that the RYR1 receptor is not mutated in thoroughbred RER [37]. Given that inhalational anaesthesia is common in equine veterinary work, but MH-like episodes are extremely rare, this seems unsurprising. Despite this, the basic research similarities between RER and MH still suggest the involvement of another protein or proteins that regulate intracellular calcium regulation in muscle. Indeed mutations in other proteins are known to cause or are implicated in human MH [38].

Currently it is not generally possible to document calcium regulation abnormalities in horses with suspected RER, because the techniques involved are invasive, technically challenging and unavailable in the clinical setting. Furthermore, muscle biopsy and histopathology, though confirming myopathy and providing information about severity, are not specific for this form of the disease (see Figure 16.1). As such, many of these cases are treated or managed without establishing the definitive diagnosis and remain in the idiopathic category.

Polysaccharide storage myopathy

PSSM or EPSM is currently definitively diagnosed by muscle biopsy. Pathognomonic changes include diastase-resistant inclusions detected by periodic acid–Schiff staining. Horses with this disorder are hypersensitive to insulin, and clear glucose from the circulation more rapidly than normal animals [39]. This disease was first reported in detail in quarter horses with exertional rhabdomyolysis in the USA. Since then, a disease with the same histopathological features has been reported in a variety of other breeds, in particular draught horses [30, 40]. Although there are sometimes clinical differences in the presentations of this disease (rhabdomyolysis in athletic animals and weakness or muscle atrophy in draught horses) these diseases share the same underlying genetic cause (genotype). Recent data suggest that the disease is inherited as an autosomal dominant trait and a mutation in a gene integrally involved in glycogen metabolism, glycogen synthase, has recently been discovered in affected quarter horses, Belgian draught horses and warmbloods [41]. Evidence suggests that in quarter horses the prevalence is between 6 and 12% [42].

Treatment of exertional myopathies

The management and treatment of exertional rhabdomyolysis in thoroughbreds depend on whether the horse is seen in the acute setting or between intermittent episodes [10]. The treatment of acute exertional rhabdomyolysis depends on the severity. Mildly affected horses (the majority) can often be managed conservatively, through controlled exercise with or without NSAIDs, whereas severely affected animals require hospitalisation, analgesics, intravenous fluids and sometimes diuresis (the last to diminish the possibility of myoglobin-induced nephrotoxicity). Various other drugs, such as acepromazine, corticosteroids and dantrolene (see below), are sometimes administered [10].

Prophylaxis is important for horses that appear predisposed to repeated episodes of exertional rhabdomyolysis. There is currently widespread use of oral dantrolene in thoroughbred racehorses. The rationale is based on two published reports that suggest some efficacy, either in thoroughbreds where calcium regulation abnormalities have been documented, or in a group of uncharacterised racehorses [43]. Dantrolene is an RYR1 receptor antagonist (although it has other less specific effects in muscle cells); as such, its main effect is probably to reduce the release of calcium from the sarcoplasmic reticulum which is required for muscle contraction. Effects of the drug on performance are currently unknown, although it has been associated with weakness in some experimental horses at high doses [44]. There is some evidence that would suggest that gastrointestinal absorption is poor without feed withdrawal. Various other treatments (such as phenytoin) and vitamin, mineral, electrolyte and hormonal supplements are administered to horses prone to repeated episodes of exertional rhabdomyolysis, but most have unproven efficacy [23].

There is, however, good evidence that episodes of exertional rhabdomyolysis in some susceptible thoroughbreds can be reduced in severity or frequency through manipulation of the diet, in particular by increasing the proportion of dietary energy derived from fat and decreasing the proportion derived from carbohydrate [45]. Similar dietary alterations are recommended for the management of PSSM [40]; however, it remains unclear why such management results in a beneficial response in these two separate disorders. Regular and consistent exercise in both groups also appears to be important.

Muscle atrophy

Atrophy of the back musculature usually falls into one of two categories: (1) generalised and symmetrical atrophy, and (2) localised and asymmetrical atrophy. In the former cases, close attention should be given to the nutritional status (and dentition) and systemic disease in animals that may have generalised weight loss. In addition, disuse atrophy (perhaps manifest as increased prominence of the tuber sacrale) may occur in horses that are rested, older or have another source of lameness. If these are ruled out, then other rarer causes, e.g. equine motor neuron disease (EMND) [46] and chronic grass sickness (in affected countries) [47], should be considered. Both of these last two conditions can usually be distinguished by other characteristic clinical signs that accompany the diseases, and the reader is referred to general medicine and neurology texts for more detailed descriptions. EMND can readily be confirmed through muscle biopsy of *sacrocaudalis dorsalis medialis* (Figure 16.6).

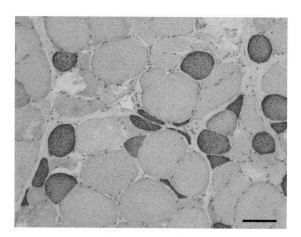

Figure 16.6 Sacrocaudalis dorsalis medialis muscle biopsy specimen: 2-year-old filly with marked muscle atrophy and weakness, labelled (immunoperoxidase) with an antibody to slow myosin heavy chain. Note the angular atrophy of particularly the darker, type I fibres, characteristic of equine motor neuron disease. Bar = 100 μm.

In horses with localised and asymmetrical muscle atrophy, a neurogenic cause or primary muscle disease should be considered. Neurogenic muscle atrophy of the back musculature may result from damage or pressure to spinal nerve roots, caused by vertebral osteoarthritis, vertebral injury or a space-occupying lesion, or by localised grey matter disease (e.g. with equine protozoal myelitis). With spinal cord lesions, additional involvement of white matter tracts may result in further clinical signs (such as asymmetrical pelvic limb ataxia or weakness). Neurogenic causes of muscle atrophy result in characteristic changes identifiable by needle EMG (see above); however, definitive diagnosis is achieved with the aid of muscle biopsy.

A primary (and presumed immune-mediated) myositis has been identified in horses with severe muscle atrophy of the dorsal musculature (and elsewhere) [48]. This may be either symmetrical or asymmetrical. Recent exposure to *Streptococcus equi equi* appears to be a risk factor and, given this organism's propensity to cause purpura, the causative agent of equine strangles may be a primary cause of immune-mediated myositis. Diagnosis in these cases is based on identification of a lymphocytic myositis by muscle biopsy and many horses appear to respond to rest, combined with corticosteroid administration.

References

1. Belcastro, A.N., Shewchuk, L.D. and Raj, D.A. Exercise-induced muscle injury: a calpain hypothesis. *Molecular and Cellular Biochemistry* 1998;**179**:135–145.
2. Gissel, H. and Clausen, T., Excitation induced calcium influx and skeletal muscle cell damage. *Acta Physiologica Scandinavia* 2001;**171**:32–334.
3. Sandri, M. and Carraro, U. Apoptosis of skeletal muscles during development and disease. *International Journal of Biochemistry and Cell Biology* 1999;**31**:1373–1390.
4. Zammit, P. and Beaushamp, J. The skeletal muscle satellite cell: stem cell or son of stem cell? *Differentiation* 2001;**68**:193–204.
5. Dubowitz, J.G. and Sewry, C., Changes in sarcolemmal nuclei. In: Dubowitz, J.G. and Sewry, C. (eds), *Muscle Biopsy: A practical approach*. Philadelphia: Saunders, 2007: 92–94.

6. Kaariainen, M., Järvinen, T., Järvinen, M., Rantanen, J. and Kalimo, H. Relation between myofibers and connective tissue during muscle injury repair. *Scandinavian Journal of Medicine and Science in Sports* 2000;**10**:332–337.

7. Toutain, P.L., Lassourd, V., Costes, G. et al. A non-invasive and quantitative method for the study of tissue injury caused by intramuscular injection of drugs in horses. *Journal of Veterinary Pharmacology and Therapeutics* 1995;**18**:226–235.

8. Harris, P.A., Marlin, D.J. and Gray, J. Plasma aspartate aminotransferase and creatine kinase activities in thoroughbred racehorses in relation to age, sex, exercise and training. *Veterinary Journal* 1998;**155**:295–304.

9. Snow, D. and Valberg, S.J. *Muscle Anatomy, Physiology and Adaptations to Exercise and Training*. Philadelphia: W.B. Saunders Co., 1994.

10. Piercy, R.J. and Lopez-Rivero, J. Muscle disorders of equine athletes. In: Hinchcliff, K.W., Kaneps, A.J. and Geor, R.J. (eds), *Equine Sports Medicine and Surgery*. London: Saunders, 2004: 76–100.

11. Leveille, R. and Biller, D. Muscle evaluation, foreign bodies and miscellaneous swellings. In: Rantanen, N.W. and McKinnon, A. (eds), *Equine Diagnostic Ultrasonography*. Baltimore, MD: Williams & Wilkins, 1998: 213–224.

12. Reef, V.B. Musculoskeletal ultrasonography. In: Reef, V.B. (ed.), *Equine Diagnostic Ultrasound*. Philadelphia: W.B. Saunders Co., 1998: 143–149.

13. Lieber, R.L. and Friden, J. Functional and clinical significance of skeletal muscle architecture. *Muscle and Nerve* 2001;**23**:1647–1666.

14. Robert, C., Valette, J.P. and Denoix, J.M. The effects of treadmill inclination and speed on the activity of three trunk muscles in the trotting horse. *Equine Veterinary Journal* 2001;**33**:466–472.

15. Licka, T.F., Peham, C. and Frey, A. Electromyographic activity of the longissimus dorsi muscles in horses during trotting on a treadmill. *American Journal of Veterinary Research* 2004;**65**:155–158.

16. Hides, J.A., Stokes, M.J., Saide, M., Jull, G.A. and Cooper, D.H. Evidence of lumbar multifidus muscle wasting ipsilateral to symptoms in patients with acute/subacute low back pain. *Spine* 1994;**19**:165–172.

17. Morris, E., Seeherman, H.J., O'Callaghan, M.W. et al. Scintigraphic identification of skeletal muscle damage in horses 24 hours after strenuous exercise. *Equine Veterinary Journal* 1991;**23**:347–352.

18. Ross, M.W. and Stacy, V.S. Nuclear medicine. In: Ross, M.W. and Dyson, S.J. (eds), *Diagnosis and Management of Lameness in the Horse*. Philadelphia: Saunders, 2003: 198–212.

19. Robert, C., Valette, J.P., Pourcelot, P., Audigié, F. and Denoix, J.M. Effects of trotting speed on muscle activity and kinematics in saddlehorses. *Equine Veterinary Journal* 2002;**34**(suppl):295–301.

20. Andrews, F. Electrodiagnostic aids and selected neurological diseases. In: Reed, S., Bayly, W. and Sellon, D. (eds), *Equine Internal Medicine*. Philadelphia: Saunders, 2004: 546–560.

21. Gerwin, R.D. Myofascial pain syndrome in the upper extremity. *Journal of Hand Therapy* 1997;**10**:130–136.

22. Gerwin, R.D. and Duranleau, D. Ultrasound identification of the myofascial trigger point. *Muscle and Nerve* 1997;**20**:767–768.

23. Beech, J. Chronic exertional rhabdomyolysis. *Veterinary Clinics of North America Equine Practice* 1997;**13.1**:145–168.

24. Proske, U. and Morgan, D.L. Muscle damage from eccentric exercise: mechanism, mechanical signs, adaptation and clinical applications. *Journal of Physiology* 2001;**537**:333–345.

25. MacIntyre, D.L., Reid, W.D. and McKenzie, D.C. Delayed muscle soreness. The inflammatory response to muscle injury and its clinical implications. *Sports Medicine* 1995;**20**:24–40.

26. Ji, L. and Leichtweis, S. Exercise and oxidative stress: sources of free radicals and their impact on antioxidant systems. *Age* 1997;**20**:91–106.

27. Brady, P.S., Ku, P.K. and Ullrey, D.E. Lack of effect of selenium supplementation on the response of the equine erythrocyte glutathione system and plasma enzymes to exercise. *Journal of Animal Science* 1978;**47**:492–496.

28. Lofstedt, J. White muscle disease of foals. *Veterinary Clinics of North America Equine Practice* 1997;**13.1**:169–185.

29. Lentz, L.R., Valberg, S.J., Herold, L.V. et al. Myoplasmic calcium regulation in myotubes from horses with recurrent exertional rhabdomyolysis. *American Journal of Veterinary Research* 2002;**63**:1724–1731.

30. Valentine, B.A., Credille, K.M., Lavoie, J.P. et al. Severe polysaccharide storage myopathy in Belgian and Percheron draught horses. *Equine Veterinary Journal* 1997;**29**:220–225.

31. Valberg, S.J., Mickelson, J.R., Gallant, E.M. et al. Exertional rhabdomyolysis in quarter horses and thoroughbreds: one syndrome, multiple aetiologies. *Equine Veterinary Journal* 1999;**30**(suppl):533–538.

32. MacLeay, J.M., Valberg, S.J., Sorum, S.A. et al. Heritability of recurrent exertional rhabdomyolysis in Thoroughbred racehorses. *American Journal of Veterinary Research* 1999;**60**:250–256.

33. Cole, F.L., Mellor, D.J., Hodgson, D.R. and Reid, S.W. Prevalence and demographic characteristics of exertional rhabdomyolysis in horses in Australia. *Veterinary Record* 2004;**155**:625–630.

34. Upjohn, M.M., Archer, R.M., Christley, R.M. and McGowan, C.M. Incidence and risk factors associated with exertional rhabdomyolysis syndrome in National Hunt racehorses in Great Britain. *Veterinary Record* 2005;**156**:763–766.

35. Dranchak, P.K., Valberg, S.J., Ohan, G.W. et al. Inheritance of recurrent exertional rhabdomyolysis in thoroughbreds. *Journal of the American Veterinary Medical Association* 2005;**227**:762–767.

36. Aleman, M., Riehl, J., Aldridge, B.M. et al. Association of a mutation in the ryanodine receptor 1 gene with equine malignant hyperthermia. *Muscle and Nerve* 2004;**30**:356–365.

37. Dranchak, P.K., Valberg, S.J., Ohan, G.W. et al. Exclusion of linkage of the *RYR1*, *CACNA1S*, and *ATP2A1* genes to recurrent exertional rhabdomyolysis in Thoroughbreds. *American Journal of Veterinary Research* 2006;**67**:1395–1400.

38. Jurkat-Rott, K., McCarthy, T. and Lehmann-Horn, F. Genetics and pathogenesis of malignant hyperthermia. *Muscle and Nerve* 2000;**23**:4–17.

39. Annandale, E.J., Valberg, S.J., Mickelson, J.R. and Seaquist, E.R. Insulin sensitivity and skeletal muscle glucose transport in horses with equine polysaccharide storage myopathy. *Neuromuscular Disorders* 2004;**14**:666–674.

40. Firshman, A.M., Valberg, S.J., Bender, J.B. and Finno, C.J. Epidemiologic characteristics and management of polysaccharide storage myopathy in Quarter Horses. *American Journal of Veterinary Research* 2003;**64**:1319–1327.

41. McCue, M.E. and Valberg, S.J. Glycogen synthase 1 mutation and polysaccharide storage myopathy in diverse horse breeds. In: *Plant and Animal Genomes*. San Diego, 2008.

42. McCue, M.E., Valberg, S.J., Byrne, K., Miller, W.B., Wade, C. and Mickelson, J.R. Identification of a glycogen synthase I mutation resulting in polysaccharide storage myopathy. Presented at the 7th Dorothy Russell Havemeyer International Equine Genome Mapping Workshop, Tahoe City, CA, 2007.

43. Edwards, J.G., Newton, J.R., Ramzan, P.H., Pilsworth, R.C. and Shepherd, M.C. The efficacy of dantrolene sodium in controlling exertional rhabdomyolysis in the Thoroughbred racehorse. *Equine Veterinary Journal* 2003;**35**:707–711.

44. Court, M.H., Engelking, L.R., Dodman, N.H. et al. Pharmacokinetics of dantrolene sodium in horses. *Journal of Veterinary Pharmacology and Therapeutics* 1987;**10**:218–226.

45. McKenzie, E.C., Valberg, S.J., Godden, S.M., Finno, C.J. and Murphy, M.J. Effect of oral administration of dantrolene sodium on serum creatine kinase activity after exercise in horses with recurrent exertional rhabdomyolysis. *American Journal of Veterinary Research* 2004;**65**:74–79.

46. McGorum, B.C. et al. Horses on pasture may be affected by equine motor neuron disease. *Equine Veterinary Journal* 2006;**38**:47–51.

47. Murphy, D. and Love, S. Diagnostic aids and prognostic indicators for chronic grass sickness: possibilities for the future. *British Veterinary Journal* 1996;**152**:497–499.

48. Lewis, S.S., Valberg, S.J. and Nielsen, I.L. Suspected immune-mediated myositis in horses. *Journal of Veterinary Internal Medicine* 2007;**21**:495–503.

17 Supraspinous Ligament and Dorsal Sacroiliac Ligament Desmitis

Luis P. Lamas

Introduction

The spinal ligaments that have been most frequently associated with clinical signs of back pain are the supraspinous ligament (SSL) and the dorsal sacroiliac ligament (DSIL). Similar to many other conditions of the equine back, injuries to these structures often cause equivocal clinical signs, and defining the cause of the injury, the significance of any ligamentous damage detected and the best management of clinically proven cases of desmitis can be equally frustrating.

Supraspinous ligament

Anatomy and biomechanics

The supraspinous ligament is a strong fibrous ligament that inserts on the summits of the dorsal spinous processes (DSPs) of the thoracolumbar vertebrae. It is the continuation of the more elastic nuchal ligament, which originates at the occipital bone, and its most caudal insertion is onto the last lumbar vertebra [1]. As it runs caudally it becomes progressively less extensible. It is also thicker in the cranial thoracic region and the lumbosacral area [2]. Important for the stabilising function of this ligament are its multiple attachments to the tendinous portion of the longissimus dorsi muscles. It lies directly beneath the skin and a variable amount of subcutaneous adipose tissue. The ventral fibres of the ligament course downwards to become continuous with the interspinous ligament, which attaches to the cranial and caudal margins of adjacent DSPs.

Aetiology of damage to the SSL

No controlled trials or models of injury to the SSL have been reported and therefore the aetiology of damage to the ligament is not known. However, there are a number of different ways in which SSL damage could occur:

- Tensile forces: the SSL will come under strain when tensile forces are applied. These forces are maximal during neck flexion and thoracolumbar ventroflexion [2]. Acute injuries usually result from this type of strain.
- Direct compressive forces: due to its proximity to the skin and saddle region the ligament is also under direct compressive forces that can induce injury; this is especially relevant over the summits of the DSPs, where the SSL could theoretically become "sandwiched" between the saddle and the bone.
- Enthesiopathies: desmopathy may occur at the ligament insertion sites on the DSP, where avulsion fractures can occur.

- Pathology secondary to other conditions, e.g. the SSL may become damaged in overriding DSPs (ORDSPs). Multiple sites of back pathology are a common clinical finding [3].

SSL injuries are reportedly more common at high levels of athletic activity. Injuries are most commonly reported in racehorses and showjumpers, although all types of horses may develop injuries to this structure [4]. A common presentation for these cases is a sudden change in behaviour during ridden exercise after a traumatic episode (e.g. fall, jump, stable cast). In less severe cases a reduction in performance or lameness might be the presenting complaint.

In the author's experience most cases of low-grade or chronic SSL injury have a concurrent site of pathology elsewhere in the back. This suggests that the change in biomechanics after a primary pathology might lead to low-grade ligament stress and damage. In the case of ORDSPs, SSL damage occurs more commonly in the interspinous space where it is probably induced by the impingement and remodelling occurring in this region.

In the author's opinion, the importance of injuries to the SSL and its poor ability to heal may be overestimated. This opinion derives from the fact that induced injuries to the SSL and the disruption of its osseous and muscle insertions, as occurs during surgical resection of the DSPs (see Chapter 14), do not cause a recognised postoperative complication. This is despite massive trauma and disruption of the SSL during the procedure.

Clinical signs of SSL desmitis

The clinical signs of injury to the SSL depend on the use of the horse and whether the injury is acute or chronic. To diagnose SSL desmitis a full clinical examination, lameness and back evaluation should be performed. The duration of clinical signs is usually long, and cases often present after other management strategies have failed and localising signs have dissipated.

Acute injuries

Acute injuries are usually accompanied by the cardinal signs of inflammation. Most cases are associated with an area of focal swelling on the dorsal midline, which can occur in any region of the back but are more common in the T15–18 region. A variable degree of pain on palpation is present; however, reactions may vary from horse to horse regardless of the severity of the lesion, depending on the horse's temperament. Local subcutaneous adipose tissue deposits or areas of fibrous tissue might cause a similar appearance to a swelling; these are non-painful but may cause a cosmetic blemish in show horses. Ultrasonography allows identification of these non-pathological changes.

A variable degree of unilateral or bilateral hindlimb lameness is occasionally present, although the relationship of this lameness to the SSL lesion is not known at the current time. This is usually exacerbated on soft surfaces and when the horse is lunged. Horses will resent tacking up and might have violent reactions similar to those seen on a "cold-backed" horse. If no change in the horse's management has occurred in the same period as the onset of such clinical signs, it is likely that this is pain related. A change in ownership or rider is often associated with a change in behaviour, and in these cases the presence of pain must be ruled out.

Chronic and low-grade injuries

Once rested and apparently recovered from acute injury, this ligament, similar to other similar structures in the body, does not recover to have the same physical properties as before injury. Thus, the ligament is stiffer than before it was injured and there is a higher chance of re-injury. A low-grade pain response is often seen. Localising signs might still be present and are usually associated with enlargement of the ligament due to fibrosis; however, painful responses on palpation are not as evident as with acute injuries. Care should be taken to identify horses that have developed a hypersensitivity at the site of a previous injury.

Enthesiopathies are often seen in association with other sources of back pathology. They often have little or no localising signs but pain on direct pressure on the summits of the DSPs might render a painful response. Many normal horses react to such a test, so this should be accompanied by diagnostic imaging of the area.

These injuries might have an insidious onset of clinical signs, are usually associated with hindlimb lameness and remain undiagnosed for long periods of time. Similar to other pathologies of the horse's back, the presenting complaint is usually a reduction in performance. In the case of jumping horses an intermittent moderate-to-severe pain response after a jump might be seen.

Diagnosis

Ultrasonography

Technique

Ultrasonographic evaluation is the most useful imaging modality for investigating SSL pathology. The technique of ultrasonography of the SSL is described in Chapter 10. The normal structure of the SSL is also described in Chapter 10 (Figure 17.1a). When SSL desmitis is suspected the SSL should be examined for the following ultrasonographic features: echogenicity, fibre pattern and size. It is considered that local thickenings of the ligament, alterations in echogenicity (hyperechoic lesions (Figure 17.1b) and hypoechoic lesions (Figure 17.1c) and remodelling of the ligament are all indicators of pathology [5].

It has been suggested that thickening of the ligament and focal hyperechoic lesions are typical of chronic lesions (Figure 17.1b), whereas hypoechogenic images (Figure 17.1c) within the SSL are more indicative of acute lesions. However, a recent study has found that variations to the normal echogenicity and pattern of the SSL can occur in the absence of back pain, and were not influenced by ridden exercise [6]. This demonstrates that changes to the normal ultrasonographic pattern correlate poorly with pain and a careful clinical examination (see Chapter 6) is the key to an accurate diagnosis.

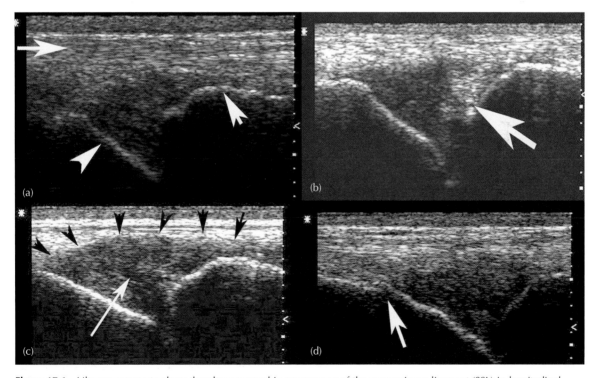

Figure 17.1   Ultrasonograms to show the ultrasonographic appearance of the supraspinous ligament (SSL) in longitudinal section. (a) The normal appearance of the ligament in longitudinal section. The ligament runs over the summits of the dorsal spinous processes (DSPs) (arrowheads) and is seen to be a horizontal structure. The fibre pattern is visible (arrow). (b) A hyperechoic lesion (whiter) within the supraspinous ligament (arrow) adjacent to a dorsal spinous process. (c) A hypoechoic lesion (blacker) within the supraspinous ligament (arrow). This hypoechoic lesion extends dorsally into the body of the supraspinous ligament (black arrowheads). (d) Enthesiopathy: the SSL has been torn away from the summit of the DSP and a small piece of bone has become detached (arrow).

Radiography

Lateral radiographs of the thoracolumbar spine should be a diagnostic step in all cases of suspected back pathology (see Chapters 6 and 8). In the case of SSL desmitis radiography can be useful in recognising avulsion fractures that may have been detected on ultrasonography (Figure 17.1d), bone modelling and sclerosis of the dorsal margins of the DSPs [7], which might be associated with SSL desmitis. Low exposures are used for this and, in the case of acute injuries, soft tissue exposures will reveal swelling of the affected area. Radiographic abnormalities present in the dorsal half of the DSPs justify ultrasonography of the SSL.

Nuclear scintigraphy

An increase in radiopharmaceutical uptake at the site of insertions onto the DSP can occur in cases of enthesiopathies. In cases of desmitis a diffuse radiopharmaceutical uptake pattern is sometimes seen on lateral views of the thoracolumbar spine. In acute cases where the horse is very painful to touch, this nuclear scintigraphy can be used to rule out fractures of the DSPs.

Thermography

Thermographic cameras used in veterinary medicine will allow detection of surface temperature differences with a sensitivity approximately 10 times higher than that of the human hand (see Chapter 12). In cases of acute injury to the SSL, the associated inflammation will cause an increase of skin temperature. As shown by Tunley and Henson, the imaging conditions should be carefully monitored to avoid artefacts [8]. The differences in temperature should be compared along the dorsal midline rather than with the surface temperature over the epaxial muscles, because there is a normal temperature difference between these two sites. Thermographic imaging measures only surface (skin) temperature, making it fairly non-specific.

Local analgesia

Infiltration of local anaesthetic around the damaged area of ligament can produce improvement in clinical signs. Approximately 5 ml 2% mepivacaine (or lidocaine) are infiltrated on either side of the dorsal midline using a 1-inch (2.5-cm) 23-gauge needle. Injection directly into the SSL should be avoided. Evaluation under ridden exercise must be performed before and after analgesia. Analgesia of a section of the SSL is often unrewarding and non-specific because other structures in the area (e.g. DSPs, see Chapter 14) can also be desensitised.

Management

Acute injuries

Similar to other acute injuries rest and anti-inflammatory therapy are paramount. In the first week after injury the horse should be box rested and systemic anti-inflammatory therapy (e.g. phenylbutazone at 2.2 mg/kg twice daily) initiated. Due to the superficial location of the SSL topical anti-inflammatory therapy can be beneficial. In the first 24 hours cold therapy and topical application of a cream of a non-steroidal anti-inflammatory drug (NSAID) [9] will help resolve the acute inflammation. Once pain on palpation is minimal, regular hand walking should be encouraged. The change in clinical signs and the ultrasonographic appearance should be evaluated regularly in order to adjust the exercise level appropriately.

Once the clinical signs have resolved, the aim should be to strengthen the epaxial muscles to provide more support to the spine. This can be accomplished, for example, by walking and trotting on soft, sandy surfaces, swimming or walking in water up to the knees (see Chapter 24). The total period of recovery can extend to a few months and care must be taken not to ride the horse too early because it may develop a "cold back". When ridden exercise is to resume, NSAIDs should be given to control any residual pain.

Chronic injuries

Apart from enthesiopathies, chronic SSL pain should be managed with a paradoxical increase in exercise in order to increase muscle support to the thoracolumbar spine. A prolonged period (up to 6 months) without ridden exercise might be required to accomplish full resolution of clinical signs. Ultrasonographic appearance may remain unchanged in the face of clinical improvement. Often if the horse has developed a significant behavioural response when being saddled, a prolonged period of turnout might be necessary and rehabilitation/retraining undertaken when the horse is brought back into work.

In the case of enthesiopathies and the more persistent cases, local infiltration with corticosteroids can be useful. A total of 18 mg/500 kg of triamcinolone should not be exceeded (to increase the volume this can be diluted in 5–10 ml of sterile saline solution). Often two or three injections a couple of weeks apart are necessary before clinical improvement is seen.

Other therapies

Extracorporeal shockwave therapy
Extracorporeal shockwave therapy (ECSWT) is used by some clinicians for the treatment of SSL desmitis. There are still conflicting results in the literature about its effect on healing tissues versus temporary post-treatment local analgesia of the area [10, 11]. However, horses undergoing treatment of SSL desmitis had a better prognosis if ECSWT was used, although this study did not include a control group [12].

Mesotherapy
This technique consists of multiple intradermal injections with a 5 mm needle of a mixture of drugs (steroid, local anaesthetic and a muscle relaxant) or a single drug over and around the lesion, the goal being to achieve a regional increase in the concentration of these drugs [13].

Prognosis

The prognosis for this condition has not been reported, and depends on the concomitant problems in the back and hindlimbs. Full resolution of clinical signs can often be achieved; however, many chronic cases have a frustrating progress with recurrence of clinical signs when the horse returns to ridden work. It is not uncommon for behavioural problems to develop unrelated to pain. Identifying these cases after an injury can be challenging.

Dorsal sacroiliac ligament

Anatomy and biomechanics

There are three pairs of sacroiliac ligaments: the dorsal, ventral and interosseous. The DSILs are divided into two parts: dorsal (or short) and lateral (or long) (Figure 17.2). The dorsal portion is a

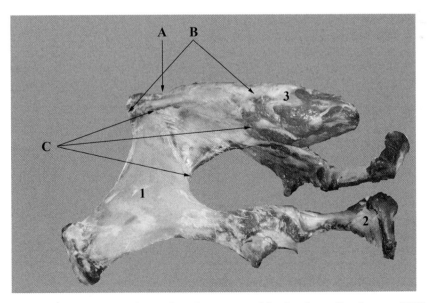

Figure 17.2   Postmortem specimen of the pelvis to show the anatomy of the dorsal sacroiliac ligament (DSIL). Arrow A points to the insertion of the thoracolumbar fascia of longissimus dorsi. Arrow B points to the insertion sites of the DSIL. Arrow C shows the triangular shape of the lateral sacroiliac ligament. (1) wing of the ilium; (2) ischium; (3) caudal sacrum.

strong cord-like structure that attaches on the dorsal aspect of the *tuber sacrale* and on the abaxial side of the sacral spinous processes [14]. Dorsally it is intimately associated with the caudal tendinous portion of the *longissimus dorsi* muscles (thoracolumbar fascia), and these two structures fuse in their caudal portion before inserting onto the abaxial surface of the sacral spinous processes [14, 15]. The lateral portion of the ligament is a triangular thin sheet that covers the sacrocaudal muscles [2]. The cranial side inserts onto the caudal margin of the proximal ilium and the ventral side onto the lateral sacral crest of the transverse processes of the sacrum and is contiguous with the sacrosciatic ligament.

The sacroiliac ligaments stabilise the connection between the spine and pelvis and, therefore, the sacroiliac joints (see Chapter 18). The DSILs prevent dorsal rotation (counternutation) of the pelvis [2]. Thus, injury to the DSIL can lead to sacroiliac joint instability.

Aetiology

Biomechanical injury to the DSIL occurs by excessive dorsal rotation of the spine. This can happen acutely after a traumatic injury such as a fall or flipping over backwards [16]. Strains can also occur during exercise as the hindlimbs transmit their propulsive force through the spine mainly by the DSIL [2]. These forces are more dramatic during jumping activities and high-speed gaits [3].

As with other joints following injury to the stabilising ligaments [17], osteoarthritis of the sacroiliac joint could occur after injury to the sacroiliac ligaments. This will aggravate the clinical signs and worsen the prognosis.

Pain or lameness originating from injury to the lateral portion of the DSIL has not yet been reported. This might reflect the difficulty in imaging this portion of the ligament. Biomechanically these two portions of the ligament come under tension with the same forces (counternutation) and, as such, injuries may occur to both of them in the same traumatic event.

Clinical signs

The severity of clinical signs depends on the amount of sacroiliac instability resulting from DSIL injury. As with other causes of back and pelvic pathology, the clinical signs of DSIL injury are variable and non-specific to the condition. Usually the presenting complaint is loss of performance or intermittent hindlimb lameness.

Asymmetry of the *tuber sacrale* is a sensitive clinical sign [18]. In one study, 33% (6 of 18) of horses with ultrasonographic abnormalities of the DSIL had a visible asymmetry [19]. If associated with acute ligament inflammation pain is usually present on palpation.

Manipulation of the pelvis to stress the DSIL can be done, placing dorsoventral pressure on the caudal portion of the sacrum. Also, when lifting one hindlimb up in a similar way to a proximal limb flexion test, the horse might become uncomfortable and the lameness might deteriorate.

No characteristic gait abnormality appears to be associated with horses with DSIL desmitis but a difficulty in maintaining a good quality canter when lunged on a soft surface can be seen. In some cases the tail may be "clamped down" and the epaxial muscles are very tense, suggesting a guarding of the lumbosacral region. Further deterioration in the gait quality is expected when the horse is ridden. Ridden exercise should be performed by the owner and another experienced rider. Different saddles should be used if clinical signs are obvious only under ridden exercise.

Diagnosis

Ultrasonography

Diagnosis is based on ultrasonographic detection of ligament disruption. The ultrasonographic technique has been described in Chapter 11 and the ultrasonographic appearance of the DSIL has been elegantly described by three recent studies [14, 15, 20].

The dorsal portion of the sacroiliac ligament and the adjacent thoracolumbar fascia (Figure 17.3) can be followed caudally in transverse section from its attachment onto the corresponding *tuber sacrale* to its common attachment with the thoracolumbar fascia onto the apices of the sacral spinous processes [14]. In its cranial portion the ligament is intimately associated with the caudal tendinous portion of the *longissimus dorsi* insertion, making them difficult to distinguish ultrasonographically.

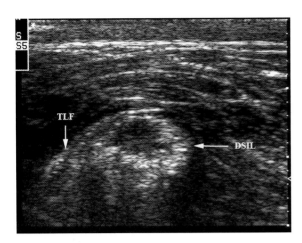

Figure 17.3 A transverse ultrasonogram of the dorsal sacroiliac ligament (DSIL). The DSIL is seen as a rounded structure (DSIL), the thoracolumbar fascia (TLF) is seen on the medial aspect of the DSIL. Note the central hypoechogeneic lesion (black) within the DSIL.

Table 17.1 The thickness at insertion and cross-sectional area of the dorsal sacroiliac ligament in different studies

Thickness at insertion (cm)	Cross-sectional area (cm²)	Study
0.4 (0.2–1.9)	1.9 (1.1–2.4)	[14]
1.09 (± 0.07)	1.1 (0.89–1.59)	[19]
0.6–1.0		[2]
0.08–0.41		[15]

They gradually fuse to form one structure as they course caudally. The caudal insertion is onto the abaxial surface of the sacral DSPs.

The cross-sectional shape of the dorsal portion of the DSIL changes as it courses caudally. At its cranial insertion it is a thin, crescent-shaped, hyperechoic structure underlying the subcutaneous tissue and the medial portion of gluteus medius. It then becomes round and, close to the caudal insertion, it becomes flattened and the lateromedial detail is lost. The echogenicity is homogeneous throughout the ligament, although a small hypoechoic area in the central portion of the ligament is a normal finding in some horses, and should not be mistaken for a core lesion within the ligament. This presumably occurs as the thoracolumbar fascia and the DSIL are fused in that region.

Values for the thickness of the DSIL have been published in different studies (Table 17.1). The variation is proportional to the size of the animal. Measurement of the cross-sectional area of the fused dorsal portion of the DSIL and the thoracolumbar fascia is subjective because of the difficulties in delineating all the borders of the medial extension of the thoracolumbar fascia on a single ultrasonographic image [14].

Pathology of the DSIL

Both an increase and a decrease in the size of the DSIL have been associated with desmitis, with the latter associated with chronic cases. In longitudinal section the normal fibre pattern is seen to be disrupted (Figure 17.4).

The fibre alignment should also be evaluated in longitudinal images. It should be homogeneous throughout the ligament and quantitative methods of assessing fibre pattern can be used to evaluate damage and healing.

At its insertion the ligament and bone interface should be carefully evaluated for signs of enthesiopathy. An irregular shape of the *tuber sacrale* with or without avulsed osseous fragments, as well as disruption in fibre pattern, can be seen in this form of pathology.

Due to the symmetry between the left and right ligaments, the normal variation of the ultrasonographic appearance of the DSIL and the low incidence of bilateral desmitis, a practical way of imaging the DSIL is by comparing left and right ligaments by sliding the probe across each one at the same level.

Lateral (long) portion of the DSIL

The lateral portion of the DSIL is visible as a thin hypoechoic line connecting the lateral portion of the sacral spinous processes and the lateral sacral crest ventrally. The lateral portion has been reported to be 4 mm thick [14]. Similar to the dorsal portion the size of the ligament is related to the size of the horse. Integrity of the ligament should be evaluated by continuity of the hyperechoic line. Although some fibre pattern is visible it is difficult to evaluate small areas of fibre disruption.

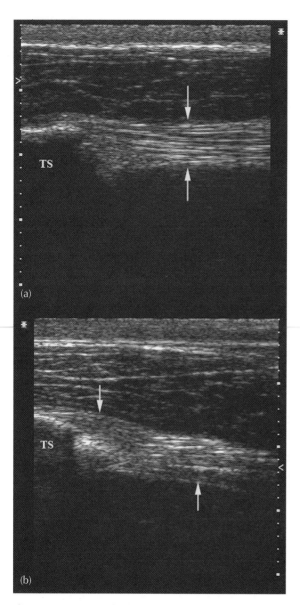

Figure 17.4 Longitudinal ultrasonograms of the dorsal sacroiliac ligament (DSIL). (a) Normal DSIL, margins delimitated by white arrows. TS: tuber sacrale. (b) Pathology within the DSIL. There is disruption of the fibre pattern and swelling close to the insertion of the DSIL (↓) and an area of fibre disruption in the body of the DSIL (↑).

Radiography

Radiography of the *tuber sacrale* for diagnosis of enthesiopathies is unrewarding because of the superimposition of both structures on lateral radiographs and difficulty in obtaining good quality images due to the film–focal distance (see Chapter 8).

Thermography

Thermographic imaging of the DSIL can be a useful diagnostic technique (see Chapter 12). One report found that 20 of 20 horses with ultrasonographic changes in the DSIL had thermographic abnormalities in the region [19], but no indication of its specificity was given. In the author's experience, thermographic imaging of the pelvic region must be carried out with care and overinterpretation avoided. An increase in surface temperature is expected in the acute stage of injury. The best way to detect this is to narrow the temperature range and compare the left and right regions for differences in temperature, rather than compare temperature differences with the more lateral portions of the gluteal region which are normally at a lower temperature.

Scintigraphy

Nuclear scintigraphic evaluation of the equine pelvis, although extremely useful, can be misleading due to the amount of soft tissue coverage of some areas [21]. Areas of increased radiopharmaceutical uptake over one tuber sacrale or any portion of the sacrum warrant ultrasonographic examination of the DSIL. Dorsal views, with the gamma camera parallel to the dorsal pelvic midline and centred over the sacrum, and with the camera parallel to the ground and centred over the tubera sacrale, are the most useful.

Local analgesia

Local analgesia of the DSIL has not been reported. It is unlikely as a result of the size and thickness, and local analgesia of the ligament may not be possible. Local infiltration may be attempted but a negative result should not rule out a diagnosis of desmitis. Local analgesia of the sacroiliac joints is, however, justified if ultrasonographic abnormalities of the DSILs are detected and sacroiliac joint laxity and dysfunction are considered to be present (see Chapter 18).

Management

Acute period

Management and treatment of DSIL injuries in the post-traumatic period are based on rest and anti-inflammatory therapy. Strict box rest with regular hand walking for 10–20 min twice a day should be continued for 2–3 weeks. NSAIDs (e.g. phenylbutazone 2.2 mg/kg) should be administered for 5–10 days. Topical NSAIDs (e.g. ibuprofen, diclofenac) can also be used during this stage. The horse should remain rugged in cold weather to improve blood flow to superficial structures such as the DSIL. A few days after injury hot therapy may be started over the area.

Long term

The long-term management should include physiotherapy aimed at strengthening the muscles of the back, pelvis and thighs. This can be achieved by walking on sand surfaces, uphill work and swimming (see Chapter 25). Ridden exercise should be delayed beyond resolution of clinical signs to avoid recurrence. The total recovery period can vary from 3 to 6 months.

References

1. Getty, R., ed. *Sisson and Grossman's The Anatomy of the Domestic Animals*, 5th edn. *Equine Syndesmology – Articulations of the Pelvic Limb*, Vol. 1. Philadelphia: W.B. Sanders Co., 1975: 362.
2. Denoix, J.M. Ligament injuries of the axial skeleton in the horse: Supraspinal and sacroiliac desmopathies. In: Rantanen, N.W. (ed.), *Dubai International Equine Symposium*. California, USA: Rantanen Design, 1996: 273–286.
3. Jeffcott, L.B. and Haussler, K.K. Equine sports medicine and surgery. In: Hinchcliff, K.W., Kaneps, A.J. and Geor, R.J. (ed.), *Back and Pelvis*, Vol. 1. Philadelphia: W.B. Saunders, 2004: 433–474.
4. Gillis, C. Spinal ligament pathology. *Veterinary Clinics of North America Equine Practice* 1999;**15**:97–101.
5. Denoix, J.M. Ultrasonographic evaluation of back lesions. *Veterinary Clinics of North America Equine Practice* 1999;**15**:131–139.
6. Henson, F.M.D., Lamas, L., Knezevic, S. and Jeffcott, L.B Ultrasonographic evaluation of the supraspinous ligament in a series of ridden and unridden horses and horses with unrelated back pathology. *BMC Veterinary Research* 2007;**3**:3.
7. Jeffcott, L.B. Back Problems in the Horse. In: 31st AAEP Annual Convention, Toronto, 1985.
8. Tunley, B.V. and Henson, F.M. Reliability and repeatability of thermographic examination and the normal thermographic image of the thoracolumbar region in the horse. *Equine Veterinary Journal* 2004;**36**:306–312.
9. Anderson, D., Kollias-Baker, C., Colahan, P. et al. Urinary and serum concentrations of diclofenac after topical application to horses. *Veterinary Therapy* 2005;**6**:57–66.
10. McClure, S.R., VanSickle, D., Evans, R., Reinertson, E.L. and Moran, L. The effects of extracorporeal shock-wave therapy on the ultrasonographic and histologic appearance of collagenase-induced equine forelimb suspensory ligament desmitis. *Ultrasound in Medicine and Biology* 2004;**30**:461–467.
11. Bolt, D.M., Burba, D.J., Hubert, J.D. et al. Determination of functional and morphologic changes in palmar digital nerves after nonfocused extracorporeal shock wave treatment in horses. *American Journal of Veterinary Research* 2004;**65**:1714–1718.
12. Crowe, O.M., Dyson, S.J., Wright, I.M., Schramme, M.C. and Smith, R.K. Treatment of chronic or recurrent proximal suspensory desmitis using radial pressure wave therapy in the horse. *Equine Veterinary Journal* 2004;**36**:313–316.
13. Denoix, J.M. and Dyson, S. The thoracolumbar spine. In: Ross, M. and Dyson, S. (ed.), *Diagnosis and Management of Lameness in the Horse*, Vol. 1. Philadelphia: Saunders, 2003: 509–521.
14. Engeli, E., Yeager, A.E., Erb, H.N. and Haussler, K.K. Ultrasonographic technique and normal anatomic features of the sacroiliac region in horses. *Veterinary Radiology and Ultrasound* 2006;**47**:391–403.
15. Kersten, A.A. and Edinger, J. Ultrasonographic examination of the equine sacroiliac region. *Equine Veterinary Journal* 2004;**36**:602–8.
16. Haussler, K.K., Stover, S.M. and Willits, N.H. Pathologic changes in the lumbosacral vertebrae and pelvis in Thoroughbred racehorses. *American Journal of Veterinary Research* 1999;**60**:143–53.
17. Simmons, E.J., Bertone, A.L. and Weisbrode, S.E. Instability-induced osteoarthritis in the metacarpophalangeal joint of horses. *American Journal of Veterinary Research* 1999;**60**:7–13.
18. Dyson, S. and Murray, R. Pain associated with the sacroiliac joint region: a clinical study of 74 horses. *Equine Veterinary Journal* 2003;**35**:240–245.
19. Tomlinson, J.E., Sage, A.M. and Turner, T.A. Ultrasonographic abnormalities detected in the sacroiliac area in twenty cases of upper hindlimb lameness. *Equine Veterinary Journal* 2003;**35**:48–54.

20. Tomlinson, J.E., Sage, A.M., Turner, T.A. and Feeney, D.A. Detailed ultrasonographic mapping of the pelvis in clinically normal horses and ponies. *American Journal of Veterinary Research* 2001;**62**: 1768–1775.

21. Erichsen, C., Eksell, P., Widstrom, C. et al. Scintigraphy of the sacroiliac joint region in asymptomatic riding horses: scintigraphic appearance and evaluation of method. *Veterinary Radiology and Ultrasound* 2003;**44**:699–706.

18 Sacroiliac Dysfunction

Leo B. Jeffcott

Sacroiliac dysfunction (SID) is a relatively poorly understood condition in the horse. Historically it has been suggested that a diagnosis of SID was a "dustbin" diagnosis – only made when no other condition could be found to explain the clinical signs of poor performance, lack of impulsion and mild hindlimb lameness exhibited by the horse (Box 18.1). However, recent studies have demonstrated a high incidence of pathological lesions within the sacroiliac region *post mortem*, which have made significant advances in our ability to establish a more definitive diagnosis of SID. A major obstacle to successful diagnosis has been the dearth of information on the biomechanics of the joint. The sacroiliac joint (SIJ) is particularly inaccessible due to its depth within the pelvis and the surrounding musculature, making it impossible to palpate the joint externally. Little is known about the three-dimensional movement of the SIJ in horses, and this has prevented the establishment of an effective model with which to study the biomechanics of this complex joint [1]. SID is most commonly seen in athletic horses. Affected horses are often older animals, and it has been suggested that larger horses are more often affected. One study demonstrated that, in the UK, horses used for dressage and showjumping are more prone to be affected with SID than general purpose or other athletic animals [2]. In addition warmblood horses are more likely to be affected, although this may purely reflect the work done by warmblood horses in the UK. There is no reported sex predilection.

Anatomy

As described in Chapter 1 the vertebral column articulates with the pelvis at the sacroiliac joints (Figure 18.1a, b). The SIJ is a highly specialised point of contact between the two flat bony surfaces of the sacrum and the ilium (Figure 18.2). The point of contact is a synovial joint with some unusual histological characteristics. The majority of synovial joints in the body are formed between two hyaline cartilage surfaces; in the sacroiliac region the joint is formed between a hyaline cartilage surface (sacral side) and a fibrocartilaginous one (iliac side) [3].

Unlike other important synovial joints in the body, the SIJ does not have the advantage of osseous contouring to aid the maintenance of joint integrity, as is found, for example, in ball-and-socket joints. The morphology of the joint indicates that it is designed for gliding movements. This is based on suggestions that the sacroiliac articular cartilage may never be subject to full weight bearing like most joints. It is subject to shearing rather than orthogonally directed compressive forces [3, 4]. The role of the SIJ is to transfer these forces from the horse's hindlimb to the

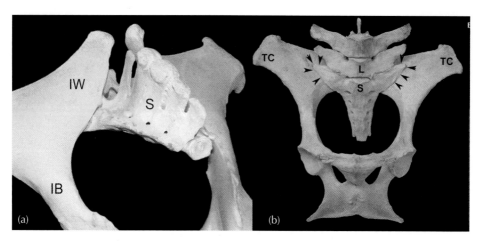

Figure 18.1   Postmortem specimens to show the anatomical position of the sacrum and ilium. (a) Caudolateral view of an anatomical specimen of the pelvis and the sacrum (S) illustrating the position of the sacrum within the pelvis, ventral to the iliac wing (IW) and medial to the iliac body (IB). (b) Ventral view of an anatomical specimen of the ventral pelvis, sacrum, sacroiliac and last two lumbar vertebrae (L) regions. The sacrum is positioned medially within the pelvis, and articulates with the iliac wing. TC = tuber coxae. The position of the sacroiliac joint is outlined by the black arrowheads. (Courtesy of M.D. Whitcomb.)

Box 18.1   List of conditions that possibly show signs attributable to sacroiliac disease in the horse

"Jumper's or hunter's bump"
Thoracolumbar damage (i.e. back problem)
Wing of ilium stress fracture (± sacroiliac pathology)
Other sites of pelvic fracture (tubera coxae, ischii, sacrale)
Fracture of wing of sacrum
Dorsal sacroiliac ligament desmitis
Sacrolumbar disc injury
Distal hind limb lameness (stifle and hock in particular)
Acute sacroiliac injury ± subluxation
Chronic sacroiliac dysfunction (SID)

---

thoracolumbar vertebral column [5]. To provide biomechanical stability to the meeting of two flat surfaces, the horse uses three strong sacroiliac ligaments (SILs): the dorsal sacroiliac ligaments (DSILs), the ventral sacroiliac ligaments (VSILs) and the interosseous sacroiliac ligaments (ISILs). These ligaments are discussed in detail in Chapter 3.

Incidence

Postmortem studies on horses have shown a high incidence (up to 100% in one study) of pathological lesions within the SIJ itself, most of which were degenerative [6]. Such a high incidence of lesions indicates that degeneration at this site is likely to be a significant clinical problem, although, at the

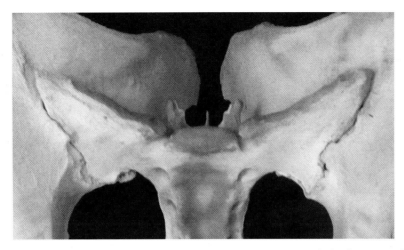

Figure 18.2   Ventral view of an anatomical specimen of the sacrum as it articulates with the ilium. Note the new bone formation at the sacroiliac interface and the irregularity of the edges of the joint.

current time, the exact progression from joint changes to pain and clinical signs is not known. Pain arising from the SIJ has long been considered to be associated with chronic mild instability of the joint, and this certainly fits with the other signs of poor hindlimb impulsion at slow paces. The pathology findings described at the SIJ [5] include enlargement of the joint surfaces, osteophyte formation, lipping of the edge of the joint and cortical buttressing (Figure 18.3). In some cases cartilage erosion is also noted, although loss of the joint space and ankylosis has not been recorded (in contrast to the situation in other low motion, high load joints, e.g. the tarsometatarsal joints). These changes have also been associated with the overriding of the thoracolumbar DSPs and the lumbar transverse processes, as well as with osteoarthritis of the articular facets of the thoracolumbar spine, suggesting that alterations within the thoracolumbar area may cause compensatory SIJ lesions or vice versa.

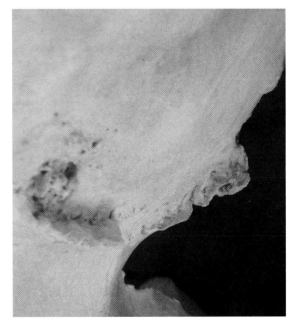

Figure 18.3   Close-up of the iliac surface of the sacroiliac joint shown in Figure 18.2. The sacrum has been removed. Note the new bone formation, bone lipping and marked remodelling associated with the sacroiliac joint. This is a degenerative joint.

Clinical signs

Horses with SID can present as either acute or chronic cases, although chronic problems are far more common. Acute sacroiliac injury is usually the result of a serious traumatic injury, e.g. falling or sustaining impact. The clinical signs of acute sacroiliac injury include noticeable lameness and localised sensitivity to palpation of the soft tissues or tuber sacrale [7].

The clinical signs of chronic SID are much more vague and non-specific, and it appears that there can be two clinical presentations. These two variations of SID may, of course, simply be different ends of a single continuum, depending on the degree of bony change that has occurred. The first occurs principally in performance horses, still in work, where the main clinical findings are pain and poor performance, with the signs usually responsive to regional analgesia [8]. The underlying pathology of these cases has not been established, but it is likely that they are associated with pain in periarticular structures rather than chronic bony changes of the SIJ. This may explain why there may be no significant asymmetry of the pelvis and the gait changes are variable.

The other, more debilitating, form of SID, resulting in poor performance and more marked gait changes with asymmetry of associated muscles and/or bone, has been reported to be associated with chronic pathological joint changes [5]. These horses show little pain response and minimal improvement to regional analgesia. The clinical signs (Box 18.2) include poor performance, a failure to engage the hindlimbs, poor hindlimb action and lameness (either unilateral or bilateral), and the clinical signs are often worse when ridden, characterised by stiffness of the back and lack of hindlimb impulsion. In addition the signs often worsen after a period of prolonged rest. Pelvic asymmetry, in particular tuber sacrale asymmetry, has long been reported to be significantly associated with SID [5]. Similarly, plaiting (hindlimb abduction before hoof placement) and dragging of the hind toes has been commonly associated with this form of SID.

This lack of consistency in what constitutes the specific clinical signs of SID underlines the difficulties associated with making a definitive diagnosis. In relation to pelvic asymmetry the following guidelines may be helpful:

- Unilateral muscle wastage from one quarter without pelvic bone malalignment: *suspect hindlimb lameness (hock or stifle) or acetabular damage.*
- Elevation of one tuber sacrale ± gluteal muscle wastage: *suspect thickening and damage to DSIL* or *stress fracture of wing of ilium on opposite side (i.e. lowered quarter).*
- Lowering of tuber sacrale associated with muscle wastage and lowering of tuber coxae on same side: *suspect chronic sacroiliac disease.*
- Lowering of tuber coxae without lowering of tuber sacrale or ischii: *suspect fracture of tuber coxae.*
- Lowering of tuber ischii without deviation of tuber sacrale or coxae: *suspect fracture of tuber ischii.*

Of these clinical signs a number have been reported to occur with more consistency in horses with SID diagnosed *post mortem*, and have been used, with anatomical features, to assign an "SID score" to horses (Table 18.1). The clinical signs that have been used as part of the SID score are plaiting of the hindlimbs, pelvic bony asymmetry (of both tubera coxae and sacrale), gluteal muscle atrophy and a positive pelvic shear.

SIJ provocation tests

A number of specific tests to identify pain in the sacroiliac region and SIJ provocation tests have been described [7, 9]. However, although these tests may well indicate that there is pain in the region of the SIJ in the horse, they are not specific for SID because other conditions, such as fractures

---

Box 18.2   The clinical signs reported to occur in horses with sacroiliac dysfunction

Reduced hindlimb impulsion
Hindlimb lameness
Stiff back
Close behind
Wide behind
Plaiting
Rolling hindlimb gait
Reduced hindlimb engagement
Poor quality canter/breaks in canter
Reluctance to work and/or work on the bit
Resistant behaviour
Poor quality lateral work
Worsening of the clinical signs when ridden

Table 18.1 The components of the SID scoring system

Clinical sign	Grades
Pelvic shear	0–1
Plaiting	0–3
Atrophy	0–3
Tuber coxae asymmetry	0–3
Tuber sacrale asymmetry	0–3
Left DSIL pain	0–3
Right DSIL pain	0–3
Left gluteal pain	0–3
Right gluteal pain	0–3

DSIL, dorsal sacroiliac ligament.

(i.e. stress or traumatic) of the iliac wing, can also give a similar response. Tests to identify SIJ pain include the following.

Manual compression of the dorsal aspects of the tuber sacrale

In this test the tubera sacrale are pushed together simultaneously. The aim is to bend the iliac wing and compress the sacroiliac articulation. Normal horses usually show no response, but SID horses show a pain response or even collapse.

"Sway test"

In this test the horse has one hindlimb raised (i.e. like a flexion test). The horse is then gently rocked from side to side by the person holding the leg in order to produce movement in the contralateral SIJ. Normal horses tolerate this procedure well, but SID horses show a pain response or will refuse to pick up the leg on the normal side (in order to avoid shearing within the affected SIJ when the normal leg is raised).

Ventral force

This test involves application of ventral force over the lumbosacral dorsal spinous processes (DSPs) in a rhythmic fashion. This test is considered to stress the ISIL. Normal horses should show no response and SID horses show a pain response.

A modified version of this test is to apply the force focally over the DSPs of the sacrocaudal junction in order to specifically stress the dorsal portion of the DSIL.

Tuber coxae stress test

This test involves application of rhythmic ventral force to the tuber coxae to induce general sacroiliac and lumbosacral joint motion. Normal horses respond with a smooth vertical motion of the lumbosacral region, SID horses have a noticeable pain response and/or gluteal muscle spasm.

Application of lateral forces to the pelvis

- Technique 1 requires that the ipsilateral tuber sacrale be pushed away from the veterinarian with one hand while the tail head is pulled towards the veterinarian with the other. This test is considered to compress the contralateral SIJ and distract the ipsilateral SIJ. Reversal of the movement distracts the contralateral SIJ and compresses the ipsilateral SIJ. Normal horses show no resentment to manipulation, but SID horses show a pain response. It has been proposed that pain on compression of the SIJ is more indicative of osteoarthritic changes, whereas pain on distraction of the joint is more indicative of ligamentous damage, although these associations have not been proved.

- Technique 2 requires that the tail head be pushed away from the operator while the contralateral tuber ischii is pulled towards the operator with the other hand, and then reversing the movement. This test is designed to stress the supporting ligaments of the SIJ. Normal horses show no resentment to manipulation.

Diagnosis of SID

The diagnosis of SID relies on a careful clinical evaluation, and the exclusion of other conditions with similar clinical signs. However, diagnostic imaging modalities and local analgesic techniques do have an ever-increasing role, particularly with the improvements in technology and experience gained with their use.

Diagnostic imaging of the SIJ region

There is a range of imaging modalities available nowadays, although all have some limitations. Radiography and ultrasonography can certainly be of some benefit, but nuclear scintigraphy is considered the most useful aid to diagnosis.

Nuclear scintigraphy

Nuclear scintigraphy provides direct visualisation of the radionuclide uptake in the SIJ region relative to other areas of the pelvis, and allows an assessment of whether there is increased uptake at other sites in the back, pelvis or hindlimbs that may be causing the clinical signs noted in the horse. Both dorsoventral and oblique views of the ilium are recommended in order to ascertain the positioning of areas of increased radionuclide uptake. The interpretation of scintigrams of the sacroiliac region is often not straightforward. Indeed, even the exact anatomical location of the SIJ on scintigrams was only fairly recently described [10] and these authors described the scintigraphic appearance of the joint in normal horses. The joint itself covers a large area of the ilium, but due to soft tissue attenuation uptake in the more lateral part of the joint may be difficult to appreciate. An oblique view of the cranial pelvis may help in diagnosis and also allow better separation of any bladder shadow and genuine uptake within the SIJ itself. Analysis of scintigrams of the sacroiliac region is complicated by the finding of pathological changes in the sacroiliac region in normal horses [6] and the findings of significant overlap in the radionuclide uptake in the sacroiliac region in groups of normal horses [11] and horses with sacroiliac pain [2]. Also, it should be noted, there is an age-related change in the sacroiliac area [12].

Notwithstanding the problems of interpretation a number of attempts have been made to quantify uptake in the SIJ region using regions of interest and computer-generated profiles (Figure 18.4) to help with diagnosis, as discussed in Chapter 9. Although it is known that scintigrams of the sacroiliac region are bilaterally symmetrical and show little or no uptake in radionuclide uptake in normal horses, it is also known that there is significant

overlap in nucleotide uptake ratios among horses affected with SID, normal horses and lame horses who do not have SID. For a detailed discussion of the interpretation of nuclear scintigraphy of the sacroiliac region the reader is referred to Chapter 9.

Ultrasonography

Ultrasonography of the SIJ region has been described by a number of authors [13] (see Chapter 11). However, in the main, they have concentrated on the easily accessible DSIL (see Chapter 10) rather than the more specific supporting ligaments of the SIL, and on the dorsal surface of the iliac wing to identify fractures of the dorsal cortices (see Chapters 11 and 13). The actual SIJ itself cannot be visualised by ultrasonography in its entirety, although transrectal ultrasonography has been used to identify remodelling along the joint margins of the ventral border of the SIJ.

The ultrasonographic appearance of the VSIL has also been described using transrectal ultrasonography. In contrast there are no ultrasonographic descriptions of the ISILs. Unlike nuclear scintigraphy, ultrasonography is not a very useful imaging modality for the identification of SID.

Radiography

Radiography of the SIJ region is difficult, unrewarding and rarely diagnostic. A number of features conspire to make SIJ radiography difficult, including the depth of the joint within the body, the soft tissues overlying the joint, the artefacts caused by the viscera within the pelvis and the overlying bone of the iliac wing. Radiography of the SIJ is best performed under general anaesthesia using ventrodorsal views. However, even when this is performed the resulting radiographs are frequently difficult to interpret in all except the smallest animals. A final complication of radiographic diagnosis of SID is that the radiographic features of chronic SID are non-specific and subtle, including non-specific increases in the joint space and enlargement of the caudomedial aspect of the joint. The use of linear tomography has been used with some success, but is really not a practical

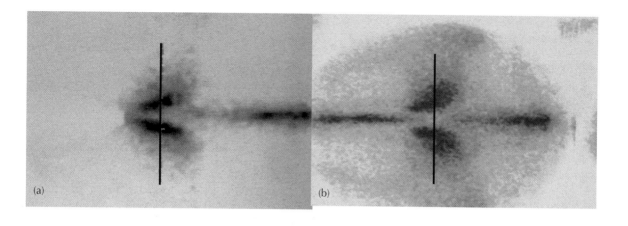

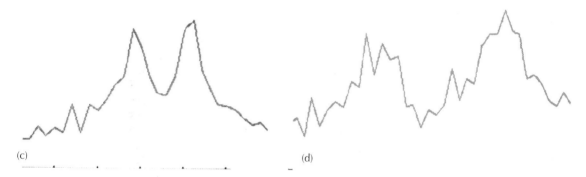

Figure 18.4 Nuclear scintigraphy of the sacroiliac region: (a, b) dorsoventral scintigrams of the cranial pelvis. (a) Normal horse: the paired tubera sacrale are seen as comma-shaped increases in radionuclide uptake either side of the midline. The black line through them is the reference line for generation of the profile of the region (c). (b) Horse with chronic bilateral sacroiliac dysfunction. In this case there is increased radionuclide uptake abaxial to the tuber sacrale at the site of the sacroiliac joint. The black line is the reference line for generation of the profile of the region (d). (c) Profile from (a): the normal profile is seen as a pair of peaks of radionuclide uptake. (d) Profile from (b): the abnormal profile is seen to have a wider peak of uptake associated with more radionuclide in the region of the sacroiliac joint.

proposition nowadays because the equipment is no longer available [14].

Local analgesic techniques

The diagnosis of joint pain in lame horses usually relies on the response to intra-articular and perineural analgesia. However, until recently local analgesia of the SIJ was not performed due to its deep anatomical location and the difficulties in targeting the small, tightly bound joint capsule. In addition, the close proximity of the greater sciatic foramen with its neurovascular contents (including the sciatic nerve) and cranial gluteal nerve

means that accurate placement of local anaesthetic solution into the SIJ is required. Inadvertent poor placement of local anaesthetic may lead to nerve damage, paresis and even marked lameness, and ataxia has been reported by a number of veterinarians.

Two approaches to the SIJ have been described [2, 7]. However, neither technique is 100% accurate in delivering local analgesia solutions to the SIJ – diffusion is seen within associated muscles and ligaments in experimental studies:

1. The dorsal approach: this approach aims to pass a needle down from dorsolateral surface of the pelvis, directly over the SIJ, to hit it just

off the edge of the wing of the ilium. The technique involves the placement of a 20–25 cm spinal needle dorsally over the iliac wing ipsilateral to the SIJ that is being anaesthetised. The needle is directed ventrally and walked off the caudal border of the iliac wing in the region of the SIJ. Local anaesthetic solution is injected. This technique is easier to perform than technique 2, but is reported to be associated with a higher risk of significant ataxia/hind limb paresis.

2. The medial approach: this approach aims to pass a needle down from just off the midline, between the divergent DSPs of L6 and S1, and into the space formed by the ventral aspect of the iliac wing and the dorsal part of the sacrum. This technique involves placement of a long (18–25 cm) spinal needle at the cranial margin of the tuber sacrale contralateral to the SIJ that is being anaesthetised (Figure 18.5). The needle is inserted along the cranial aspect of the tuber sacrale, directed towards the greater trochanter of the femur of the opposite limb (at approximately 20° to the vertical). The needle is advanced along the medial aspect of the iliac wing (on the affected side), in a caudolateral direction until contact is made with bone. This should be near the SIJ margin. Local anaesthetic solution is then injected (20 ml). The response to the local analgesia is assessed at 15–20 minutes.

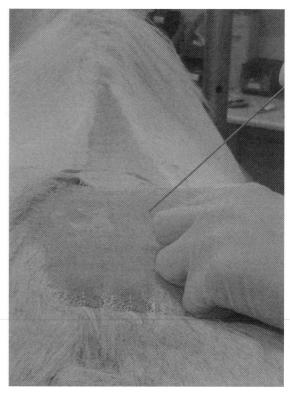

Figure 18.5 The site of injection for local analgesia of the sacroiliac joint via the medial approach. This technique involves placement of a long (18–25 cm) spinal needle at the cranial margin of the tuber sacrale contralateral to the SIJ that is being anaesthetised.

Management of SID

The treatment of SID remains largely empirical because of the lack of understanding of its primary pathogenesis.

Acute SID

In cases of acute SID the aim of treatment is to reduce inflammation at the damaged site and promote effective healing. It is recommended that the horse have a period of prolonged rest including a period of strict box rest for 4–6 weeks followed by hand walking. Restricted turnout is advised. During this initial period it is recommended that systemic non-steroidal anti-inflam-matory drugs (NSAIDs) be given. There is no documented evidence for the efficacy of any other medical treatment of this condition.

Affected horses should be allowed 6–12 months to recover from acute injuries (analogous to the time required for healing in other ligaments and tendons in the body). The injection of anti-inflammatory medication, such as corticosteroids, into the joint (or at least around the joint) is also a logical option after the first repair phase has passed.

Chronic SID

Management of SID in horses should be based on clinical presentation, but includes use of rest, and anti-inflammatory medication, and exercise [7]. Reduction of pain associated with SID is important, but it should be noted that complete rest may be contraindicated due to the possible adverse effects of reduced pelvic and hindlimb muscle function and worsening functional instability of the SIJ [7]. NSAIDs can result in temporary improvement in performance [5, 8]; however, it is ideal to rehabilitate the horse so improvement is consistent and lasting. A specific rehabilitation programme based on biomechanical findings may achieve this. Exercise to build up the muscles of the back and hindquarters [5] is more appropriately recommended. However, the use of exercise to manage SID has generally been non-specific, and there is a clear need for more specific muscle re-training to enhance functional stability of the region, and ultimately improve performance, in individual cases. An understanding of the biomechanics and neuromotor control of the equine SIJ region is needed to approach that of the human SIJ. This may lead to the development of manual mobilisation and/or manipulation techniques, which can be applied to the equine pelvis and SIJ, to improve joint kinematics.

In some cases, some veterinarians have described the injection of sclerosing agents at the site of the SIJ to aid management of the condition [1, 12]. Chronic cases may well improve when the musculature around the SIJ strengthens.

Conclusion

Although sacroiliac dysfunction is still something of an anathema to equine veterinarians, many of the difficulties relating to diagnosis and management have greatly improved in recent years. Much progress has been made in research, and there is a better appreciation of the functional anatomy of the SIJ and the type of pathological lesions that can develop. This is complemented by the improvements in clinical evaluation, local analgesia and the use of modern diagnostic imaging modalities. The current thrust of research in biomechanics, kinesiology and various forms of physiotherapy bode well for the future.

References

1. Goff, L.M., Jeffcott, L.B., Jasiewicz, J. and McGowan, C.M. Structural and biomechanical aspects of equine sacroiliac joint function and their relationship to clinical disease. *Veterinary Journal* 2008;**176**:281–293.
2. Dyson, S., Murray, R., Branch, M. and Harding, E. The sacroiliac joints: evaluation using nuclear scintigraphy. Part 2: Lame horses *Equine Veterinary Journal* 2003;**35**:233–239.
3. Dalin, G. and Jeffcott, L.B. Sacroiliac joint of the horse. 1. Gross morphology. *Anatomia, Histologia et Embryologia* 1986;**15**:80–94.
4. Dalin, G. and Jeffcott, L.B. Sacroiliac joint of the horse. 2. Morphometric features. *Anatomia, Histologia et Embryologia* 1986;**15**:97–107.
5. Jeffcott, L.B., Dalin, G., Ekman, S. and Olsson, S-E. Sacroiliac lesions as a cause of poor performance in competitive horses. *Equine Veterinary Journal* 1985; **17**:111–118.
6. Haussler, K.K., Stover, S.M. and Willits, N.H. Pathology of the lumbosacral spine and pelvis in Thoroughbred racehorses. *American Journal of Veterinary Research* 1999;**60**:143–153.
7. Haussler, K.K. Diagnosis and management of sacroiliac joint injuries. In: Ross, M. and Dyson, S. (eds), *Diagnosis and Management of Lameness in the Horse*. St Louis, MO: Saunders, 2003: 501–508.
8. Dyson, S. and Murray, R. Pain associated with the sacroiliac joint region: a clinical study of 74 horses. *Equine Veterinary Journal* 2003; **35**:240–245.
9. Goff, L.M., Jasiewicz, J., Jeffcott, L.B. et al. Movement between the equine ilium and sacrum – in vivo and in vitro studies. *Equine Veterinary Journal* 2006;**36**(suppl):457–461.
10. Erichsen, C., Eksell, P. and Berger, M. The scintigraphic anatomy of the equine sacroiliac joint. *Veterinary Radiology and Ultrasound* 2002;**43**:287–292.
11. Dyson, S., Murray, R. and Branch, M. The sacroiliac joints: evaluation using nuclear scintigraphy. Part 1: The normal horse. *Equine Veterinary Journal* 2003;**35**:226–232.
12. Dyson, S.J. Pelvic injuries in the non-racehorse. In: Ross, M.W. and Dyson, S.J. (eds), *Diagnosis and Management of Lameness in the Horse*. St Louis, MO: Saunders, 2003: 491–501.
13. Denoix, J.M. Ultrasonographic evaluation of back lesions. In: Haussler, K.K. (ed.), *Veterinary Clinics of North America Equine Practice*. Philadelphia: Saunders, 1999: 131–139.
14. Jeffcott, L.B. Radiographic appearance of equine lumbosacral and pelvic abnormalities by linear tomography. *Veterinary Radiology* 1983;**24**:204–213.

Section 4

Back Pathology in Specific Disciplines

19 Dressage Horses

Svend E. Kold

To identify sports horse injuries, veterinary surgeons must possess knowledge of the particulars of each different sport, no more so than with dressage. By watching large numbers of "normal" horses train and compete, the veterinary surgeon learns about the demands from the sport on the horse, which structures are most vulnerable and to understand the language involved.

Dressage horses are the epitome of the well-balanced athlete with their gaits expressing balance, suppleness and highest level of activity and proprioception (Figure 19.1). All this requires a strong and supple back, so some horses may be destined for a career in dressage but do not have the requisite in terms of an anatomically correct back. Too many owners believe that good training can make an anatomically inferior horse into a top dressage horse, but, unfortunately, not all horses are athletes! Certain anatomical requirements are needed for natural balance and self-carriage with the head and neck positioned sufficiently high to facilitate "working uphill" as the centre of gravity moves backwards. "Cadence" is the term used to describe balance, suppleness and power, and is intimately associated with working "over the back" and self-carriage, reflecting a change in point of gravity in order to balance not just itself, but also the rider, which is achieved only if the centre of gravity of the horse and the rider become confluent and move backwards,

which assists in freeing the front end of the horse off the ground, thereby creating more uphill, airborne movements (Figure 19.1).

The back and the withers must also facilitate placement of the saddle in the correct position. Positive correlations between conformation and movement and orthopaedic health have been proved [1], although positive anatomical traits such as joint angles and range of positive diagonal advance placement (the spatial difference between the contralateral forelimb and the hindlimb contacting the ground) have also proved to be of significant positive value [2]. The positive diagonal advance placement does not change with more collection (i.e. advanced training) and may therefore become a useful selection criterion in younger horses for future potential [2]. However, despite all such criteria being fulfilled, temperament and ability to cope, not just physically but also mentally, with the demands of training and competition may be the ultimate limiting factor.

The German equestrian terminology describes the aims of the correctly trained dressage horse as follows:

* *Takt* (rhythm)
* *Losgelassenheit* (looseness and suppleness)
* *Anlehnung* (contact with the bit)
* *Schwung* (energy, swing and elevation from the hindlimb)

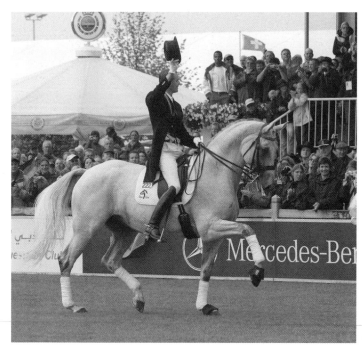

Figure 19.1   World-class dressage horse showing collection and suspension.

- *Geraderichten* (straightness)
- *Versammlung* (collection via engagement of the hindlimbs).

It requires only minimal understanding of dressage and its requirement in terms of athleticism to realise how essential a normally functioning back is to the fulfilment of every one of these six key descriptions, with the common denominator being "balance" – a healthy back is essential for optimal balance. A restricted back, on the other hand, will not allow collection, will often prevent the horse being straight, will prevent looseness and suppleness, and will not allow the horse to obtain the all-important contact with the bit. Without a strong back no movements will be produced! The rhythm to the paces will be absent and in many cases associated with a slight hindlimb gait irregularity. If unbalanced, the horse will hang on its front end with more weight on the bit, using the rider's arms as a fifth leg in order to pull itself forward with its forelimbs rather than pushing with its hindlimbs. Both the back and neck are integral to maximum performance and, as clinical symptoms are not always easy to separate, both areas should be kept in mind and investigated if necessary.

Even correct dressage applies additional and sometimes unusual strains to the back, particularly because the horse, in certain movements, e.g. shoulder-in, half pass, renvers and travers, is bent evenly in its neck and body, but moves on two tracks. These movements create a rotational strain on the horse's back and an additional twisting movement on the appendicular joints. A recent debate in the dressage world has centred on the so-called "rollkur" (hyperflexion of the neck, also referred to as *tief eingestellt*), which includes working the horse low, deep and round with the nose well behind vertical and what the Federation Equestre Internationale (FEI) accepts for international competitions, i.e. that the front of the head be positioned in or in front of the vertical plane. The debate centres on the possible requirement (or not) of maximum stretching of the muscles of the neck and back to their fullest during active work in order to lift the back, or whether stretching of the muscles should be a passive and relaxing exercise between work and that lifting of the back can be performed without stretching of the neck's nuchal ligament in particular. This debate will continue, but it highlights the attention to and importance of maximum strength and flexibility of the back in the dressage horse.

Assessment of the dressage horse at exercise/competition

Observing dressage horses for possible back pain is not only a question of confirming back pain, but also of ruling out other related or non-related appendicular skeletal problems such as primary or secondary lameness. It is particularly important to watch the horse exercise both with and without a rider in order to assess any alterations occurring to the gait when ridden because many horses investigated reproduce only the perceived problem, often no more than a hardly visible resistance, when ridden through certain movements. The non-ridden work could, for example, be an assessment of the horse's paces when lunging on surfaces of different firmness and texture. It is always most useful to have the usual rider trying to "recreate" the difficulties encountered, but it should be remembered that good riders can (and will) often involuntarily "hide" the consequences of back pain (i.e. imbalance, unlevelness) while an impression of gait asymmetry/lameness and therefore an inherent suggestion of back pain may, on the other hand, be the result of a less experienced rider "creating" an imbalance, noticed as a lameness. It is also worth reiterating that not all horses are athletes, just as only a very limited number of schoolchildren have the physical (and mental) toughness to become top athletes. Unfortunately, many owners think that their horse can be *trained* to become a top dressage horse, where the truth is that missing athleticism cannot be overcome by training or veterinary intervention.

The veterinarian must not forget to look out for the obvious but also be imaginative and able to approach an investigation from an unusual angle if necessary. It is essential to focus not just on the limbs when watching the horse, but also on the whole horse, and to observe changes such as the horse grinding its teeth, working in an irregular rhythm (e.g. four-beat canter) as opposed to being overtly lame or the rider commenting on the

horse taking more contact with one rein than the other (often noticed as the horse lathering on one side of the mouth only). The tack should always be checked, in particular the saddle (for size and fitting), but also the bit and its position in the mouth. Listen to the horse's breathing; once the horse has relaxed through its back and obtained straightness, rhythm and contact with the bit, its breathing will immediately relax and often be encountered as a quiet rhythmical expiratory blowing of its nostrils. Many dressage horses defecate during training only once tension has been overcome.

As a very generalised rule of thumb, horses with back pain, almost irrespective of underlying type of pathology, find it more difficult to canter than to trot, even unridden. The trot is often surprisingly big and well suspended and may be helped by the rider changing the weight-bearing diagonal (of the horse), whereas the canter is on the forehand, often fast and frequently accompanied by swishing or clamping of the tail and/or constant changing of the leading hindlimb at the canter.

Listen to the rider's observations, have an open attitude and be prepared for some surprises.

Common conditions

Overriding dorsal spinous processes

Although overriding dorsal spinous processes (ORDSPs) or "kissing spines" are, in the author's opinion, more commonly seen in horses jumping at speed, in particular eventers, hurdlers and steeplechasers, it remains a significant problem in all athletic horses. From postmortem examination of young horses it has been suggested that, rather than necessarily being the consequence of a primary anatomical problem, ORDSPs may be the consequence of superseding normal adaptive processes in young horses as the result of repeated non-physiological descent of the spine, possibly associated with the onset of ridden work [3]. The consequence of this is shearing of the ventral parts of the supraspinous ligament at its insertions, which in turn leads to formation of osteophytes and consequent narrowing of the interspinous spaces (Figure 19.2). However, the earliest regressive changes of ORDSPs may occur in the ligaments and are not therefore demonstrated on radiographs. Randelhoff [3] also believes that repeated excessive descent of the spine results in change of the position of the vertebral bodies, which occurs around a centre of rotation in the small vertebral joints and subsequently leads to incongruence of the articular facets and osteoar-

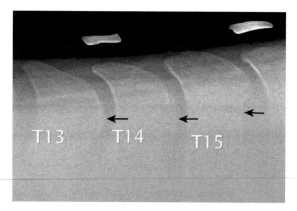

Figure 19.2 Lateromedial radiograph of mid-thoracic region of 10-year-old thoroughbred (NZ) gelding used for jumping. The arrows point to areas of mineralisation/ossification within the interspinous ligament.

thritis. This may explain the not infrequent observations of facet joint osteoarthritis in the lower thoracic spine in cases of severe, longstanding ORDSPs, an observation that inevitably reduces the prognosis for a return to an athletic career, but may alternatively be improved by the mechanical gains expected following selective spinous process removal.

It is therefore possible that excessive training, without full development of the strength of the back in young horses, may result in ORDSPs at a very early age, as is frequently seen. Moderately severe ORDSPs can be seen in thoroughbred horses as young as 2 and 3 years, in some cases after only a few months of light ridden work (Figure 19.3). Against this theory is the occasional observations of severe "kissing spines" in horses that have never yet been ridden (Figure 19.4).

It has been suggested that as many as 34% of normal horses without back pain may show radiographic changes suggestive of ORDSPs [4]. An inherent problem with that and similar studies is to define what comprises a group of normal horses *without* back pain. The author's clinical impression has been that there is poor correlation between radiographic signs and clinical signs in horses

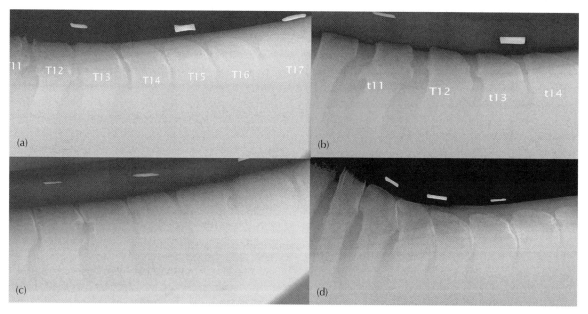

Figure 19.3 Lateromedial radiographs of mid-thoracic of different horses showing a range of changes in the dorsal spinous processes. In (b) changes are clearly evident in a 4-year-old thoroughbred mare (Figure 19.4).

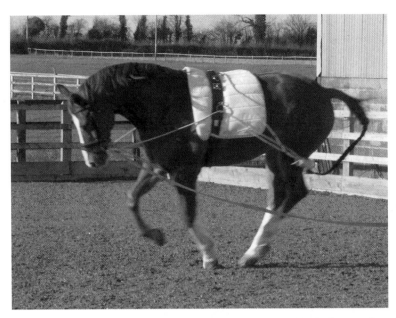

Figure 19.4 Thoroughbred mare that, after only a few weeks' lunging work, was already showing clinical symptoms of back pain. There are significant radiographic changes throughout the mid-thoracic region (Figure 19.3b)

with milder degrees of ORDSPs in particular. This statement is not least based on the subsequent outcome of surgery in horses with mild radiographic signs, but noticeable reduced performance before surgery, and a successful return to full function at the same or higher performance levels after surgery (S. Kold, 2008, unpublished data).

Although nuclear scintigraphy may show increased radionuclide uptake in some cases of ORDSPs, both false positives and false negatives occur (see Chapter 9), and selection of the successful surgical candidate must be based on multiple confirmatory observations, including radiographic changes of a severity believed to be incompatible with a continued athletic career, as well as strong clinical evidence of back pain. Infiltration analgesia is used but may provide both false positives and negatives and at the most will confirm that there is a painful condition in the injected *region* of the back. The anatomical specificity is probably poor.

The surgical technique involves resection of the proximal half of non-consecutive DSPs (see Chapter 14), if possible through numerous, individual, single, minimal-sized incisions. Rehabilitation post-ORDSP surgery is of particular

importance and consists of unlimited ascending walking in hand for 6 weeks, followed by 6 weeks' intensive working from the ground, using a Pessoa training aid to ensure that the horse is "fixed" in a frame with hyperflexion of the neck for maximum elevation of the back, although stronger abdominal musculature is encouraged by trotting over a series of caveletti. Return to ridden training begins at 12 weeks.

Desmitis of the supraspinous ligament and dorsal sacroiliac ligaments

Soft tissue injuries often occur as the result of single, acute traumas and are not surprisingly common in dressage horses just as they occur through training or competition in any other athlete, equine or human. The complex nature of the supraspinous ligament (SSL) ligament, with its functional origin as the nuchal ligament from the base of the skull and functional contributions from epaxial back muscles in the lower back, predisposes this complex structure to injury. Recent work has suggested that, functionally and biomechanically, the SSL should be categorised as a

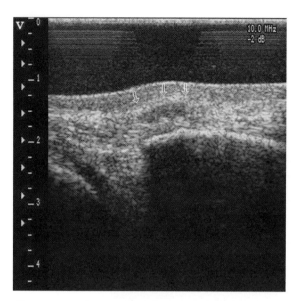

Figure 19.5   Ultrasonogram of supraspinous ligament (SSL) in the mid-back region (10 MHz linear probe, longitudinal scan). An area of SSL pathology is seen above the summit of the dorsal spinous process (outlined by arrows).

structure somewhere between a ligament and a tendon [5].

Most injuries to the SSL occur in the mid-thoracic region, approximately T13–16, and are often recognised as low-grade back-related loss of performance and tension during ridden work. Occasionally, but not consistently, such patients are sore to direct digital pressure to the ligament. Ultrasonograms reveal regional thickening and changes in infrastructure of the ligament, in particular approaching the proximal margin of one or more spinous processes (Figure 19.5), occasionally accompanied by ultrasonographic (and radiographic) evidence of a double contour to the process.

Pain from the dorsal sacroiliac ligament is often unilateral and can be associated with severe pain to deep digital pressure. In unilateral cases, mild lameness may be present, whereas bilateral cases may show reluctance to elevate the back and stretch the neck into a soft contact due to the reciprocal arrangement of the nuchal, supraspinous and proximal sacroiliac ligaments. Unilateral cases occasionally show severe osseous irregularities along the interface with the ipsilateral tuber sacrale; injection of corticosteroids at this interface can produce excellent results.

References

1. Lundquist, K., Kvalitetsbedömming av unge ridhäster, samband mellam bedömningsresultat och fremtida brukbarhet. PhD thesis, Swedish University of Agricultural Sciences, Uppsala, 1983.
2. Holmström, M. Quantitative studies on conformation and trotting traits in the Swedish warmblood riding horse. PhD thesis, Swedish University of Agricultural Sciences, Uppsala, 1994.
3. Randelhoff, A. Pathologische – anatomische und – histologische Untersuchungen zum Pathogenese von Wirbelsaülenveränderungen bei Pferden. PhD thesis, Berlin, 1997.
4. Jeffcott, L.B. Radiographic examination of the equine vertebral column. *Veterinary Radiology* 1979;**20**:135–139.
5. Nørgaard, J.K. and Krogh-Rasmussen, S. Det equine ligamentum supraspinale: et mikroanatomisk og biomekanisk studie. Royal Veterinary and Agricultural University, Copenhagen, Denmark, 2006.

20 Showjumpers

Frances M.D. Henson

Showjumping horses, in my opinion, are among some of our hardest working equine athletes. They repeatedly lift themselves over large obstacles, without the advantage of speed that their racing and eventing counterparts have. From the author's experience, and from the literature, showjumping horses do seem to suffer a high incidence of clinical back pain.

The jumping effort

To identify where the stresses and strains of jumping occur it is first necessary to examine how the back moves when jumping. Jumping can be divided into five phases [1] (Table 20.1).

The orientation of the spine changes during jumping relative to the ground. In phase A there is an upward rotation of the spine combined with a raising of the withers and a lowering of the lumbosacral region; during phase B the upward angle of the spine increases. During phase C the spine is horizontal to the ground and then, during phase D, the vertebral column starts to rotate downwards. Within the spine itself, clearly some of the articulating structures do have to move, in order to rotate the trunk high enough to clear the jump. Studies on the movement of individual segments of the spine have been reported [2]. These studies have shown that most of the movement occurs in the thoracolumbar and the lumbosacral regions. Indeed, in poor jumpers, these two regions have to move more than in a good jumping horse, in order to compensate for the trunk not getting high enough from the hindlimb thrust. It is likely that the movement seen in the thoracolumbar and lumbosacral regions is a composite movement from a number of different articulations, because it has been shown that individual dorsal spinous processes could be moved only a mean 1.1–6.0 mm on maximum ventroflexion and 0.8–3.8 mm on dorsiflexion. The overall flexibility of the back was found to be 53.1 mm [3].

Conformation of the showjumper

The conformation of showjumpers is obviously similar to other horses in most respects. However, it is important to be aware that short-backed horses are considered by many riders/owners/trainers to be good jumpers. Thus the showjumper may well be predisposed to overriding dorsal spinous processes (ORDSPs). In addition, another conformational 'extreme' favoured by showjumping people is the prominent tuber sacrale/sloped sacral region conformation – the so-called 'jumper's bump'. This conformation, although noticeably different to other horses, has not been proved to be associated with any pathological conditions,

Table 20.1   The phases of the jump

Phase	Description
A	Last approach stride before hindlimb take-off
B	Take off; hindlimb stance phase
C	Jump suspension
D	Forelimb landing
E	First departure stride

although there are suggestions that it may predispose to sacroiliac dysfunction (see Chapter 18).

Clinical examination

Before the clinical examination of the jumping horse it is important to take a detailed history. Information on the level of jumping that the horse is doing, its recent jumping record and the nature of the clinical problem should be ascertained. The horse may have a varied jumping-related history (see also Chapter 6). Often there is a history of starting to refuse jumps when it would not normally do so, having the back rail down over spread fences, having problems in combination fences, jumping flat (to avoid spinal movement) or just resistance to enter the ring/leave the collecting ring. In the author's opinion, many jumping horses will continue to try to jump even when they have significant pathology.

The clinical examination of the jumping horse should be based on the normal clinical examination for back pain (see Chapter 6). In addition to the normal examination in hand and when ridden, it is advisable, where possible, to see the horse jumping over the normal size of fences that it would be jumping.

Diagnostic imaging

To identify the presence of back pathology in the jumping horse radiography, nuclear scintigraphy, ultrasonograpy, thermography or diagnostic analgesia can be used as discussed in earlier chapters.

It is recommended that a thorough diagnostic imaging investigation be performed on these horses, particularly the high value performance horses.

Specific back pathology in the showjumper

There is no specific back condition that is found exclusively in showjumpers; however, there are a number of different conditions that have been described as occurring more frequently in the showjumper. These include ORDSPs (see Chapter 14), supraspinous ligament (SSL) desmitis (see Chapter 17) and sacroiliac dysfunction (see Chapter 18).

Treatment of the showjumper

Treatment of the jumping horse depends on the clinical condition that the horse is suffering from, the timescale over which the treatment is to be attempted and the aim of the treatment long term. In some horses with mild back pain/pathology, the aim of the treatment may not be to treat the pathology itself, but rather to manage the pain using a combination of medication and physiotherapy in order to provide temporary relief in the short term. This will allow the horse to compete and meet its competition schedule and targets. In other horses with more severe pathology, the aim of the treatment will be to remove the horse from training and competition, and allow a full recovery from the pathology to take place. In these horses a complete investigation/diagnostic imaging survey should be performed.

When treating the jumping horse, the demands of the competitive sport that it is undertaking, with regard to the medications permissible and the drug withdrawal times, must be considered. Thus non-invasive treatments that do not involve prohibited substances will be beneficial in cases in which they are expected to compete in the near future. These include, for example, the use of physiotherapy, Sarapin and extracorporeal shock wave therapy for cases of ORDSPs and SSL desmitis.

References

1. Clayton, H. and Back, W. *Equine Locomotion*. Philadelphia: Harcourt Publishers Ltd, 2001: 156–161
2. Cassiat, G., Gegueurce, C., Pourcelot, P. et al. Influence of individual competition level on back kinematics of horses jumping a vertical fence. *Equine Veterinary Journal* 2004;**36**:748–753.
3. Jeffcott, L.B. and Dalin, G. Natural rigidity of the horse's backbone. *Equine Veterinary Journal* 1980;**12**:101–108.

21 Eventers

Andrew P. Bathe

Introduction

Eventing is the most all-round test of the competitive horse with speed, flatwork and jumping ability being assessed. Back pain is most commonly the limiting factor during the dressage and showjumping phases, as there is a high level of adrenaline during the cross-country phase. Low-grade back pain is a common finding in event horses [1], but is generally not as much of a limiting factor as it is in pure jumping or dressage horses. Event horses tend to suffer from the common problems seen in other sports horses, the main difference being that they are more prone to external traumatic damage when falling.

Saddle fit can contribute to back pain in the horse (see Chapter 24) and it can be more of an issue for event horses than other horses because different saddles are required for the different phases of the competition. It can be difficult to get one saddle to fit perfectly, let alone two or three. Also rider security in the saddle may be a primary concern in the cross-country phase rather than its fit on the individual horse, which can lead to problems with the horse in the saddle region. In addition, the event horse's condition and leanness also tend to vary considerably during the season as the more advanced level horses are normally aimed at competing in two 3-day events per year, with the 1-day events mainly being used as training. Thus the back of the horse is constantly changing and it is likely that the horse will experience poor saddle fit at some stage during the season.

Diagnostic approach

Low-grade back pain is relatively common in the event horse. However, the rider, groom or regular physiotherapist may notice the back soreness upon palpation in normally competing horses, and this would normally be managed conservatively or with physiotherapy, with no veterinary involvement.

In cases of more serious back pathology, the level of diagnostic investigation will vary depending upon the severity of the problem. The horse that presents with mild signs of back pain will normally just be assessed clinically and the response to short periods of rest, anti-inflammatory drugs, physiotherapy and changes in saddle fit assessed. More in-depth investigations will employ radiography, ultrasonography, scintigraphy and diagnostic local analgesia depending upon the significance of the problem and the finances available. If the presenting problem is relatively subtle, the response to specific treatment, such as medication of impinging dorsal spinous processes, may be used to determine the significance of such findings.

The clinical examination of the event horse

The clinical examination of the event horse should be based on the standard clinical examination as detailed in Chapter 6. A number of discipline specific differences do, however, exist. In terms of the response to palpation, the varying temperament of event horses can make interpretation of behavioural responses challenging and, at the stage of the season where sitting trot is recommenced, event horses normally go through a transient period of back soreness.

When performing the dynamic evaluation, the degree of spinal flexibility should be assessed when the horse is trotted. Note, however, that the more thoroughbred eventing lines will often have limited flexibility in comparison to the more expressive warmblood types. The quality of the canter should be critically assessed, as should the spinal flexibility at this gait. The horse should then be assessed and ridden by its normal rider with its normal tack. This allows the saddle fit and quality of equitation to be assessed. It is easy for back pain to be blamed for a lack of ability in either the horse or the rider. Back pain during riding may manifest as a poor quality of movement or behavioural signs of resentment, particularly at trot/canter transitions, and as poor jumping technique.

When performing the clinical examination, the horse should be closely assessed for any lameness as hindlimb lameness is commonly found in association with back pain. In many cases this may be the cause of back pain without any primary pathology in the back region being identified. In some cases it will exacerbate an otherwise manageable mild back problem and in others there may just be concurrent and unrelated lameness and back pain. Simply treating back pain in horses with significant hindlimb lameness is often unrewarding, and attention to both problems is likely to be most effective.

Further diagnostic work-up

Radiography of the dorsal spinous processes (DSPs) (see Chapter 8) will be commonly undertaken to rule out the presence of impingement (overriding DSPs or ORDSPs). Interpretation of these radiographs is often difficult, as discussed in previous chapters, because many event horses will have impinging spinous processes that do not cause a clinical problem. Thus, the significance of any finding should be assessed along with the response to diagnostic local analgesia by infiltrating the affected spaces, or in more subtle presentations by assessment of the response to trial medication of the region.

Thermographic evaluation (see Chapter 12) is helpful in a small number of cases in identifying any soft tissue inflammation, but any findings should be interpreted with care and in conjunction with other imaging modalities.

Ultrasonographic examination of the supraspinous ligament (see Chapter 10) can be helpful, particularly in horses with an acute onset of severe back pain. Again interpretation is complicated by the fact that there is a wide degree of variation in the appearance of the supraspinous ligament and injuries do not tend to improve ultrasonographically during the healing process. Again diagnostic local analgesia should be used to determine the significance of any findings. Arthritis of the thoracolumbar articular facets does not appear to be a particularly common limiting problem and is most accurately assessed by the combination of oblique radiographs, scintigraphy and ultrasonography.

Treatment

Many actively competing event horses have their backs monitored on a frequent basis and the response to various treatments assessed. If the problem is severe or persists, it is sometimes helpful to assess the case from scratch and take a more aggressive imaging approach to fully assess the case. The principles of treatment are the same as for any other horse. For actively competing horses, medication control regulations will prohibit the use of long-acting depot steroids such as methylprednisolone acetate. As a general principle for low-grade back pain, prolonged periods of rest are inappropriate. For a fairly acute, mild problem, a short period out of ridden exercise can be beneficial but it is helpful to keep maintaining the musculature in the back region in the long term. Lunging in a Chambon or similar device can be helpful to encourage the appropriate muscling over the top line. Many event riders use equipment such as electromagnetic rugs and massage (e.g. Equissage) machines on a regular basis.

Impinging DSPs are commonly treated with local injection with corticosteroids such as triamcinolone in combination with small doses of local anaesthetic and drugs such as Sarapin (see Chapter 14). Extracorporeal shock wave therapy can be useful as adjunctive analgesic treatment in many horses and I recommend an initial course of three treatments at 2-weekly intervals initially and then maintenance treatments at approximately 5-monthly intervals. In horses that are limited by impinging DSPs, surgical resection can be extremely effective. These horses can return to competing at a high level.

Supraspinous ligament injuries are more frustrating to treat and a long period of rest is often necessary. Ligament splitting may have a role in management of non-responsive cases. Arthritis of the articular facets should be managed by appropriate exercise, intravenous infusion of tiludronate and ultrasound-guided injection of the affected areas.

Physiotherapy and other complementary treatments can be extremely helpful once veterinary treatment of any significant underlying problems has been effective. These are often employed at competitions to maximise performance (Plate 33) but the most important work is to treat any underlying conditions before arriving at the competition.

Conclusions

Veterinary monitoring and treatment of back pain can enable event horses to have an improved level of comfort and performance. The close monitoring of management in terms of exercise and saddle fit should also be performed. With client education the number of back problems can be significantly reduced and certainly I see more low-level event horses presented for evaluation of back pain than those ridden by more élite riders. A team approach by the rider, groom, physiotherapist and vet is recommended.

Reference

1. Bathe, A.P. Lameness in the three day Event Horse. In: Ross, M.W. and Dyson, S. (eds), *Diagnosis and Management of Lameness in the Horse*. Philadelphia: Saunders, 2003: 984–996.

22 Racehorses

Marcus J. Head

Introduction

Thoroughbred racehorses in the UK commonly suffer back injury. This injury can arise from a number of areas including:

- direct trauma, e.g. "soft" saddles, ill-fitting tack, poor riders, falls during jump racing
- athletic endeavour, e.g. stress fractures, soft tissue strain
- a combination of the above along with unknown factors, e.g. impinging dorsal spinous processes (DSPs)
- secondary effect of hindlimb lameness.

Many trainers employ physiotherapists or a variety of variably qualified "paraprofessionals" to treat these horses and the "back man" usually holds a position of seniority in the yard, considerably above that of the veterinarian. The recognition of specific injury to the spine relies, as always, on careful examination, diagnostic imaging and, occasionally, diagnostic anaesthesia. Treatment regimens used in this group are dependent on the type of racing for which the animal is used, the value of the horse, the time available for drugs to be clear before competition and the willingness of the trainer/owner to address the primary problem.

Most common diagnoses of back pathology in the racehorse

- Management problems leading to superficial injury
- Back pain secondary to hindlimb lameness
- Impinging DSPs
- Pelvic fractures
- Lumbar laminar stress fractures
- Other spinal stress fractures
- Traumatic fractures to the thoracic DSPs/ sacrum, etc.
- Soft tissue injuries (dorsal sacroiliac ligaments; muscle tears)
- Congenital/developmental defects.

Approach to clinical cases

The clinical examination of the back can be difficult in these horses – most young racehorses exhibit tenderness on palpation of the epaxial musculature, and the response to manipulation of the spine and to pressure applied across the back or pelvis can be highly variable. It is vital to take time to ensure the repeatability of findings.

Many cases present with a vague, universal history of reduced performance or "cold-backed" syndrome. Reduced performance in racehorses often manifests as a reluctance to exercise – the trainer may complain that the horse refuses to canter or "jump off". Some primary lesions of the spine will be intensely painful and cause guarding of the affected area: mild lameness is often seen with such lesions, affecting the ipsilateral hindlimb. Mild elevations in muscle enzyme levels in venous blood samples may, erroneously, lead to a diagnosis of rhabdomyolysis, but the clinical signs are usually more severe, and one sided, than the degree of creatine kinase (CK) and aspartate transaminase (AST; also known as aspartate aminotransferase) elevation would suggest. Stress fractures of the pelvis almost always have a history of obvious lameness, but can mimic rhabdomyolysis or back pain, particularly if bilateral. The horse should be examined walking and trotting in straight lines and on the lunge on hard and soft surfaces (unless the clinical examination or history suggests a possible fracture), paying particular attention to "tracking up" and hindlimb action. Oddly, many racehorse vets seem reluctant to use lunging as part of their assessment – it is as useful in this group of athletes as in any other group of horses. Ridden assessments are performed rarely, the clinician usually relying on the reports of the rider and trainer, but this should be considered, particularly if the problem is reported to worsen during ridden exercise.

In all cases, unless the signs are so obvious that primary back or pelvic pathology must be present, assume that the horse is lame. Bilateral hindlimb lameness is the most common cause of back pain in the racehorse, often resulting in considerable discomfort caused by secondary muscle spasm. In our clinic, the classic "back pain" horse will trot with a restricted action, often showing marked plaiting (crossing) of the hindlimbs: many cases exhibiting such signs will actually be suffering from metatarsal stress reactions. As hind fetlock lameness is so common in racehorses, and even if overt lameness is not evident, it is strongly recommended that a "low six-point" nerve block (perineural analgesia of the plantar and plantar metatarsal and dorsal metatarsal nerves) is placed in one hindlimb. This will often result in lameness becoming obvious in the contralateral hindlimb. Unless treatment is aimed at the primary lesion, rather than the secondary back pain, the outcome is, clearly, unlikely to be satisfactory.

Main differential diagnoses for back pain in the thoroughbred racehorse

- Bilateral hindlimb lameness
- Pelvic stress fracture
- Recurrent rhabdomyolysis.

The role of diagnostic imaging in the detection of back pathology in the racehorse

Nuclear scintigraphic imaging (see Chapter 9) is, undoubtedly, the gold-standard technique for

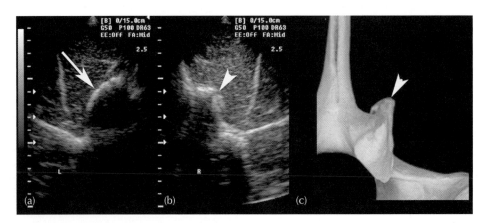

Figure 22.1 Two ultrasonograms and a postmortem specimen of the articular facets. (a) Transverse ultrasonogram of the articular facet region to demonstrate the ultrasonographic view of new bone formation at the articular facet (arrow). (b) Normal ultrasonographic appearance of the articular facet on the other side of the horse at the same level. The sharp angle of the articular facet is seen (arrowhead), as it is on the postmortem specimen (white arrow) (c).

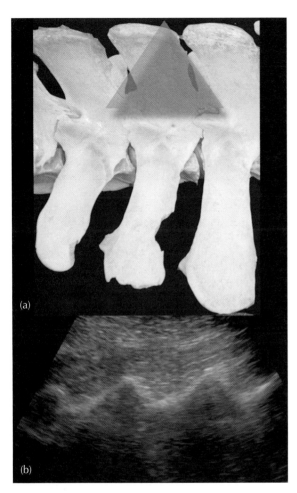

(a)

(b)

Figure 22.2 (a) Photograph of a postmortem specimen of transverse processes of the lumbar vertebrae. The direction of the ultrasonographic beam for longitudinal scanning of the transverse processes is shown. (b) An ultrasonogram of the normal appearance of transverse processes in longitudinal section.

investigation of musculoskeletal injury in the racehorse. The high incidence of stress fractures and stress reactions in these athletes means that, even if a pathognomonic "hot spot" is not identified, a large number of differential diagnoses can be ruled out with a bone scan. The author recommends the use of approximately 4.5 GBq of technetium-labelled methylene diphosphonate ($[^{99m}Tc]MDP$) per patient and acquires the images using a rectangular, large field-of-view camera, 2–3 hours after injection (Plate 34). Even if primary spinal pathology is suspected or known, it is con-

sidered standard practice to image the entire back, pelvis and hindlimbs – many cases have several areas of injury in the ipsilateral or contralateral hindlimb that may have resulted in the main, currently pertinent, injury. The back should always be imaged from both sides (see Chapter 9). Other views are possible, although, in the author's clinic, dorsoventral views are obtained only to further characterise pathology identified on the lateromedial and/or oblique views. The pelvis is always imaged from both sides and from above.

Radiography (see Chapter 8) is usually used as a follow-up to nuclear scintigraphy to assess lesions of the back and distal limbs. Lateromedial radiographic views are useful to highlight the DSPs and vertebral bodies. The addition of radio-opaque markers attached to the skin above the summits of the DSPs allows precise anatomical location of diseased bone, so that treatment can be administered accurately. Other views are also useful. As discussed in Chapter 8, dorsomedial–ventrolateral–oblique (DMVLO) projections of the thoracic and lumbar facet joints can be useful, but are technically demanding and require large exposures. Ultrasonography of the lumbar region may be more useful and it is certainly easier to obtain reasonable images of this region with this imaging modality (see Chapter 10). The conditions that can be identified using radiography of the back are detailed in Chapter 8. Overriding DSPs (ORDSPs), osteoarthritis of the articular facets and fractures are all seen. In addition, ventral spondylosis of the thoracic vertebrae is occasionally identified scintigraphically and radiographically (Plate 35). Interpretation of these imaging modalities in this condition is difficult; in the author's opinion (and in the opinion of many others) it is assumed that the lesions are painful while scintigraphically active.

As described by the author in Chapter 10, ultrasonography of the articular facets (Figure 22.1 and see Figure 10.4 in Chapter 10) of the thoracolumbar spine is an extremely useful and informative procedure. Ultrasonography may also be useful in identifying the integrity of the transverse processes of the lumbar vertebrae (Figure 22.2).

The identification of pathology of the articular facets (Figures 22.1 and 22.3) does not always signify the presence of pain. Unfortunately, once enlarged, the joints will continue to appear

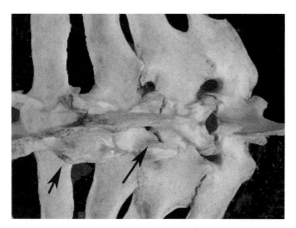

Figure 22.3   A photograph of the dorsal view of a postmortem specimen of the lumbar vertebrae, taken from a racehorse with no history of back problems. Note the enlargement and virtual fusion of the joints on the left side (arrows), compared with the right.

abnormal on ultrasonography long after they have ceased to become a painful problem, so nuclear scintigraphy is often required to ascertain the significance of ultrasonographically detected abnormalities. In significant cases there is an increase in radionuclide uptake associated with the articular facets. In addition, it has been demonstrated that articular facet joint disease is a common finding *post mortem* of thoroughbreds (California-based studies have identified thoracolumbar joint degeneration in 97% of animals examined and stress fractures in 50% [1]). The author does not believe that the incidence of disease is as high in the UK, but the possibility of identifying an old, no longer significant lesion using ultrasonography should be borne in mind. Horses affected with lumbar injuries often trot on three tracks, with a pronounced scoliosis and mild ipsilateral hindlimb lameness. Stress fractures occur in other parts of the spine (e.g. the sacrum, Figure 22.4) but are rare. Ultrasonography also permits assessment of

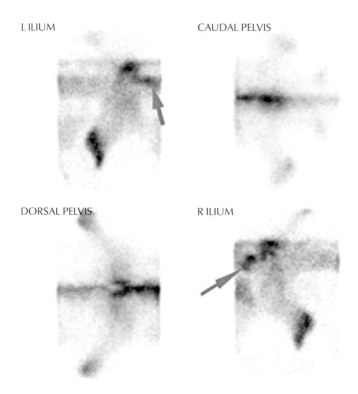

Figure 22.4   Nuclear scintigrams to show the scintigraphic appearance of a stress fracture of the sacrum in a racehorse (arrows) – an unusual site for stress fractures in the racehorse.

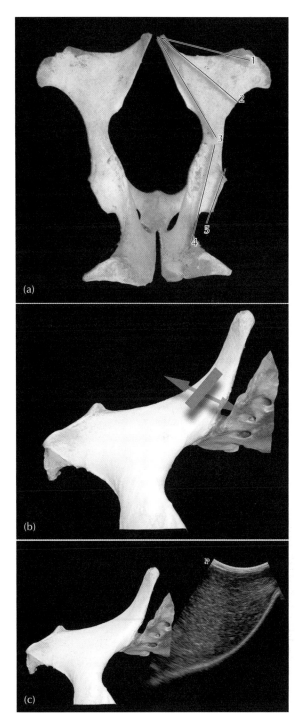

Figure 22.5 Ultrasonography of the pelvis. (a, b) Photographs of the dorsal and lateral views of a postmortem specimen of the pelvis. Lines have been drawn upon the specimen to demonstrate the sites for ultrasonography of the pelvis. The transducer is moved along each of the planes in turn to acquire information regarding the iliac wing (1–3), the iliac shaft (4) and hip joint (5). In (c) the normal ultrasonographic appearance of the iliac wing is shown. The iliac wing is seen as a smooth, curved bony surface.

the supraspinous ligament and dorsal sacroiliac ligaments (see Chapters 10 and 11), but these injuries are either very, very rare, or hugely underdiagnosed in racehorses.

Ultrasonography of the pelvis is a well-documented method for identification and follow-up of iliac wing fractures (see Chapter 11). The author uses pelvic ultrasonography as a first-line imaging modality, but pelvic fracture cannot be ruled out with ultrasonography. Again, using a low-frequency convex probe, the iliac wings can be imaged – as the probe is moved caudally along the lumbar facet joints the next structure to be seen is the wing of the ilium. It appears as a sweeping curve running from the tuber sacrale to the tuber coxa. The easiest and most systematic method for examining the ilium has been described previously [2] and involves imagining three lines drawn from the tuber sacrale to the tuber coxa, representing three planes of imaging along the iliac wing, from cranial to caudal. The transducer is moved slowly along each of these lines in turn, starting towards midline and moving outwards, holding the probe at 90° to midline (Figure 22.5). The most important aspect of the ilium to image is the caudal edge, because this is the region that most stress fractures affect first. Changes may be subtle in early damage. Be aware of edge artefacts produced by the many large vessels within the muscles – these can give the impression that there is discontinuity in the surface of the bone. Stress fractures often have a degree of new bone production evident ultrasonographically by the time that they are clinically evident, so look for callus formation as well as a break in the bone surface (Figure 22.6). Immature callus will appear irregular and allow some of the ultrasound beam to pass through; mature callus is smooth and of equal echogenicity to the adjacent, normal, bone (Figure 22.6). Remember that a normal ultrasound scan does not rule out iliac wing stress fracture: false negatives can occur. Rotating the probe to image the iliac wing in a parasagittal plane is sometimes interesting, but its main use is to identify the iliac shaft easily – the smooth caudal edge of the wing becomes the long smooth surface of the shaft and can be followed down to the hip joint. Catastrophic fractures of the iliac shaft will be seen as a step in this smooth contour (Figure 22.7). Young animals can suffer "green stick" fractures of the iliac shaft.

Traumatic injury

Racehorses relatively commonly suffer traumatic injury to the back and pelvis (see Chapter 13), usually as a result of a fall while racing (national hunt horses) or when rearing over backwards (Figure 22.8). Occasionally, unusual fractures will cause poor racing performance. One example of this is a horse that had a fractured rib, detected

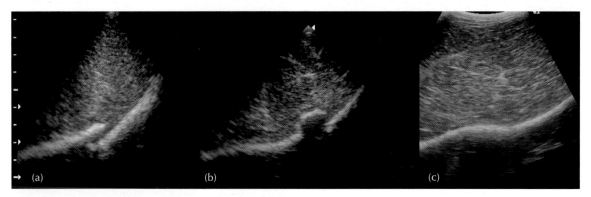

Figure 22.6 Ultrasonography of the iliac wing: (a) the ultrasonographic appearance of a complete iliac wing fracture. Note the 'step' in the contour of the ilium. (b, c) Ultrasonographic images of the iliac wing at two stages of repair. In (b) the callus bridging the fracture gap is irregular and allows transmission of ultrasound: this is immature callus. (c) Ultrasonographic appearance of an iliac wing fracture that has almost completely healed. There is now only a gentle convexity in the bone surface that has the same appearance as the adjacent bone. This will soon disappear altogether and the ilium will appear normal

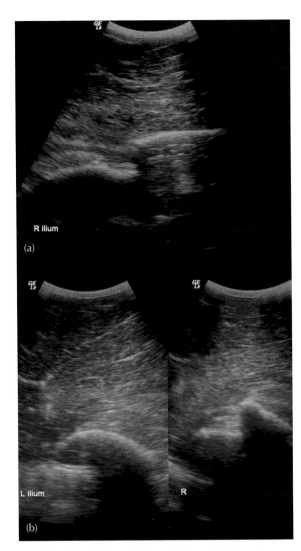

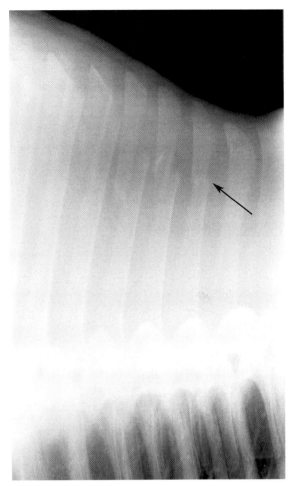

Figure 22.7 Ultrasonography of an iliac shaft demonstrating the radiographic appearance of a fracture affecting a 3-year-old thoroughbred filly. A distinct gap can be identified in the normally smooth contour of the shaft in both (a) the longitudinal and (b) the transverse plane (the normal side is included for comparison).

Figure 22.8 A lateromedial radiograph to show multiple fractures of the dorsal spinous processes (DSPs) secondary to a fall – this racehorse reared over backwards on the way out of the yard to exercise one morning. The arrow shows the most caudal fracture.

during a bone scan being performed for investigation of poor jumping (Figure 22.9). Management of these traumatic injuries is usually a period of rest. The prognosis is, broadly speaking, better for racehorses than other horses because any minor gait abnormalities or asymmetry that results from this type of accident is less of a concern than it would be for, say, a dressage horse.

Congenital/developmental defects

Spinal abnormalities producing scoliosis and lordosis/kyphosis are very rare but do occur (see Chapter 15). In the author's opinion they can be surprisingly difficult to detect clinically, unless severe, and milder cases will go undetected until early training. If the affected segment is mid-thoracic, radiography can be useful to localise the lesion and assess the severity of the lesion (Plate 36). Nuclear scintigraphic evidence is also often

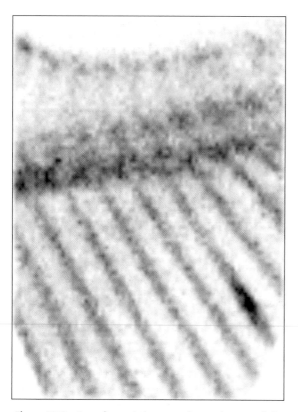

Figure 22.9 A nuclear scintigram to show a fracture of rib 14 in a racehorse – an unusual cause of poor performance. The fracture is seen as a focal increase in radionuclide uptake down the shaft of the rib. Callus associated with this fracture was confirmed ultrasonographically.

helpful (Plate 36b, c). There is no treatment for these congenital conditions and their management depends on the severity of the deformity.

Management problems leading to superficial injury

Saddle area trauma

Thoroughbreds are ridden with "soft" treeless saddles – exercise saddles are similar to racing saddles but a little bulkier and more robust. Saddle fit issues are a common cause of back problems in other disciplines and it is likely that the racing thoroughbred is no different, although this is difficult to quantify. Attempts to exercise racehorses in "proper" saddles are usually met with extreme resistance, but this option should be borne in mind if it is felt that the direct application of the rider's weight to the midline may be contributing to a problem. Direct trauma to the skin of the saddle area can lead to several common problems including the following.

Haematoma/Seroma formation

The formation of a haematoma or seroma is a frequent event (Plate 37a). These are usually very painful in the initial stages and surrounded by oedema. They can be treated by injection of a small amount of triamcinolone acetonide (2–5 mg) into the swelling, after draining some of the fluid away.

Nodular collagen necrosis

Although not unique to the racehorse, nodular collage necrosis is usually more of a cosmetic issue for the trainer than a painful one for the horse (Plate 37b). Once again, injection of corticosteroid subcutaneously can help reduce the number and size of the swellings but is rarely curative. Some clinicians advocate surgical removal, but the author believes that this is very rarely indicated.

Patchy sweating in the saddle region

In some individuals patchy sweating can also occur, presumably due to damage to the sympathetic supply to the sweat glands (Plate 37f).

Girth galls

Girth galls are the result of the girth being over-tightened and appear as firm swellings on the ventral chest (Plate 37c). They can be extremely painful, mimicking colic when they form acutely, but resolve with systemic and topical non-steroidal anti-inflammatory drugs.

Miscellaneous causes

In addition to these more commonly recognised causes of injury in the saddle region, occasionally unusual injury does occur, e.g. the author has encountered an outbreak of erosive, painful back lesions in one yard (Plate 37d). This was found to be caused by poor management: the horses were allowed into a sand-filled pen after exercise. Unfortunately they were not washed off properly afterwards, so sand was left in the hair and then rubbed into the skin by the saddle during exercise the following morning.

Staphylococcal folliculitis

Staphylococcal folliculitis occurs commonly in young racehorses (Plate 37e). They are usually very painful and associated with "runners" – engorged lymphatics that can be seen radiating from the lesion. They are most common over the neck, back (particularly the saddle region) and chest, and respond well to a short course of intravenous antibiotics, although will usually resolve spontaneously if given enough time.

Treatment and management of back pathology in the racehorse

Common to other disciplines, the biggest factors dictating management are cost and time. Generally speaking, flat racehorses have short careers (the majority start as 2 year olds and finish by the time they are 4), whereas hurdlers and steeplechasers have longer athletic lives. This means that, for example, surgical intervention for DSP impingement is rare in flat racehorses because the recovery time is too long. Most trainers and owners want amelioration of the clinical signs so that training and racing can be continued in the short window of opportunity available.

Injection of *corticosteroids* around impinging DSPs or the supraspinous ligament is often effective, transiently, but care should be exercised regarding withdrawal times – the author's group use triamcinolone acetonide, up to 30 mg per horse, per treatment, and advise a withdrawal for racing of *at least* 21 days, although positive tests have been returned on horses treated 42 days earlier. Side effects, such as laminitis or dystrophic mineralisation, are very rare, but should be considered, especially when repeated treatments are

necessary. Ultrasound-guided, perilesional injection of diseased lumbar facet joints has been spectacularly successful in a handful of cases, but should be used with caution so that horses are not trained on and worsen the injury.

Extracorporeal shock wave therapy is popular among many of our trainers and, anecdotally at least, has had some very favourable results. For the treatment of impinging DSPs the author's group use up to 5000 cycles, at 3 bar, with a 10 or 15 mm diameter applicator (Dolor Clast Vet), applied to the DSPs and surrounding epaxial muscles.

Physiotherapy is useful for the management of horses that are being trained in the face of minor injuries, and the increased use of such *qualified* professionals in yards is testimony to their perseverance and skill. Trainers should be encouraged to utilise these services on a regular basis, and not just when a horse has already succumbed to an injury necessitating veterinary intervention.

Unfortunately, if significant damage to the bones, joints or ligaments is present, a period of time out of training is inevitable. Strict box rest is rarely indicated unless normal activity is likely to destabilise the injury – this is more likely with pelvic than spinal damage but, even so, complete iliac wing fractures can resume walking and restricted turnout within a few weeks. Most people are too conservative in their management of back and pelvis stress fractures, giving the horse weeks or even months of rest, when controlled exercise is far more effective and reduces the risk of succumbing to another injury on resumption of training.

Diagnostic imaging is of limited use in the follow-up of injury to the spine – in the author's opinion bone scans will reveal increased radionuclide uptake even when sufficient healing has occurred to allow full work to be resumed. Ultrasound scans of the pelvis are very useful after iliac wing/shaft fracture (much more so than repeat bone scans), to ensure bony union is progressing with each increase in exercise level. Radiographs of DSP impingement do not, in the author's experience, ever improve, and often reveal deterioration with time, or dystrophic mineralisation of the soft tissues after surgery. A gradual return to exercise should be based on clinical findings.

Reference

1. Haussler, K.K. and Stover, S.M. Stress fractures of the vertebral lamina and pelvis in Thoroughbred racehorses. *Equine Veterinary Journal* 1998;**30**:374–381.

2. Pilsworth, R.C., Holmes, M.A. and Shepherd, M. An improved method for the scintigraphic detection of acute bone damage to the equine pelvis by probe point counting. *Veterinary Record* 1993;**133**:490–495.

Section 5

Complementary Therapy and Rehabilitation

23 Complementary Therapies in the Treatment of Back Pain

Mimi Porter

Introduction

Pain control is a primary concern in human sports medicine but, after surgery or injury, pain in horses often goes unacknowledged. It is difficult to determine the degree of pain that a horse is experiencing and people can fail to observe the circumstances and the horse's body language that would provide early information about its discomfort.

Circumstances that could lead to the horse becoming painful include, among many things:

- over-training of the horse
- condition of the training surface
- change in training surface
- change in hoof care
- increase in the intensity of the training.

A good equine therapist is a good horseman and a good horseman is a good observer: one who recognises early evidence of discomfort, when problems are most easily remedied.

The horse's body language

The horse uses body language as its primary means of communication with humans. Many of the postures and facial expressions of the horse are subtle and often overlooked by grooms, handlers, trainers and veterinarians. The more easily recognised expressions of equine body language are included in Box 23.1.

Knowing that the horse is a prey animal and genetically coded to conceal pain and dysfunction, the horseman must be observant and sensitive to early signs of pain, when it is most successfully treated.

Difficulties in the clinical diagnosis of back pain

The problem with diagnosing back pain in its early stages is that it typically does not cause overt clinical signs, e.g. lameness. The horseman must therefore be able to read the more subtle signs of the horse's body language and realise that any change in behaviour or attitude may indicate a change in physiological status. Examples of the difficulty encountered in the diagnosis of back pain/pathology using standard veterinary techniques and diagnostic imaging are encountered throughout the veterinary literature, e.g. ultrasonography of the soft tissue structures of the back is often used to identify sites of pathology; however, ultrasound evaluation of the supraspinous ligament in a group of 39 horses revealed that every horse in the study had at least one site of desmitis. This

---

Box 23.1   Summary of the easily recognised expressions of equine body language

Muscle tension
Tail carriage and movement, e.g. clamping down of the tail, tail swishing
Head carriage
Ear position
Tension around the eyes or mouth
Facial expression
Unwillingness to stretch/give to pressure during exercise or work-outs
Alterations of rhythm of the hoof strikes with each stride

---

study found no correlation between the ultrasonographic findings and clinical symptoms of back pain or pathology [1]. Similarly, a Norwegian study examined the back of 33 non-symptomatic riding horses using radiographic and nuclear scintigraphic techniques and found that 26 of these animals had scintigraphic or radiographic evidence of pathology. The pathology detected included sclerosis, radiolucencies, abnormal spacing of the dorsal spinous processes and increased radiopharmaceutical uptake within the spine. Most of these findings were located between T13 and T18 and were mild. The researchers concluded, as did those in the previous study, that the presence of some radiographic and scintigraphic changes cannot be interpreted as clinically significant [2].

In addition to diagnostic imaging techniques, regional anaesthesia is commonly used by veterinarians when evaluating musculoskeletal injuries, particularly in the lower limbs. When used in cases of equine back pain, however, the results are thought to be somewhat subjective. A recent study showed that clinically sound horses responded to infiltration of a local anaesthetic solution into the interspinous spaces between T16 and L2 with increased range of motion in both dorsoventral flexion–extension and lateral bending of the back [3]. The results of these studies indicate that, although pathologies may be present in the structures of the dorsal aspect of the horse, the use of local analgesia as a means of objectively locating and measuring these changes clinically in their early stages has not been validated.

Given these problems with the diagnosis of back pathology using conventional veterinary approaches, the equine therapist is in an ideal position to understand the source and extent of a horse's back pain because of both the hands-on nature of this profession and the level of horsemanship necessary to be a skilled equine therapist.

In the author's opinion, the job of the equine therapist is not to diagnose the problem causing equine back pain, but rather to locate regions of discomfort and dysfunction through palpation and observation, and then to provide non-pharmacological means of managing the problem through the use of physical agents such as electrical stimulation, therapeutic ultrasound, therapeutic laser, magnetic fields, ice, heat, the many manual therapies, stretching and ground exercises. Through the early application of these tools, discomfort is managed and mobility is maintained. The equine therapist's information, derived from palpation and observation, coupled with the veterinarian's diagnostic procedures, will provide the optimal therapeutic approach.

Communication and relaxation

A horse's behaviour and body language are driven primarily by biological triggers. If a horse feels well, it performs well and any change in behaviour or performance indicates a change in its physical health. Chris Irwin, internationally renowned equestrian coach and author, points out that the horse's body shape will illustrate the "frame of mind" of a horse [4].

Two shapes that are important to the equine therapist are the high-headed with an inverted back and the low-headed postures (Table 23.1). The consequences of a high head carriage are as follows:

• Thoracic spine is in extension. The horse is robbed of the power and balance that it should get from the *longissimus dorsi* and middle gluteal muscles. It uses muscles of the front quarters to pull itself along, rather than

Table 23.1 Summary of the changes that occur in the back, stride length and hindquarter impulsion in a horse with high and low head carriage

	High head carriage	Low head carriage
Thoracic spine	Extension	Flexion
Spinal flexion	Dorsiflexion	Ventroflexion
Stride length	Shortened protraction and retraction	Normal protraction and retraction
Hindquarter impulsion	Significantly reduced	Maximal

pushing itself from the more powerful hindquarters.

- As spine is in dorsiflexion there is a shortening of the stride in both protraction and retraction of the front and back legs.

This posture is often seen at the racetrack with the horse galloping around the track braced against the bit while the rider is "skiing" with the reins and stirrups, bracing against the horse. The inverted, bracing posture creates adrenaline production and a tense, reactive horse. Although being in a frame of high-headedness and spinal dorsiflexion may not be a cause of injury, it contributes to the discomfort that is already there. As Chris Irwin states: "Head position not only indicates the problem but is an integral part of it."

The consequences of a low head carriage position (head held at or below the plane of the withers) are as follows:

- Thoracic body will ventroflex.
- Muscles of the abdomen are strengthened when the horse exercises in this posture and the limbs can move through a greater range of motion.
- Horse is naturally calm. Relaxing neurotransmitters are reported to be produced when a horse's head is down, allowing the muscles to release tension. The presence of increased circulation of sedating neurochemicals may be reflected in the horse's facial expression and lowering of the ears.

Relaxation

One of the great benefits of the equine therapist's treatment is the resulting relaxation response. The use of electrical stimulation for relaxation, as well as for pain relief, in humans dates back to the 1940s. Low-frequency electrical stimulation, at 4 p.p.s. (pulses per second), is reported to release β-endorphin in the brain and met-enkephalin in the spinal cord, whereas high-frequency stimulation of 100 p.p.s. and above mediates pain through dynorphins in the spinal cord. These complex chemical messengers are produced in the brain and in many other body tissues, but production is altered or slowed with age, when injury occurs or chronic pain is allowed to persist. Neurochemical assays taken from blood samples before an electrical stimulation treatment, after 20 minutes of treatment and 24 hours after the treatment revealed that the neurotransmitters β-endorphin, serotonin and others were increased during treatment and for at least 24 hours after treatment [5].

Practical horsemanship skills are a vital part of accomplishing the analgesia and relaxation sought in equine therapy treatments. When the handler puts a chain over the horse's nose, under the chin or over the gums in an attempt to control or discipline the horse, the horse's fight-or-flight mechanism is stimulated. The horse invariably assumes a high-headed posture and cannot relax. The equine therapist must recognise and remedy this situation in order to maximise the benefits of the therapeutic session. The handler should be instructed to put gentle but steady pressure on the halter chinpiece to bring the horse's head down, releasing the pressure the instant the horse comes down. This will put the horse in a more relaxed frame of mind. Jerking movements and tension in the handler's arms and hands conveys to the horse that it is captured, so it braces for flight and produces adrenaline. This is counterproductive to the production of inhibitory neurotransmitters, relaxation and pain relief. Skills of observation and horsemanship are crucial to success of equine therapy treatments.

Pain and performance

The equine therapist must have an advanced understanding of musculoskeletal pain and its effects on equine performance. An article in the University of Kentucky College of Agriculture's *Equine Disease Quarterly* provides a useful way of classifying pain using a numerical system [6]. The author describes type I pain as sharp and intense. Its purpose is to warn of impending tissue damage and initiate responses to limit or prevent that damage. Type I pain is triggered by very hot, very cold or strong mechanical stimulation. Ideally, the animal is able to make use of protective reflexes and withdraw from the cause of this type of pain. In the circumstance of training for a race or a show, overuse or over-training by the rider and trainer prevents the horse from voluntarily limiting its exposure to damaging exercise.

Type II pain often follows type I pain after an injury. It is triggered not only by intense thermal or mechanical stimuli, but also by chemical changes occurring in damaged tissue. Type II pain is carried by slower speed neural pathways and is often described as dull or aching; it normally persists until damaged tissues heal. The purpose of type I pain is to provoke avoidance whereas the purpose of type II pain is to encourage rest and disuse to avoid further injury. Tonasic states that to completely suppress the pain response with pharmacological therapy and then continue training is to put the horse on a dangerous path towards a third type of pain that can end its athletic career [6].

It is clear that an injury that is not allowed to heal completely or a trauma that is repeated can lead to actual damage to the sensory nerve axons and type III pain. With type III pain the horse will muscle splint and immobilise the painful areas. These areas cease normal, symmetrical, coordinated muscle function and will de-condition. Disuse muscle atrophy, muscle contracture and periarticular tissue contracture can ensue. This is all too often seen in the racehorse or the performance horse with atrophied *longissimus dorsi* and gluteal muscles, creating the "roof peak-like" conformation of the back and hips.

Most equine injuries should be considered a process – not an event. When a horse becomes lame, we are observing the results of type III pain.

The compensatory mechanisms that have served in a supportive role have fatigued and physical dysfunction is now recognisable. Looking at a population of 805 horses engaged in dressage, showjumping and trot racing, it was observed that, of the horses with back problems, 74% were lame [7].

The effect of the training/competition surface

The recent introduction of artificial surfaces for racetracks, arenas and horse exercise machines has given rise to a new overuse syndrome that includes the suspensory ligaments, gluteal muscles and sacral joint. High-speed video of horses running on artificial surfaces showed that the forward slide that normally occurs with hoof-to-ground contact does not occur on the artificial surface. As pointed out by Rooney in 1981, the forward slide of the foot prevents over-dorsiflexion of the fetlock joint [8]. Repeated over-dorsiflexion puts stress on the suspensory ligament. This ligament contains a small amount of muscle tissue that serves to control vibration in the ligament as it stretches. According to Rooney, the suspensory ligament is the first structure to receive the force or take up the weight of the body when the horse is moving. Fatigue in this structure allows kinetic energy generated by the hoof impact to focus higher up in the body, especially in the sacroiliac joint. When the hindfoot impacts and cannot slide, the sacrum rotates caudally whereas the iliac rotates in the opposite direction, tearing ligaments of the sacroiliac joint. This syndrome has been associated with the new track surfaces and farriers are evaluating the shoeing requirements for them. Equine therapeutic intervention for this problem could include the use of therapeutic ultrasonography applied to the ligaments of the sacrum and to *longissimus dorsi* as well as laser to the suspensory ligaments, bilaterally.

The consequences of persistent pain

Abnormal posture and gait can lead to overuse of ipsilateral and the opposite diagonal joints and musculature, and can lead to pain in previously uninjured areas of the body. Persistent pain can result in immune suppression, neural synaptic depletion and hormone imbalance in the horse. Persistent tension in the perispinal muscles results from non-functional spasmodic contractions that splint or guard the vertebral joints, interfering with their normal movement. When the perispinal muscles function normally, they act to lift the back against gravity and to provide a strong platform against which the legs work when the horse is moving. A force vector moving through longissimus dorsi parallel to the long axis of the back compresses the vertebrae together creating stability. Without this stabilisation, vertebral joints are subject to vibrational forces and stress. The pain–spasm–pain cycle perpetuates, the back muscles atrophy and joints degenerate. In a study using 15 sound horses, electromyographic (EMG) analysis of the long back muscles showed that stress from a rider is less apt to cause back muscle stiffness than are problems in the distal limbs [9]. Surely, there would be much less equine back pain if trainers and riders could identify orthopaedic problems in their early stages when they are easier to remedy?

The effect of saddlery

According to a recent study, the saddle is seen as a significant contributor to equine back pain and a possible aetiological factor in the development of "kissing spine" syndrome (overriding DSPs or ORDSPs, see Chapter 14) [10]. This study points out that carrying a saddle with weight simulating a rider caused an increase in back extension, which may contribute to soft tissue injuries and to ORDSPs. This study underscores the importance of horsemanship that maintains a more ventro-flexed body posture in the horse, whether during work or during therapy treatments. Saddle fit is extremely important in the management of the equine back (see Chapter 24).

Pulse signal therapy

The label "kissing spine" syndrome or ORDSPs is often given to any pain in the lumbar area of both humans and horses, although it is likely that much

of the pathology comes from osteoarthritis and soft tissue damage in the region. Pulsed signal therapy (PST), a device that has been developed over the last 20 years, has been tested in double-blind clinical trials and has shown effectiveness and safety in horse and human patients suffering from osteoarthritis of the cervical and lumbar spine. Data were collected over a 10-year period in the USA, Canada, France, Italy and Germany, at major medical centres. The PST device produces a pulsed magnetic wave, which induces a weak electrical signal that mimics the physiological signalling normally occurring in healthy tissue. PST has been shown to restore normal cell differentiation and stimulate joint cartilage maturation by means of passively generating streaming potentials that emulate chondrocyte activity in the healthy joint under load [11]. This device is easy to use because it requires only proper placement of the magnetic coil pads and activation of the unit. This device is relatively new to the equine world, but shows promise of efficacy in the treatment of osteoarthritis.

The role of the equine therapist

There is considerable evidence that pre-emptive pain management can be effective in decreasing the development of chronic pain states and is beneficial to the health, recovery and quality of life of horses. The role of the equine therapist is to identify the site/area of the pain and to apply the appropriate therapy. There are a number of different therapies available to the equine therapist. The following are, in the author's opinion, the most useful in the treatment of the equine athlete.

Therapies

Ice

A simple and effective intervention in the pain–spasm–pain cycle is the use of ice massage directly on the area of inflammation. To create a handy tool for ice massage, fill a Styrofoam cup with water and freeze it. Remove the lip of the cup to expose half of the ice block, keeping the rest of the cup intact to insulate your fingers from the ice.

Massage the affected area for 5–10 minutes, depending on the depth of the involved tissue. The area should feel quite cold to the touch. This will interrupt the pain–spasm cycle and cause local capillary constriction, reducing the leakage of fluid and blood from the damaged capillaries, and reduce the release of harmful chemicals involved in prolonged inflammation. Ice massage and a reduction in training intensity can provide effective therapy in the acute phase of injury development.

Therapeutic ultrasound

Therapeutic ultrasound makes use of the kinetic energy of particle vibration within the high-frequency sound wave. Absorption of this energy takes place at the molecular level with protein in the tissue acting as the absorbing agent. Therapeutic ultrasound is delivered as either a thermal (continuous wave train) or a non-thermal (pulsed or intermittent wave train) application, generally at frequencies of 1 MHz or 3 MHz. A topical transmission gel must be applied to the hair coat to eliminate air, which is a deterrent to ultrasound transmission. Determination of frequency, duration and whether to use pulsed or continuous application depends on the nature of the injury, its acuteness or chronicity, and the depth of the injured tissue. Ultrasound delivered at 1 MHz will penetrate to deeper-lying soft tissue and bone, whereas 3 MHz ultrasound is absorbed superficially. It is the sound wave frequency that determines the depth of ultrasound energy penetration, not output intensity. Increasing the intensity setting when delivering ultrasound at 3 MHz could cause over-heating of the superficial tissues and will not drive the sound wave deeper. Continuous wave ultrasonography of over $1.5 \, \text{W/cm}^2$ can cause a significant rise in tissue temperature, even beyond the therapeutic range. Used correctly this modality can benefit the horse through:

- increased elasticity of collagen in tendons, joint capsules and scar tissue
- increased motor and sensory nerve conduction velocities, which assist in reducing pain
- altered contractile activity to skeletal muscle, which reduces muscle spasm

- diminished muscle spindle activity, another factor in muscle spasm reduction
- increased blood flow.

Therapeutic laser

Therapeutic laser, also known as phototherapy, was introduced to the arena of equine health care in the 1980s. At that point collimated, monochromatic light devices did not have approval from the US Food and Drug Administration (FDA) for use on humans, so these devices were marketed to the horse industry. As the devices commonly used in the horse industry are not true lasers, the name phototherapy is a more accurate identifier. Many phototherapy devices in use today use a combination of light-emitting diodes and infrared-emitting diodes.

Research on the effects of phototherapy has shown that it stimulates cell growth, increases cell metabolism, improves cell regeneration, induces an anti-inflammatory response, reduces oedema, fibrous tissue formation and levels of substance P, stimulates production of nitric oxide, decreases the formation of bradykinin, histamine and acetylcholine, and stimulates the production of endorphins.

Phototherapy must be applied in contact and perpendicular to the skin surface. The horse's hair coat can absorb and scatter the energy, so diodes that protrude from the pad are better suited to contact the skin surface. The number of sessions required varies according to disorder, length of time that the disorder has been present and its severity.

Electrical stimulation – the longitudinal muscle channel system

Electrical stimulation is a tool available to the equine therapist for many purposes, such as tissue repair, reduction of swelling and mental relaxation, as well as for pain relief. A treatment strategy that the author has found to be particularly successful involves the use of the traditional Chinese medicine concept of the longitudinal muscle channel system combined with the western approach of the use of dermatome patterns.

Dermatomes are areas of skin that are innervated, essentially, by one spinal nerve. Sensory fibres and nociceptors from the skin, muscles, joints and viscera enter a specific spinal cord segment via the dorsal nerve root. These dermatomal patterns correspond loosely with the longitudinal muscle channels, as described in traditional Chinese medicine.

The longitudinal muscle channel system is an adaptation of the more familiar meridian system of acupuncture. Similar to the acupuncture meridians, each of the muscle channels has its own pathway, which generally follows the acupuncture meridian pathway but is much wider, covering larger areas of the body. All muscle channels start in the extremities and go to the trunk or head. Dermatome pathways begin in the extremities and go to the spine.

Electrical stimulation, using four electrodes, provides a convenient agent for applying this system of pain control for the horse. The equine therapist begins by identifying the dermatome and spinal segment involved. An electrode is then placed on the lesion site or on a distal area of the dermatome. A second electrode is placed on the related spinal segment.

The next step is to determine the muscle channel involved and to place an electrode on a significant point along the muscle channel. This trigger point may be a muscle–tendon junction, or a point that is significant acupuncturally. A fourth electrode is placed on the association point of the channel; these association points are found along a line running parallel to the spinal cord on the horse's back.

The electrical stimulation protocol is supported by a generally accepted model of pain control mechanisms, i.e. large sensory fibres in the area of pain are stimulated to block nociceptor transmission in ascending pathways in the spinal cord – a modified Wall's gate control theory. In contrast another commonly used therapy available to the equine therapist, acupuncture, relies on the stimulation of peripheral sites in the body to activate descending influences on pain transmission. The stimulation of acupuncture sites enhances the release of endogenous opiates for prolonged pain relief.

Twelve muscle channels are described in traditional Chinese medicine, each covering a specific area of the body. By incorporating these transmission pathways into an electrical stimulation treatment protocol, the equine therapist has the opportunity to combine a traditional western therapeutic approach with an eastern therapeutic paradigm that has stood the test of time.

Association points

If "the eyes are the windows to the soul", for the equine therapist the thoracolumbar region of the horse is a window to pathology in the body. This is due to the existence of acupuncture points, called association points, that lie on both sides of the spine in a line parallel to the spine about 7 cm from the spinous processes. This pathway is called the bladder meridian and can be thought of as a thread that runs through the fabric of the horse's fascia. Palpation anywhere along this thread causes a response at some other place in the body. The local twitch response is due to a burst of electrical activity which consists of action potential spikes of high amplitude and short duration. There is no discharge in the rest of the muscle, which is at rest.

Acupuncture theory is based on the concept that action taken on an acupuncture point on the surface of the body affects metabolic and disease processes inside the body and that these reactive surface sites offer reliable information for identifying where a problem exists in the limbs, hooves or body. These points are reactive to pressure when a problem exists in the associated body part, reactivity in association points may also indicate local back pain. This emphasises the need for a complete veterinary evaluation to understand the true nature of the discomfort. The list of association points in Table 23.2 and their descriptions come from the video, *Equine Veterinary Acupuncture*, created by Dr Meredith Snader [12]. Location descriptions are from the *Equine Atlas of Acupuncture Loci* by Peggy Fleming [13].

Association points can be an aid in understanding the origin of thoracolumbar pain and they can be used to treat it. There are a number of studies in the literature that support the use of acupunc-

Table 23.2   The anatomical site of association points and the condition that might be indicated by activity at the site

Association point	Anatomical site	Condition that might be indicated
BL13	Eighth intercostal space just caudal to the scapula	Medial splint
BL14	Ninth intercostal space	Foot or medial forelimb problem
BL15	Tenth intercostal space	Medial forelimb problem
BL16	Eleventh intercostal space	Back problems
BL18	Thirteenth and fourteenth intercostal spaces	Body soreness
BL20	Seventeenth intercostal space	Medial stifle or body soreness
BL21	Just caudal to the last rib	Stifle soreness
BL22	Intercostal space L1–2	Gynaecological problems – ovarian/testicular
BL23	Intercostal space L4–5	Contralateral forelimb problem
BL27	Lumbosacral space	Contralateral forelimb problem or sacroiliac joint
BL28	First interosseous foramen of the sacrum	Ovarian problems

ture in the treatment of back pain. A trial was conducted at the University of Florida to determine the value of electroacupuncture for treatment of horses with chronic thoracolumbar pain [14]. Horses with signs of chronic back pain received electroacupuncture while another group received phenylbutazone, a non-steroidal anti-inflammatory drug. Results provided evidence that three sessions of electroacupuncture treatment can successfully alleviate signs of thoracolumbar pain in horses. The analgesic effect induced by electroacupuncture can last at least 2 weeks. Phenylbutazone did not effectively alleviate signs of thoracolumbar pain in horses in this study. A study of the effects of acupressure (applying pressure with the thumbs or fingertips to the same points on the body stimulated in acupuncture) on human back pain concluded that acupressure was effective in reducing chronic low back pain in terms of disability, pain scores and functional status. Each of the 129 participants received six acupressure sessions within 1 month. One senior acupressure therapist gave each session of acupressure treatment to ensure a uniform technique and consistent experience. The benefit was seen not only in the short term, but was sustained for 6 months [15]. Reactivity in acupressure points can be reduced with the use of therapeutic laser and ultrasound, as well as electricity and tactile pressure.

A treatment example – "taut band" or muscular knotting

Local back pain is often manifested in a muscular condition referred to as a taut band. Taut muscle bands are regions within the muscle of increased pain and tension on palpation. They are described as fibrocystic nodules, ropiness of the muscle or knots in the muscle. A taut band is also known as a contracture. Contracture in the muscle makes it feel thick or hardened and tense compared with the surrounding tissue.

Muscle fibres in the taut band show no EMG activity at rest. Although the muscle feels tense and resists stretching, the absence of EMG activity means that the muscle is not in spasm; it is shortened for other reasons. Taut bands have been observed to persist after death, but can be released by acupressure or other equine therapy modalities applied to the area of most sensitivity, called the trigger point.

Normally, contractile activity of a muscle fibre is controlled by the rapid release and reabsorption of calcium from the sarcoplasm in the muscle. Release of calcium initiates contraction and return of calcium terminates contractile activity. The release of calcium is normally triggered by an action potential but, if trauma has damaged the sarcoplasm and spilled its calcium, the sarcomeres exposed to the calcium would sustain contractile activity as long as their ATP energy supply lasted. So the contractile activity would persist despite the absence of action potentials. The uncontrolled contractile activity of this portion of the muscle causes uncontrolled metabolism. Vasoconstriction in the region is needed to control excessive local metabolism. Stretching and acupressure consistently help to relax a taut band by providing brief anoxia to the local cells through stimulation of the release of neurotransmitters. Cortical recognition of back pain is blocked by the superficial tactile stimuli. Other means of deactivating the trigger point in a taut band include the use of therapeutic ultrasonography at a low intensity of $0.5\,W/cm^2$, 20% or 10% pulse rate, or with electrical stimulation, gradually increasing the intensity until it is just below the discomfort threshold. Laser therapy and ice massage are also effective.

Therapeutic exercise

The equine therapist's model of rehabilitation is based on that of the human athletic trainer. The therapeutic aspect is aggressive in terms of symptom relief and exercise plays an equally important role. Ground exercises improve musculoskeletal flexibility and increase the horse's kinaesthetic awareness, a factor in prevention of re-injury. Experimental and clinical studies demonstrate that early, controlled movement is superior to immobilisation for treatment of acute musculoskeletal soft tissue injuries and postoperative management. There are many books and videos that provide examples of ground exercises for the horse. Rehabilitation is dealt with in detail in Chapter 25, but three ground exercises that are of particular value to the horse with a stiff and painful back are described here.

Lateral flexion–extension exercise

Begin with the horse moving around the handler on a long rope, at least 8 feet (2.5 m) long. If the horse is moving in a clockwise direction the rope is in the handler's right hand. The handler reaches with the left hand to grasp the rope and direct the horse to bend its torso to the left and change directions on the circle. The handler must not step back to offer the horse a bigger space in which to turn. The horse must demonstrate lateral flexion–extension of the thoracolumbar spine to complete the movement. This exercise could be called "the waltz" because, when it is done correctly and repeatedly going from one direction to the other, it should be fluid and smooth like a dance.

Hip disengagement exercise

Using the long rope, bring it from the head down the right side of the body around the horse's hips to its other side. Gently pull the rope to direct the horses head to the right until the rear legs move in an abduction adduction motion. Continue until the horse faces the handles. This creates lateral flexion and extension throughout the entire spine, strengthens the adductor/abductor muscles in the hips, and gives the equine therapist clues to the functionality of the rear hip joints.

Dorsiflexion–extension exercise

Downward fingertip pressure on the horse's back alternates with upward pressure from the fingertips on the belly. A clinical manifestation of back pain results in diminished flexion–extension movement at or near the thoracic lumbar junction. Carrying out this exercise with several repetitions daily will enhance spinal mobility over time.

Conclusion

The equine therapist has much to offer the horse in terms of detecting, treating and, ultimately, avoiding back pain. Physical agents are used to reduce the symptoms of discomfort and to enable the horse to move more freely through the full range of joint movements in the spine and in the limbs. Beyond pain relief, physical agents support the repair process through stimulation of neurochemical agents that cause relaxation, or activate vasodilatation, and increase metabolism at the injury site. The addition of functional exercises completes the therapy session, leaving the horse more comfortable and more mobile.

References

1. Henson, F.M.D., Lamas, L., Knezevic, S. et al. Ultrasonographic evaluation of the supraspinous ligament in a series of ridden and unridden horses and horses with unrelated back pathology. *BMC Veterinary Research* 2007;**3**:3.
2. Erichsen, C., Eksell, P., Holm, K.R. et al. Relationship between scintigraphic and radiographic evaluations of spinous processes in the thoracolumbar spine in riding horses without clinical signs of back problems. *Equine Veterinary Journal* 2004;**36**: 458–465.
3. Holm, K.R., Wennerstrand, J., Lagerquist, U. et al. Effect of local analgesia on movement of the equine back. *Equine Veterinary Journal* 2006;**38**:65–69.
4. Irwin, C. *Dancing with your Dark Horse*. New York: Harlowe & Co., 2005.
5. Mossanen, A. The use of synaptic 1000 in the treatment of chronic pain in a neurological setting. Toronto East General Hospital, Ontario, Canada, 2002.
6. Tonasic, M. The bane that is pain. *Equine Disease Quarterly* 2004;2–3.
7. Landman, M.A., de Blaauw, J.A., van Weeren, P.R. et al. Field study of the prevalence of lameness in horses with back problems. *Veterinary Record* 2004;**155**:165–168.
8. Rooney, J.R. *The Mechanics of the Horse*. New York: RE Krieger Publishing, 1981.
9. Peham, C. and Schobesberger, H. Influence of the load of a rider or of a region with increased stiffness on the equine back: a modelling study. *Equine Veterinary Journal* 2004;**36**:703–705.
10. de Cocq, P., van Weeren, P.R. and Back, W. Effects of girth, saddle and weight on movements of the horse. *Equine Veterinary Journal* 2005;**37**:231–234.
11. Markoll, R., Da Silva Ferreira, D. and Toohill, T. PST: An overview. *Journal of Rheumatology* 2003;**6**:89–100.
12. Snader, M. *Equine Veterinary Acupuncture*, 2007. Available at: www.equinehealthcare.com.
13. Fleming, P. *Equine Atlas of Acupuncture Loci*. Dade City, FL: Florida Equine Acupuncture Center, 2000.
14. Xie, H., Colahan, P. and Ott, E.A. Evaluation of electroacupuncture treatment of horses with signs of chronic thoracolumbar pain. *Journal of the American Veterinary Medicine Association* 2005;**227**:281–286.
15. Hsieh, L.L.-C., Kuo, C-H., Lee, L.H. et al. Treatment of low back pain by acupressure and physical therapy: randomised controlled trial. *British Medical Journal* 2006;**332**:696–700.

24 Integrative Therapies in the Treatment of Back Pain

Joyce Harman

Introduction

Back pain is an important cause of loss of performance and economic loss in the horse industry. Conventional medicine may help treat back pain, but integrative medicine, also known as complementary and alternative medicine, can offer, in the author's opinion, many more solutions. The successful treatment of back pain requires multiple modalities, time and patience to achieve the best results. In most cases a return to the previous level of comfort and performance can be achieved. In many cases the level of comfort exceeds expectations, with the horse better able to perform than before being sidelined due to back pain.

The major integrative modalities used in the treatment of back pain include acupuncture, spinal manipulation (chiropractic, osteopathy), massage and the physical therapies (e.g. heat, cold, laser, ultrasonography, electrical stimulation) discussed in Chapter 23. Herbal and homoeopathic medicines are also used as adjunctive therapies. It is critical to check saddle fit and important to use various rehabilitation exercises.

The successful treatment of back pain, whether done with conventional or integrative therapy, requires a combination of treatment modalities and management changes. Management practices that directly influence back pain are saddle fit, feet, teeth, bitting, training styles, training aids and, of course, the rider's influence on the horse. When all aspects related to the back are corrected, the horse often returns to a higher level of performance than before it was diagnosed with a back problem.

Integrative approach to diagnosis of back pain

The symptoms of back pain can range from mild to intolerable and some symptoms are not as specific for back pain as others. In the author's opinion sinking down as the rider mounts is likely to be a symptom of back pain, while refusing a jump could be due to back or orthopaedic pain, as well as rider interference, or just that the horse hates to jump. However, many of the persistent difficulties encountered in training horses can be traced to back pain or back and neck pain.

The integrative practitioner uses similar techniques to those used by the veterinarian to make a diagnosis of back pain. However, the emphasis of the clinical examination is slightly different with closer attention paid to the way of moving and muscular function. A complete history needs to be taken, followed by observation of the horse at rest and in motion, with and without tack. The muscles and joints are palpated thoroughly. Standard diagnostic procedures such as nerve blocks and diagnostic imaging can be used. Therapies mentioned in this section, such as acupuncture and chiropractic, are discussed in more detail later in the text.

History of the horse with back pain

Pertinent history questions to focus on are:

- What is the primary complaint?
- When does the problem show up?
- What makes the problem better?
- What makes the problem worse?

Many riders want to blame their problems on the horse's attitude rather than back pain. Boxes 24.1 and 24.2 summarise common behavioural and performance-related symptoms of back pain.

Observation of the horse

Observe the shape of the back for muscle development or atrophy. Also note if there are any visible physical signs of trauma from the saddle. Trauma from an ill-fitting saddle almost invariably leaves some degree of back pain, even if the problem occurred with the previous owner (Box 24.3).

The horse should be observed standing at rest with no saddlery on. Note the natural stance of the horse, because many horses develop a compensatory positioning of the legs at rest when there is pain present. Some horses stand stretched out or "parked out" to rest their back, whereas others

---

> ### Box 24.1   Summary of behavioural problems related to back pain
>
> Objects to being saddled
> Hypersensitive to brushing
> Exhibits a "bad attitude"
> Difficult to shoe
> Bucks or rolls excessively
> Rearranges the stall bedding constantly
> Displays repetitive behaviours
> Piles up bedding in stall to stand on or leans
>   on the wall

> ### Box 24.2   Summary of performance problems that may indicate back pain
>
> "Cold backed" during mounting
> Slow to warm up or relax
> Resists work
> Reluctant to stride out
> Hock, stifle and obscure hindlimb lameness
> Front leg lameness, stumbling and tripping
> Excessive shying, lack of concentration on rider
>   and aids
> Rushes downhill, or pulls uphill with the front
>   end (exhibits improper use of back or
>   hindquarters)
> Demonstrates an inability to travel straight
> Is unwilling or unable to round the back or
>   neck
> Displays difficulty maintaining good stride
> Falters or resists when making a transition
> Bucks or rears regularly

---

stand with their limbs underneath their bodies. Look at the shoeing, because unbalanced feet lead to alterations in stance, movement [1] and upper body pain. Does the horse always rest one foot, or place one foot in a certain position? Can the horse stand square if asked?

Look at the horse from all angles for symmetry and asymmetry. Many horses' shoulders are uneven. Stand the horse squarely on level ground and look at the points of the shoulders, the carpi and slope of the distal metacarpals, as well as the shape of the feet. Stand directly behind the horse, noting asymmetries in the pelvic structure, muscle mass over the hindquarters and in the gaskins, and the shapes of the feet. Make a note of the differences.

Place a stool behind the horse and stand above the horse's back, looking down. Be sure that the horse is standing square, though it may be impossible to be square in front and behind at the same time due to discomfort. The shoulders often appear asymmetrical from differences in muscle tension. This can lead to saddle-fitting problems, stiffness and imbalances in movement. Observe the entire spine up into the neck for asymmetries.

Observe the horse walking and jogging in hand, while being lunged and with a rider mounted.

Many horses move freely on the lunge line, but with a rider the horse loses its free movement, or adversely changes its movement, a strong indication of back pain.

Biomechanically, the head, neck, back and hindquarters are connected and move together, so, if a horse carries his neck in a raised "upside-down" (dorsiflexed), hollow position, the back is also going to be hollow. The hollow position of the back will alter the position of the pelvis, making it impossible to engage the hindquarters correctly underneath its body. To allow the horse to use its back properly the *rectus abdominis* muscles, *iliopsoas*, *tensor fasci latae* and *quadriceps* (all protractor muscles of the hind limbs) must contract.

As the horse's back becomes hollow or stiff, the hindlegs cannot engage properly, and the front feet tend to hit the ground hard. Unnatural strain is placed on the stifles and hocks, creating lameness or soreness. Common incorrect back movement leads to horses with an attractive headset, a motionless back and relaxed abdominal muscles.

The rider may feel that the horse is "off" or just not quite right on a particular limb. To the observer, the main sign is often stiffness or resistance in one direction or another, but the horse is not lame enough to warrant the use of local analgesic techniques to localise pain in the suspect limb. In some horses, multiple limbs may be involved, which may well manifest as a general stiffness. A stiff spine means that the horse is not moving correctly and the muscles of the back are painful or in spasm. In other cases it is clear that the horse is protecting a painful part of the body, often the back. As the horse moves stiffly and incorrectly, over time, the distal limbs may become affected secondarily, slowly resulting in overt lameness. In the author's opinion, correct treatment during the back pain stage may prevent distal limb lameness.

Palpation of the back

Palpation skills are enhanced by learning acupuncture and chiropractic approaches to treating horses. The information gathered by specific palpation allows the practitioner to make a complete diagnosis and treatment plan.

The first palpation is a gentle passing of the practitioner's hands over the entire neck, back and thorax, looking for muscle tension, sensitivity, flinching or discomfort. A light touch often reveals more than a heavy touch and much practice is needed to develop the light touch.

Acupuncture palpation and diagnosis

The next stage is the acupuncture palpation and diagnosis. This involves palpation of the acupuncture meridians looking for pain or tension. The most common meridian to palpate for back pain is the bladder meridian. The section of the bladder meridian used is about 10 cm lateral to the midline of the spine in an average-sized horse, beginning in the pocket just behind the shoulder blade and ending near the tail. This meridian is one of the most important pathways in the body and is easily affected by ill-fitting saddles.

As the practitioner's fingers gain experience palpating for acupuncture points, subtle changes can be found. Any sensitivity found along the back will cause the horse to alter its gait. Pain in the back and neck acupuncture points may, in the author's opinion, be the origin of distal limb problems.

Chiropractic examination

The chiropractic examination is the next stage. All joints in the body including the spine should move smoothly through their entire range of motion. Many horses have lost normal motion throughout their spine, resulting in stiffness and pain. To examine the range of motion, the practitioner gently moves the spine through its normal range, looking and feeling for stiffness. A carrot can be held by the horse's hip, stifle and down between the front limbs to check neck mobility (the "carrot stretch"); then the back can be raised (ventroflexion) by pressing on the ventral midline to contract rectus abdominis ("sit-ups" for horses).

A normal horse can reach its hip and close to its stifle, as well as reach down well between its forelimbs. The back should be able to rise up easily, resulting in the horse extending and lowering its neck. A horse can become very upset if raising its

> **Box 24.3   Physical evidence of poor saddle fit**
>
> Obvious sores
> White hairs
> Temporary swellings after removing the saddle
> Scars or hard spots in the muscle or skin
> Muscle atrophy on the sides of the withers
> Friction rubs in the hair

back is painful. If the horse cannot raise its back while standing still, it will not be able to raise its back with a rider in place, which is the goal in many sports. Loss of normal motion at the junction of the ribs and the sternum, or loss of motion through the withers, mid-thorax or the thoracolumbar area, usually produces pain when raising the back.

The practitioner then does a specific motion palpation of the individual joints of the spine and extremities looking for restrictions. Healthy joints move freely and have spring to them, whereas problem joints often feel stiff.

Muscle palpation is also important, starting with a light touch and moving deeper to assess muscle quality. A healthy muscle will feel soft and springy; the horse will not object in any way to the palpation. A muscle under tension will feel tight and hard, and have little spring. A muscle in spasm will be more likely to become injured and will take a long time to warm up, because there is less blood flow through the spasm. Sometimes a horse will "splint" its back, or hold it rigidly in place while being examined, to avoid moving it. This reflects pain.

As the palpation is being done, if signs of saddle-induced injuries are found, they indicate that there has been a problem with a saddle, either past or present (Box 24.3). If a poorly fitted saddle has been used on a horse for any length of time, there will be residual back pain and probably loss of normal motion of the thoracic and lumbar vertebrae.

The use of diagnostic imaging

When evaluating horses for back pain, diagnostic imaging of all types can be used to complete the picture. However, as noted in other chapters, it is common to have minimal or non-specific radiographic and scintigraphic changes. This is partly because considerable back pain in the horse and indeed other species is often due to soft tissue injury rather than to the degenerative bone and joint disease that radiography and nuclear scintigraphy provide information about. A diagnostic imaging modality that can provide information on soft tissue inflammation is thermography (see Chapter 12). Thermography detects areas of increased and decreased blood flow and, in horses that have inflammatory processes causing pain, an increase in body surface temperature may be detected. In contrast chronic pain, in many cases, shows up as decreased blood flow and cool areas in the muscle [2]. Anti-inflammatory therapy will not affect the cool areas; manual therapies such as acupuncture, chiropractic, osteopathy and massage will increase blood flow and reduce pain, and may be useful in these cases.

Saddle fit

Poor saddle fit is perhaps one of the primary contributors to back pain and must be addressed in an examination for back pain (Box 24.4). Saddle fit should be considered as important as, and similar to, shoe fit in a person.

Saddle structure

Saddle structure is extremely important and the manufacture of saddles has seldom included quality control. Many new saddles are purchased with serious defects such as panels and flaps installed asymmetrically and/or twisted trees. The initial cost of the saddle seems to have no bearing on the number or severity of structural defects to be found. Examine the saddle carefully from all angles to check for balance and symmetry. Minor differences from one side to the other can be tolerated, but most differences that can be easily seen will create pain or cause the rider difficulty in finding the correct position in the saddle.

Box 24.4   Considerations when assessing saddle fit in a horse with suspected back pain

The structure of the saddle

The position of the saddle on the back

The contact of the bars or panels against the horse's back; absence of bridging

Must have enough rocker and twist to the bars to conform to the horse's back (western)

Whether the panels are wide enough for good support (English)

Whether the gullet is wide enough to clear the spine completely (2.5–3 inches or 6.4–7.5 cm) (English)

Whether the gullet is the correct width and tall enough to clear the withers (western)

The fit of the tree to the horse's back, especially across the withers

Whether the saddle sits squarely in the centre of the back

The levelness of the seat

The placement of the girth

How the rider fits in the saddle

Position of the stirrup bars or stirrup placement

Saddle position

Saddle position is the most critical aspect of saddle fit. Commonly, the saddle is placed too far forward. This position places the rigid tree over the top of the shoulder blade, which significantly restricts the movement of the front legs. If the saddle is moved back to the correct position the stride will generally lengthen immediately. When an English saddle is placed too far forward, the pommel is too high. This causes the seat to slope down towards the cantle and places the rider's legs too far forward in an unbalanced position. The rider then tries to level the seat with pads under the back of the saddle.

Western saddles, when too far forward, exert enormous pressure on the top of the scapula. Moving the saddle back to the correct position frees the scapula but can put the rider and the saddle too far back. Saddles with shorter bars –

such as those used in barrel racing or for Arabians – can be easier to move back into the correct position due to the shorter bar. The shorter bar may still be too straight.

If the saddle, no matter what type it is, does not fit, no change in position will correct the problem.

Saddle panels and bars

The saddle must sit squarely down the middle of the back supported by the bars or panels sitting evenly over longissimus dorsi. The dorsal spinous processes have no muscle covering, so there is little soft tissue to protect them from saddle pressure.

A bar or panel should conform to the shape of the back. If it is too flat or long, a bridge will be created with pressure on the shoulders and the back of the saddle. The weight becomes distributed on four points, one on each side of the withers/shoulder blade and one on each side of the back at the rear of the saddle. Some flexible panelled endurance saddles cannot follow the contour, while a treeless saddle naturally follows the shape of the back.

English panels need to be wide enough to offer good support. The gullet needs to be wide enough (2.5–3 inches or 6–7.5 cm) to allow the spine both complete freedom from pressure and to bend slightly laterally during movement. The angle of the panels needs to follow the angle of the horse's back under the cantle. Saddles can have too acute an angle, putting pressure on the outer corner of the panel.

English saddles need to be reflocked (restuffed) every year or even more frequently. Finding a competent saddler to do this can be a challenge. Wool stuffing is very useful because it is resilient and offers a smooth surface to the horse's back. High-quality foam-stuffed panels can be excellent, whereas low-quality ones lose their resilience in a few years' time. Foam is hard to adjust and replace but does not need restuffing.

Western bars should put pressure only on the ribcage; any part of the saddle extending past the eighteenth rib should not put any pressure on the loins. Bars need to have enough rocker (curve to the bottom) and flair (curve at the ends) so that the bar shape conforms to the shape of the horse's back. Very few trees have enough shape. Skirts need to be short and flared so that they do not interfere with the shoulders or loins.

Saddle trees

The tree must follow the contour of the withers without the use of pads. If the tree is too narrow for the withers, the front will sit up high, unbalancing the rider. If the rider then places pads under the back of the saddle to raise it, more pressure is placed on the withers. If a saddle is too wide across the withers the rider will be tipped forward and the saddle may make contact with the withers.

Unfortunately many saddles are poorly designed. Cheap western saddles may have the bar grooved too deeply for the stirrup leathers, leaving what appears to be a bulge at the base of the fork. English close-contact jumping saddles may have an outward flare in the tree where the withers are flat in shape. Other saddles, especially dressage and a few western/endurance saddles, have pressure points underneath the stirrup bars or attachments.

The importance of a level seat

An important aid in determining saddle fit is that the seat must be level when viewed from the side and the rider must be placed in the centre of the seat. If the seat is not level or the lowest point is incorrectly placed, the rider will be out of balance, either tipped forward, if the saddle is down at the front, or tipped back into a chair seat, if the saddle is too high at the front. Roll a pill bottle on the seat to see where the lowest point is.

Position and shape of the girth

The girth will always finish the ride in the narrowest point of the ribcage. It must drop naturally perpendicularly into this space or the saddle will move either forward or back as the girth finds its natural spot. Some horses' girth spots are close to

the elbows, whereas others are one to two handbreaths behind the elbow. An otherwise well-fitting saddle can become a poorly fitting saddle just by having the girth attached in the wrong place.

Short girths (both the western girths and the short dressage girths) can cause discomfort. The correct length is to have the buckle or rigging just below the saddle, out of the rider's way and away from the horse's elbow.

Rider fit

If the saddle does not fit the rider, the rider becomes the saddle-fitting problem. The most common fault is having the seat too small for the rider, forcing him or her to sit at the back of the saddle.

The position of the stirrup attachment is critical to the comfort and balance of the rider. Stirrup leathers placed too far forward will cause the rider's legs to drift forward, leaving them in a chair-seat position.

On western saddles in particular, the ground seat is made too wide for the rider's legs to drop comfortably down to the side. The wide seat pushes the thigh out to the side so that the knees cannot lie against the horse's side. This rolls the pelvis back and prevents the correct use of the lower leg.

Locating pressure points

The most obvious way of ascertaining whether chronic pressure points have been experienced under a saddle is if white hairs appear under there – indicating that there is a pressure point above them. On a western saddle the sheepskin covering of the panels will become worn down over the pressure points. One way to locate pressure points is to ride with a thin, clean, white, saddle pad. Dark spots that appear after 15 or 20 minutes will usually be pressure points. Light areas or areas with no sweat are generally from a lack of pressure, but, be careful, these can also be caused by excess pressure which decreases the amount of sweat produced.

Measuring the back for saddle fitting

To measure the horse's back for some assistance in fitting saddles, a flexible ruler from an office supply store is a tool that is easy to use and works well as a rough guide to the fit of the tree. Such a ruler can be moulded to the shape of the horse's withers; then a drawing can be made on cardboard and cut out. If this is done at 4-inch (10-cm) intervals along the saddle area, a basic diagram of the horse's back can be constructed. By holding the cut-out shapes of the back inside a saddle, a very general idea of whether the saddle may fit can be obtained. Several new methods, including computerized pressure analysis and thermography, are available to help with fitting saddles.

Rider variables

The rider, by virtue of the fact that he or she is sitting on top of the horse, has an enormous influence on the horse's back. Sally Swift and her concept of "centred riding" [3] has demonstrated very clearly that, if a part of the rider is stiff, that stiffness will be reflected in the horse directly. Most riders have some degree of back pain or other old injuries that create stiffness in their body; this is transferred directly to the horse.

As veterinarians, making suggestions about the rider is the most difficult aspect of the problem to solve, because most riders do not want to hear that they need to change; they have hired the veterinarian to "fix" their horse. Riders must be handled carefully, because if they are offended they will look elsewhere for someone to "fix" their horses.

The use of therapeutic pads

Therapeutic pads are often used to try to solve saddle-fit problems. Much of the time the pads provide only temporary relief and may cause more problems than they solve in the long run. The addition of the pad to a saddle is similar to a person adding an extra sock to his or her shoe. If the tree of the saddle is wide enough the pad may help. If the tree is already too narrow, and this is the most common scenario, the addition of the pad causes more pressure on the withers, the pommel may sit higher in front, which unbalances the rider, who then adds some more pads under the back of the saddle, raising the back of the saddle and driving more pressure onto the withers. Muscles will atrophy along each side of the withers from increased pressure.

The addition of a pad may cause a dramatic improvement in a horse's performance. This may last for a short time, but the same problems usually return, because the pad changes the fit of the saddle and moves the pressure points slightly but seldom eliminates them. Over time pressure points find their way through the pads.

A saddle properly fitted with a pad to act as an interface and shock absorber can be a big help. Many pads are useful; the secret is to select the pad with care and fit it with the saddle, just as you would fit a shoe with the type of sock that it will be worn with. For long distance horses it is especially important that the pads breathe due to the long hours in the saddle.

Shims are thin pads that can be placed under a part of the saddle to make a temporary change in fit. If shims are used carefully they can solve many problems. Be sure that they do not interfere with saddle fit.

Teeth, mouth pain

Pain in the mouth, either from poorly cared for teeth or bit pain, can mimic or cause back pain. Mouth pain will cause a horse to travel with its head high and neck hollowed, which leads to a hollow or dropped down back. As the back hollows muscle tightness is created, altered gait patterns occur and back pain is the result. Mouth pain must be corrected, with quality teeth care, a change in bits or an improvement in rider skill.

Additional management factors influencing back pain

Many other management and training practices can, in the author's opinion, cause back pain:

- *Ponying racehorses:* torques the muscles and vertebrae in the neck and back; primarily done in America.

- *Lunging, round pen work*, especially for long periods of time, or at a fast pace as is done in round pen training with young horses.
- *Training aids* range from benign to abusive. These cause at least one joint to brace against the device. The best way to use them is to interval train for a few minutes, then release and reconnect after a few minutes of rest.
- *Mechanical hot-walkers* place the horse in a hollow position with the head and neck up in the air causing the back to hollow also. Old-fashioned hand walking or caged hot-walkers are much better
- *Swimming* has an excellent place in the rehabilitation of lameness. However, the hollow position of the back tightens back muscles and can increase back pain.
- *Blankets* are an important source of back and wither pain. Blankets cut out over the withers cause a vice-like tightness between the caudal aspect of the withers and the points of the shoulders. The cranial thoracic vertebrae with their long dorsal processes often become subluxated, as do the attachments of the first few ribs to the sternum. The shoulder muscles become compressed, and the stride shortens significantly. To compensate, the horse then tightens up the entire back and shortens the stride. Blankets should be selected to fit as loosely over the shoulder as possible so that, after the horse has been turned out all night, it should still be easy to open the buckles. The most effective shape is one that comes over the withers and up onto the neck. Use new lightweight and durable materials. An old blanket can be adapted by adding darts in the centre of the neck area; this pulls the blanket away from the shoulder [4].

Treatments for back pain

Acupuncture

In this author's practice, acupuncture is an extremely useful treatment for back pain. Approximately 85–90% of the horses treated return to their previous level of performance in one to four treatments given about 1 month apart. When clients are unwilling or unable to correct management issues or the horses are in hard work, the horse must be maintained with regular preventive treatments. Human athletes have discovered that it is necessary to maintain some regular form of musculoskeletal therapy to keep maximum performance with minimum injury because continued athletic activity puts a certain degree of strain on the musculoskeletal system.

Acupuncture is best known for its treatment of back pain and arthritis. It is best performed by a veterinarian with advanced training in the technique. Practitioners who just pick a few standard points or follow a single formula will find that their results are inconsistent. A significant improvement with one to three or four treatments is considered a normal response. If a significant positive response (not necessarily a cure, but a definite improvement) is not achieved in horses after four treatments, the diagnosis was wrong, the pathology is too far advanced or the treatment is incorrect. Maintenance treatments can often slow the progression of degeneration and give pain relief even if no cure is possible.

Acupuncture operates on the concept that there is another system in the body in addition to the cardiovascular and neurological systems [5]. Similar to vessels in the cardiovascular system, and the nerves in the nervous system, there are pathways along the body through which there is a flow of energy, or as the Chinese call it "chi" or "qi". Along these pathways, called meridians, are acupuncture points. Acupuncture points are real structures with arterioles, venules, fine nerve endings and mast cells [6]. The points have a lower electrical resistance than the rest of the body so it is possible to measure the points with a modified ohmmeter [7].

It is easiest to understand the acupuncture system if it is compared with an electrical system. The points are like dimmer switches in that, if the flow of qi becomes blocked, it is similar in concept to turning the dimmer switch down and not allowing much electricity through. If a point is treated with acupuncture, it is like turning the dimmer switch back on and allowing qi to flow again. Sometimes qi gets backed up behind the blockage or the dimmer switch, and treating the point allows a more even flow of energy.

Acupuncture points can be stimulated in many ways, including by needles, electrical stimulation, moxa (a herbal form of heat), injection of vitamin B$_{12}$, cold laser stimulation, and massage or acupressure. Horses are generally very receptive to the treatment. Several excellent textbooks are available on the subject [5, 6] and courses are taught internationally (see Organisations and courses at end of chapter).

Chiropractic and spinal manipulation

Restricted motion in a joint may primarily be due to osseous pathology or, conversely, in the author's opinion, lead to pain, reduced performance and osseous pathology. As described elsewhere in this book, significant spinal pathology is well recognised in the horse. Restoration of normal spinal movement is the goal of spinal manipulation [8]. Full range of motion in all joints allows the horse to perform comfortably, and with flexibility in its back [9, 10].

During motion palpation of the back the chiropractic practitioner locates joints with restricted motion, and aims to restore motion to that segment of the spine.

Spinal manipulation of horses is usually performed using chiropractic manipulation or osteopathy. These are different modalities although their goal is to restore function to the spinal cord and nerve supply. Training is critical before a practitioner is qualified to work on a horse and cannot be accomplished in a weekend or through a correspondence course. Courses are available worldwide, and only qualified practitioners should be referred to.

Chiropractic is often misunderstood partly due to the use of the word "subluxation". The traditional medical definition of a subluxation is a partial dislocation. Modern chiropractic terminology uses the vertebral subluxation complex (VSC) to describe all the manifestations of the biomechanical and neurological components of the alteration of normal dynamics, anatomical or physiological relationships of contiguous articular surfaces in the spine – the term does not necessarily refer to a partial dislocation. The research behind chiropractic techniques is extensive, although only a few studies have been done directly within the equine field [11, 12].

The physiological stages of the VSC show that symptoms (pain) do not begin to manifest until kinesiopathy, myopathy, neuropathy, vascular abnormalities, connective tissue disorders and inflammation have all begun. Once signs of pain are present the next stage is degeneration of the joints [8]. Consequently, the reason for regular chiropractic adjustments is to prevent getting to the stage of pain.

A chiropractic adjustment is a short-lever, high-velocity, controlled thrust, by hand or instrument directed at a specific articulation in a single motor unit (two vertebrae and the associated nerves, tendons, ligaments and soft tissue) [8]. Chiropractic adjustments do not require great strength, just skill in making the short, sharp thrust, and knowledge of how to direct that thrust. This author adjusts all sizes of horses from ponies to draft horses with her hands with no difficulty.

A manipulation, as is frequently done in the name of chiropractic or osteopathy, is a non-specific, forceful passive movement of a joint beyond its active range of motion, generally done with a long lever by jerking a leg or twisting the entire neck. Manipulations can result in damage to the joint capsules and the joints themselves. Initially improvement in flexibility and performance is often seen, so these practitioners stay in business, but the long-term joint damage starts immediately. The effects of manipulations may not show up for several years. This style is most common with lay practitioners, but is unfortunately seen with trained veterinarians, chiropractors and osteopaths who should know better.

Untrained practitioners can use some simple exercises, such as the carrot stretches and belly lifts described below, find restricted or abnormal areas of motion, and begin to restore that motion to the spine; owners can continue those exercises.

Stretching

Stretching is one of the simplest, most effective ways to enhance back pain treatment, aid in rehabilitation after injury or help locate areas that may be of concern. Stretching can be performed by the owner on a regular basis or by the veterinarian as part of an examination and treatment. In this author's experience horses who are stretched on a regular basis (daily or at least two to four times a week) are generally more flexible through their back and stay sounder than horses who are not stretched.

Stretching must be done correctly and carefully to avoid injury. The use of force can damage muscles and joints. Any joint can be stretched safely to restore its full range of motion if the handler holds the leg in position and waits for the horse to release and relax the muscles. The stretch can be taken further as the horse continues to release muscle tension. A horse is always stronger than its handler, so, if force is applied and the horse pulls back, it will only tighten the very muscle that the handler is trying to loosen. The following stretches are used:

- *Carrot stretch:* the horse is asked with a carrot or other treat to reach to the tuber coxae and down between the front legs. A horse with normal flexibility can reach its tuber coxae by moving its head and neck directly around without twisting it down. This stretch restores flexibility to the neck, withers and thoracic area, with some muscle stretching as far as the lumbar area. Often a horse has restricted motion in its neck and cannot complete the stretch. Some horses may need spinal manipulation to restore complete motion.
- *Belly lifts:* these stretches (regular and lateral) restore dorsoventral and lateral motion through the thorax and are perhaps the most important stretches for the back. Many horses are incapable of performing all or parts of this stretch without significant pain and will kick or bite, so caution must be used. Perform this stretch very gently and carefully, to try to keep the horse comfortable and relaxed so the muscles stretch rather than contract:
  - Dorsoventral belly lift: the handler places the fingertips on the midline of the sternum behind the elbows and presses upwards. The fingers can be moved along the midline to the centre of the abdomen to raise and stretch different parts of the back. Start with a light touch and increase pressure until the back rises. In some cases a blunt plastic tool such as a needle cap or plastic writing pen may be needed to raise the back.
  - Lateral belly lift: stand on one side of the horse and reach across the midline up into

the girth area behind the elbows on the opposite side. Pull the ribcage diagonally upwards towards the withers on the side on which the handler is standing (towards the handler's head). When belly lifts are comfortable for the horse, the abdominal muscles should contract, the longissimus muscles should fill out and relax, the withers should rise, and then the head and neck should stretch forwards and down. With the lateral belly lifts the ribcage should move easily laterally, the same on both sides. The withers on the side that the handler is standing should fill with relaxed muscle, while the opposite side should form an even concave bend. The head and neck should stretch down and forward, curved slightly away from the handler. When there are pain and tension, parts of the *longissimus* group of muscles will contract, which can be seen by depressed areas or muscle spasms in the muscle as the back is raised. Pain may be from muscle tension or as a result of the loss of motion or arthritis, which may be present throughout the spine and may require chiropractic care to restore. When back pain is present the head and neck usually rise up during this stretch.

- *Withers stretch:* this can relieve tension and pain through the cranial thorax. The handler places his or her hands over the withers, and leans back, gently pulling on the withers. Start at the cranial edge (T3–4) and move towards the caudal part (T9–11). When the stretch is ended, the handler should release the withers slowly. If there is little pain, and the horse is enjoying the stretch, it will pull against the handler and relax into the stretch. If there is significant pain, muscle fasciculations and spasms may be felt under the handler's hands and the horse will not pull into the stretch. Proceed gently if this reaction should occur and hold the stretch until the muscles relax. This stretch is especially useful for horses wearing tight blankets.
- *Psoas stretch:* this is one of the most important stretches for the back and can be combined with a stretch for semimembranosis and semitendinosis (hamstring). When the psoas muscle

is tight it prevents the caudal stretch of the hindleg. This stretch is performed by holding the leg either caudal (psoas) or cranial (hamstring) to the vertical at the limit of the range of motion, then waiting for the horse to release the leg a bit. As the muscle relaxes, the stretch can go further until the leg reaches the back of the knee (hamstring stretch) or can touch the ground behind the vertical (psoas). If force is used, the horse will pull back and tighten the muscle. If the horse is comfortable with the stretch, it will release the leg quickly: if uncomfortable, it may release only small amounts at a time.

- *Psoas release:* an excellent therapeutic release for the psoas, sacroiliac and lumbar muscles can be performed. The leg is held up a few inches off the ground in a comfortable position for the horse; gentle movements are made in a circular fashion for a minute. Then, for the next 2 minutes, the leg is brought progressively higher until it is flexed much as the leg would be for a regular flexion test. The gentle movement is kept and, if the horse needs to put the leg down, set it gently on the ground vertical or forward of vertical, not in a caudal position. This is not a daily stretch as much as it is used as therapy for the caudal part of the back. The activity is performed daily for about a week, then two to three times a day for another week or two, to be repeated if necessary.

Massage

Massage therapy consists of manipulation of the muscle using a variety of techniques depending on the problem and the background of the practitioner. Massage can be very specific to treat a small area such as trigger point therapy (also known as myotherapy or neuromuscular therapy) where the practitioner applies concentrated finger pressure to "trigger points" (painful irritated areas in muscles) to break cycles of spasm and pain. Trigger points can commonly occur in any muscle, but are common in the gluteal muscles and longissimus dorsi over the last few ribs and lumbar muscles.

Massage techniques can be used to treat specific muscle injuries, for prevention of injuries, pre-event preparation and post-event recovery. Damaged, contracted muscle has less blood flow through the capillaries than healthy muscle. If an injury to a muscle is recent, massage techniques are used to enhance the clearing of lymphatic fluid and blood from the area of damage and to reduce swelling. Once the injury is older and has become chronic, massage is used to restore circulation and flexibility. Massage is currently routinely used on many human athletic teams to prevent and treat muscle injuries and should be used more routinely with equine athletes.

Massage is performed, in most cases, by laypeople, many of whom have little training other than a 1-week course. At the present time, the best way to find a qualified person is to locate someone who has completed a full 500-hour human massage course and who has then taken one of the more extensive equine courses offered. Veterinarians would be well advised to locate a few top quality massage therapists for client referrals so that effective therapy is performed.

Homoeopathic treatment of back pain

Homoeopathy is a branch of complementary medicine [13] that is perhaps the least well understood of the modalities, yet it is useful in the treatment of back pain, especially that caused by injury. Homoeopathic remedies can be used in conjunction with any conventional treatments, although, as a practitioner becomes more comfortable with this type of therapy, faster results can be achieved by using the remedies alone, along with any required supportive care.

Homoeopathic medicine approaches disease in a different manner to allopathic (conventional) medicine. Conventional thinking considers each disease to have a consistent, recognisable set of signs and symptoms that should then be treated with a specific drug or therapy. In homoeopathy symptoms are regarded as an expression of an imbalance present in the body, which can be from internal weakness or an external force that disturbs the workings of the body. The symptoms are the result of the body trying to correct the imbalance.

Allopathic treatment of a disease such as arthritis asks questions about how much pain the patient has and whether the current treatment is helping. Treatment usually includes one of a variety of similar-acting anti-inflammatories or a cyclo-oxygenase 2 (COX-2) inhibitor type of drug. As the disease progresses, the drug dosage is usually increased in order to counteract the symptoms.

Homoeopathic treatment of the same disease examines the patient from a broader perspective and asks questions about the type of pain (sharp, dull, stiff) and the modalities – what makes the pain better, worse (weather, season of the year, motion or lack of motion), and whether there are visible changes to the shape of the joints. The treatment is tailored to the individual, with a different remedy for each presenting set of symptoms. This variability in treatment plan, depending on the individual's response to a disease, is what makes it difficult to perform traditional double-blind research studies [14].

Homoeopathic remedies are usually supplied in small tablets or sand-sized granules listed with a potency (strength) of 6X, 12X, 12C, 30X, 30C or 200C. The standard dose for an adult horse is six to eight tablets, or one half-teaspoon of granules, three to five for a pony or foal. The remedies can be given once or twice a day (for the 200C), or two to three times a day for the 30X or C potency, and can be fed with small quantities of food or placed directly in the mouth.

Homoeopathic remedies are prepared by diluting the original substance, so they will not test positive in a drug test during competition in the strengths described here. They are prepared according to exacting standards and are regulated by the FDA (*Homeopathic Pharmacopoeia*). Several remedies are particularly useful in treating back pain.

Arnica montana is a homeopathic remedy used by this author very successfully to decrease the pain, swelling, stiffness and healing time in many traumatic injuries of the back. Arnica, in this author's experience, is useful in helping chronic or long-standing back pain. The remedy can be given one to three times daily, with the more frequent dosing used when the injury is more severe. Arnica can be administered at any point in the healing process to improve the healing; however, if it is started at the time of the injury, the results are quicker than if started later [15].

Ruta graveolens (Ruta grav) is a remedy that has particular affinity for injuries to the periosteum, tendons and ligaments. The back contains many small joints and associated structures. In cases of chronic back pain, Ruta grav can be given two to three times a week for several weeks, followed by the next remedy (Rhus tox).

Rhus toxicodendron (Rhus tox) is indicated when an injury to muscle, tendon, ligament or joint has healed to the point where the horse is stiff when starting out, but warms up and moves much better. Rhus tox can be given for 2–5 days in a row, then may be given one to three times a week for a few weeks. Rhus tox is also commonly used for arthritic conditions of any joint, because the most common complaint is that the condition is better after being warmed up.

Ledum palustra (marsh tea)

Ledum is a remedy that is well indicated for arthritic pains of the small joints including those in the back, with or without inflammation and worse with motion. The pains associated with Ledum may move from place to place, as is often the case in Lyme disease. Pain is better with cold hosing, and can be worse after bandaging.

Traumeel

Traumeel is a combination of many homoeopathic remedies, used in low potencies. It is available as a topical, internal and injectable format in most countries. Clinical studies in Germany have shown Traumeel to be useful in treating muscle pain. Clinically this author has found Traumeel to be a helpful adjunct in treating back pain.

Herbal therapy for back pain

Herbs have been used for centuries to treat various injuries and, in China, the martial arts practitioners used herbal preparations to strengthen tendons and ligaments also. Herbs can be used internally (as powders or teas) as well as externally as an ointment, liniment or poultice. Herbs contain active ingredients and certain herbs can cause a positive in blood tests for drugs, mainly when ingested. Practitioners should become aware of herbs that may test positive (yucca, white willow bark, for example) and use caution when prescribing.

Arnica montana can used as a poultice, ointment, body wash or liniment, as a topical treatment for bruising, or muscle, tendon and ligament injuries, as well as overworked and tired muscles. Arnica should never be used on broken skin because it is irritating. Its primary action is anti-inflammatory; however, it is not powerful enough to mask pain as a non-steroidal anti-inflammatory would.

Internally, dried herbs or liquid extracts of devil's claw, meadowsweet, white willow bark and yucca are all known for their anti-inflammatory action. In general herbs such as these take several days of feeding or longer for the effects to be seen, so they are usually more effective when given for chronic problems rather than acute ones. Products containing anti-inflammatory herbs can be used in acute situations. However, for more immediate results, the practitioner may wish to try the homoeopathic remedies listed above. Please note that some "herbal" supplements may contain additives that are not permitted by the governing council under which the horse competes and the veterinarian must consider this before recommending a remedy.

Conclusion

Treatment of back pain requires a whole-horse approach to be consistently successful. The rewards are great because performance often improves to better than the previous level. There are many causes of back pain that need to be identified, followed by an individually tailored programme to best aid in the recovery.

References

1. Chateau, H., Degueurce, C., Jerbi, H. et al. Normal three-dimensional behaviour of the metacarpophalangeal joint and the effect of uneven foot bearing. *Equine Veterinary Journal* 2001;**33**:84–88.
2. von Schweinitz, D.G. Thermographic diagnostics. In: Haussler, K.K. (ed.), *Veterinary Clinics of North America: Back pain*. Philadelphia: W.B. Saunders Co., 1999;161–173.
3. Swift, S. *Centered Riding*. North Pomfret: Trafalgar Square Books, 1985.
4. Harman, J.C. *The Horse's Pain Free Back and Saddle Fit Book*. North Pomfret: Trafalgar Square Books, 2008.
5. Xie, H., Colahan, P. and Ott, E.A. Evaluation of electroacupuncture treatment of horses with signs of chronic thoracolumbar pain. *Journal of the American Veterinary Medicine Association* 2005;**227**:281–286.
6. Schoen, A. *Veterinary Acupuncture: From ancient art to modern medicine*. 2nd edn. St Louis, MO: Mosby, 2001.
7. Steiss, J.E. Neurophysiological basis of acupuncture. In: Schooen, A.M. (ed.), *Veterinary Acupuncture: From ancient art to modern medicine*, 2nd edn. St Louis, MO: Mosby, 2001;342–343.
8. Haussler, K.K., Chiropractic evaluation and management. In: Haussler, K.K. (ed.), *Veterinary Clinics of North America: Back problems*. Philadelphia: W.B. Saunders Co., 1999;195–209.
9. Denoix, J.M. and Audigié, F. The neck and back. In: *Veterinary Clinics of North America Equine Practice: Equine locomotion*. Philadelphia: W.B. Saunders Co., 2000;167–192.
10. Denoix, J.M., Audigié, F., Robert, C. and Pourcelot, P. Alteration of locomotion in horses with vertebral lesions. Presented at Conference in Equine Sports Medicine Science, Taormina, Italy, 2000.
11. Haussler, K.K., Bertram, J.E.A., Gellman, K. and Hermanson, J.W. Dynamic analysis of in vivo segmental spinal motion: An instrumentation strategy. *Veterinary and Comparative Orthopaedics and Traumatology* 2000;**13**:9–17.
12. Haussler, K.K., Bertram, J.E.A., Gellman, K. and Hermanson, J.W. Segmental in-vivo vertebral kinematics at the walk, trot and canter: A preliminary study. *Equine Veterinary Journal* 2001;**33**(suppl):160–164.
13. Kleijnen, J., Knipschild, P. and ter Riet, G. Clinical trials of homeopathy. *British Medical Journal* 1991;**302**:316.
14. Birnesser, H., Klein, P. and Weiser, M.A. A modern homeopathic medication works as well as COX 2 inhibitors for treating osteoarthritis of the knee. *Der Allgemeinarzt* 2003;**25**:261.
15. Macedo, S.B., Ferreira, L.R., Perazzo, F.F. and Carvalho, J.C. Anti-inflammatory activity of Arnica montana 6cH: preclinical study in animals. *Homeopathy* 2004;**93**:84–87.

Organisations and courses

Association of Chartered Physiotherapists in Animal Therapy

Nimrod House, Sandy's Road, Malvern, Worcs WR14 IJJ, UK

Options for Animals International Global Headquarters and Options for Animals International Academy of Animal Chiropractic

4267 Virginia Rd, Wellsville, KS 66092, USA
Tel: +1 309 658 2920, fax +1 785883 4710, website: www.animalchiro.com

International Veterinary Acupuncture Society (IVAS)

PO Box 271395, Ft Collins, CO 80527-1395, USA
Tel: +1 970 266 0666, fax: +1 970 266 0777, email: office@ivas.org, website: www.ivas.org

Chi Institute of Chinese Medicine

9708 West Highway 318, Reddick, FL 32686, USA
Tel: +1 352 591 5385, fax: +1 352 591 2854, website: www.tcvm.com, email: admin@tcvm.com

25 Rehabilitation

Mary Bromiley

Introduction

The processes of physiotherapy and rehabilitation should complement each other. In terms of personnel, in some cases the physiotherapist undertakes both but rehabilitation is very time-consuming and a specialist trainer – the rehabilitation trainer (RT) – is the best person to effect rehabilitation. The RT should work together with the physiotherapist and any other involved professional, e. g. the vet, osteopath, chiropractor, acupuncturist or masseur.

At the outset of rehabilitation there are some important factors to be recognised. Following a diagnosis of the cause of the symptoms displayed by the horse, musculoskeletal problems should never be addressed as a single entity with attention focused only on the identified problem. It is widely acknowledged that disruption of normal function in one area leads to a cascade of interrelated problems. When considering pain arising within the vertebral column, the core of the axial skeleton, secondary limb dysfunction is a common finding. Unfortunately, these secondary complications are often those targeted by the owner or untutored RT.

One major problem when initiating back rehabilitation is to identify which of the epaxial muscle groups is affected. Until recently visualisation has been the only method to assess muscular integrity

(Plate 38a). Significant atrophy of superficial muscles is usually obvious, seen as increased prominence of the dorsal spinous processes (DSPs), either in localised sites or throughout the thoracic and/or lumbar areas. Unfortunately, atrophy of deep-sited muscles, like the scalene group (leading to instability at the cervicothoracic junction), is not usually visually obvious in the early stages. However, the ability to diagnose muscle problems at this site is very important because loss of stability leads to impaired neck function and this area, probably after L6–S1, is the most important junction within the vertebral complex.

In addition to the problems of assessing muscular atrophy or loss of function, other structures such as tendons and ligaments are very important in the back, as loss of nuchal ligament support affects the entire back leading to secondary loss of traction throughout the supraspinous ligament with consequent muscle atrophy in the longissimus group of muscles.

To improve the diagnosis of both muscle and ligament damage, the use of ultrasonography has become widespread in the veterinary profession (see Chapters 10 and 11) and in the field of rehabilitation. In addition to providing primary information on the presence of pathology, the technique is useful for rehabilitation, as it is useful for determining the relative size of the epaxial groups before and after rehabilitation. In addition a quantitative comparison of response to treatment might allow a more selective use of appropriate techniques.

The back

Anatomically the vertebral column, each described individually for convenience, rather than the structure being considered as a whole. In most descriptive literature the term "back" is generalised, then discussed as though it comprises only the section from the withers to the lumbosacral junction.

When undertaking rehabilitation, it is essential, for a successful outcome, to consider the vertebral column as a whole; stability and normal function throughout the complete structure determine efficient locomotion of the entire body mass. The RT needs to appreciate that the skeletal and soft tissue components of all sections (cervical, thoracic, lumbar, sacral and pelvic) form an interdependent, interreliant mechanism. In addition it must be appreciated that the function of the appendicular skeleton relies on stability of the axial skeleton. To deliver effective rehabilitation for the equine back it is therefore necessary to consider not just the section from the withers to loins, but also the cervical, sacral and pelvic areas. In rehabilitation, therefore, the cause of the malfunction must be addressed; there is little or no benefit gained in removing back discomfort, and restoring mobility and stability, if the primary cause has not been addressed. One of the complicating functional consequences of the intercommunication and interdependence between all body parts is that disuse muscle atrophy (secondary to loss of proprioception) occurs after all traumatic incidents, be they as a result of accident, direct injury, a musculoskeletal condition or any form of disease.

When examining the horse, a broad approach should be adopted, with significant attention being paid to the skeletal and soft tissue components of the body. In addition the following all require consideration before designing an appropriate rehabilitation programme in order to achieve a successful outcome and restoration of pre-injury function: neural and circulatory supply; the feet, teeth and general health of the horse, including nutrition; the age of the horse; the breed; and the discipline and eventual level of activity required by the rider.

Anatomy

To achieve acceptable results an understanding of the interaction of the varied tissues and a detailed knowledge of the anatomy and physiology of the components involved in locomotion are required, in addition to an appreciation of the function of proprioceptors (the receptors that provide information on where the body is in space and relative to the ground; this information is used to adjust and correct imbalance).

Anatomical understanding should include:

* skeletal components
* ligaments
* individual muscles, origin and insertion, and the functional nerve supply
* the neural supply of dermatomes
* the range of movement expected under normal circumstances, within and appropriate to the area targeted.

It should be appreciated that the anticipated range of movement, will also, to a degree, be governed by age, conformation, muscle tone and underlying bone pathology.

Vertebral ligaments

Back rehabilitation necessitates an understanding of the ligament support structure of the back and the ligament/muscular interactions that occur in the back, in particular the specialist activity of the nuchal and all associated ligaments. From a functional perspective, when considering the back, the vertebral ligaments can be imaged as two interacting chains influencing the dorsal and ventral sections of the whole.

Ligaments influencing the dorsal section of the body

Of great importance dorsally are the nuchal ligament and its direct continuation, the supraspinous ligament (SSL, see Chapter 10). In situations in which the nuchal ligament is affected, if the musculature of the neck (intimately connected to the nuchal ligament) is compromised, or there is pain in the mouth that affects the correct positioning of head and neck, nuchal ligament tension will be affected. Alterations in nuchal ligament tension lead, in turn, to SSL dysfunction with consequent minute changes in vertebral positioning. The interspinous ligaments and the ventral ligament of the spinal column work as stabilisers, and are closely associated with the multifidus muscles, the deep muscles sited on the dorsal aspect of the entire vertebral column.

Muscles influencing the dorsal and ventral sections of the body

Just as with the ligament chain, the dorsal (epaxial and hypaxial muscles, see Chapter 2) and ventral muscle chains contribute to the positioning of the back, and their functional development influences the "top line" and "bottom line", terms adopted by the riding fraternity.

Dorsal section

The dorsal section is comprised primarily of the longissimus dorsi system which functions to extend the vertebral column. The system extends from the pelvis to the cervical spine. Thus, an unidentified problem in the cervical segment of

the muscle can affect other areas; conversely problems in the lumber segment of the muscle will affect the cervical area.

The muscles that make up the longissimus dorsi system and the effects of loss of function of these dorsal muscles are shown in Table 25.1.

Ventral section

The "bottom line" comprises the cervical ventral muscles and continues, extending from sternum to pelvis via the abdominal musculature. Without synergistic interaction of the dorsal and ventral musculature, the vertebral column is compromised with subsequent malfunction, so rehabilitation must also be targeted to involve the muscular chains.

In the lumber region, the ventral placement of iliopsoas creates an important bridge assisting the ventral ligament. The abdominal muscles complete the muscular part of the chain.

The muscles that make up the ventral muscle system and the effects of loss of function of these muscles are shown in Table 25.2.

Back pain

Pain actually *originating* in the back appears, from field experience, to be less common than is generally supposed by the lay public. True primary back pain is usually associated with a known incident, the horse getting a cast, a travel accident, a

Table 25.1 The muscles that make up the longissimus dorsi system and the effects of loss of function of these muscles

Muscle	Effects of pathology	Notes
Iliocostalis cervicis and thoracis	Reduction in stability of the lumbar spine	
Longissimus, lumborum, thoracis, cervicis, capitis et atlantis	Reduction of vertebral stability	
Spinalis, thoracis, cervicis	Reduction of stability of the cranial thoracic and caudal cervical areas	
Multifidus muscle system, lumborum, thoracis, cervicis	Reduces vertebral stability	Deep muscles. Span up to six vertebrae in lumbar area. Lumbar atrophy manifests in a roach back appearance, often unilateral, associated with atrophy of contralateral gluteus muscles

Table 25.2   The muscles that make up the ventral muscle system and the effects of loss of function of these muscles

Muscle	Effects of pathology
Abdominal muscles	Reduces vertebral stability
Iliopsoas	Reduces stability of the lumbar spine and sacroiliac joint

fall or identified pathology. In the author's experience back pain, disuse, muscle atrophy and skeletal changes are often secondary to a seemingly often remote primary cause.

Possible causes associated with back discomfort

There are many possible causes of back discomfort including the following:

- *Inappropriate training/preparation*: can be considered a "chain malfunction". When evaluating the effects of inappropriate training, consider the breed characteristics of the horse as well as the muscle characteristics of the breed.
- *Limb dysfunction* resulting in abnormal vertebral stresses; consider foot balance, conformation, adductor muscles.
- *Interrupted neural supply*: consider dermatome responses to identify nerve involved, and so identify muscles compromised.
- *Muscle imbalance* within the ring of muscle groups supporting the axial skeleton; consider the abdominals, neck and hindquarter musculature; test for possible power asymmetry, agonist/antagonist balance.
- *Mouth discomfort* with associated incorrect head carriage; consider teeth, bit position, type and size.
- *Poll discomfort*: often associated with a history of the horse pulling back when tied or rearing and falling over backwards. Test movement of the atlanto-occipital and atlantoaxial joints.
- *Restricted respiratory function*: this can cause, in the author's opinion, a reluctance to flex at the poll or break over-correctly; consider narrow jaw angle, oedema of parotid glands.

- *Metabolic malfunction*: consider diet, to include water, inappropriate protein levels, azoturia, gastric ulceration. Does the horse lack the necessary dietary balance to maintain a competent musculature? Attention should be paid to trace minerals in particular.
- *Mares*: although not generally accepted, ovarian cysts or uterine discomfort can, in the author's experience, give rise to back discomfort.
- *Saddle fit*: the greater the area of back covered by the under panel, the more evenly distributed is rider weight; many modern saddles create a fulcrum at approximately T12, T13, T14, causing a seesaw motion at trot with consequent local bruising (see Chapter 24). Note that the purchase of a new expensive saddle, endless pads or re-flocking to suit the shape of the back is often the unsuccessful route chosen by the rider to alleviate back pain.
- *Rider position*: consider disparity of leg length, a common cause of rider imbalance necessitating adaptive repositioning of the vertebral column of the horse to counteract asymmetrical weight distribution.

Rehabilitation programmes

The aims of a rehabilitation programme are first to restore muscle competence in affected groups and then to re-train normal movements. However, the RT must be aware that it should never be assumed that the normal, pre-injury pattern of movement will be automatically restored after muscle recovery.

In the human model, electromyography (EMG) has determined the role and level of activity of muscles during selected movement patterns, including athletic tasks. It is also possible, in the human model, to isolate an individual or number of individual muscles by incorporating apparatus to fix body parts. After isolation and EMG identification, experimentation has resulted in appropriate choice of activities in order to recruit and so influence selected muscles.

When trying to determine appropriate activities in order to rebuild the musculature in specific areas of the horse, and although currently work to determine muscle recruitment is ongoing, with some undertaken having been published, it should be remembered that the work is far from complete and unfortunately somewhat inadequate, particularly as experimentation is generally undertaken utilising a treadmill.

Movement isolation in the horse is not possible as it is in the human model, so general activity must form the basis of rehabilitation; however, by careful positioning of head and neck, choice of appropriate movement patterns and creating situations to increase load, at the same time influencing and targeting normal limb activity, it is possible to partially localise muscle recruitment.

Only with underpinning knowledge of the functional role of individual muscles, insofar as is currently known, and utilising group muscle activity, can the RT select appropriate exercises and activities to ensure that the muscles that need to be influenced are exercised effectively, both to recover their pre-injury tensile strength and to ensure restoration of their pre-injury capability.

After re-establishment of muscle competence, it is necessary to select appropriate activities to re-establish the cortical pattern of natural balanced movements.

Rebuilding muscle

A programme incorporating progressive resistance is considered to be the most efficient means of improving muscle but consideration of fibre type is also necessary. From the human model it has been demonstrated that type I fibres (slow twitch) respond to exercises incorporating slow repetition against a load, whereas type II fibres (fast twitch) respond to exercises involving rapid repetitions against a lesser load. It has also been established in the human model that fibre type can, to a small degree, be changed; this change is influenced by the type of muscle activity demanded.

Each breed of horse, before cross-breeding was introduced, retained its own specific characteristics, including that of muscle fibre type; this made the choice of an exercise regime relatively simple, e.g. the Arabian, with muscles predominantly endurance-type fibre, responds best to slow work against a load.

The crossing of a warmblood (slow twitch/endurance) to a thoroughbred (fast twitch/speed) can result in a thoroughbred-type frame and appearance but with predominantly warmblood-type muscle. Many problems arise from a lack of appreciation of this fact, with inappropriate muscle training often resulting in poorly prepared muscles leading, among other problems, to back pain.

The body musculature needs to be considered as consisting of stabilising or postural muscles, which function to stabilise the axial skeleton; the latter achieve movement and are concerned in the main with the appendicular skeleton.

Postural muscles are considered to consist, predominantly, of endurance (slow-twitch)-type fibres. The deep postural muscles, adjacent to the vertebral column, are linked functionally, as previously described, to the supporting ligaments; these and the joint capsules are all richly enervated. The role of the postural muscles throughout the vertebral column is to ensure correct positioning of individual vertebrae; their rich innervation also contributes to balance and stability throughout the entire axial skeleton.

Stability is the essence of recovery, so early work in any rehabilitation programme should be aimed at rebuilding the stabilising musculature of the back. This is achieved through the use of long reins, and necessitates slow work, with the back unencumbered by rider weight. With experience, it is possible to observe restoration of muscle activity. The musculature appears to "ripple" as the horse is worked from the ground.

The basic exercises of the classical school were designed to "strengthen" a horse before the introduction of ridden work, although it is unlikely that the exponents of these basic schooling activities appreciated that they were achieving axial stability.

The RT should incorporate such exercises in the daily routine, because, when the horse subconsciously appreciates that it possesses a stable frame, it will automatically begin to increase the range of appendicular movement.

A recent, much discussed schooling position, "rolkur", undoubtedly focuses, by subtle positioning of head and neck, on activating and so strengthening the "bridge" of muscles spanning the important junction of the base of neck to thorax. Stability of the cranial portion of the thoracic cage is achieved, which allows exaggerated forelimb extension, the horse instinctively realising that the forelimbs are attached to a firm underlying frame.

When the horse can work in long reins at both walk and trot, a gradual introduction of appropriate loading is required. Loading is achieved by the use of a weight boot, heavy shoe, suitably arranged poles in the arena, blocks, varied surfaces and, later, slopes.

If available the walker, water treadmill or water walker can be incorporated to vary activity. Only when back stability has been restored, a process that often takes up to 6 weeks, should the programme be advanced to include ridden work.

When riding is introduced, working diagonally across a slope, wading in the sea and working in sand all achieve muscle loading.

Throughout the programme the discipline of the horse must be considered. Although the thoroughbred requires, in the early stages, exercises involving slow work to influence postural recovery, as rehabilitation progresses the speed and type of activity should be varied, to ensure fibre-type recruitment, appropriate to discipline. Little benefit is gained if the rehabilitation programme produces endurance muscle in a horse that requires only speed.

Long reins

Tack required for successful work in long reins (Plate 38b):

* snaffle bridle
* cavesson
* roller with at least three sets of side rings
* pair of side reins with a rubber couple adjustable at both ends
* pair of long reins, medium weight.

Horses take 2–3 days to become accustomed to being driven.

The side reins are used when the horse is first introduced to long reins; acting as an essential control aid, they run from cavesson to roller, not bit to roller. The side reins can also be utilised, for very short periods, to position the head and neck in order to influence body position and so influence muscle recruitment (Plate 38c).

Why rehabilitate in long reins, rather than lunge?

The horse's back was designed to suspend the weight of the abdominal contents and resist gravity, not to carry weight. To achieve muscle recovery it is sensible to exercise the horse, by working it, as nature intended, riderless. Down the ages, and until quite recently, horses "broken" in the old-fashioned manner in long reins were subjected, probably without the nagsman appreciating the fact, to the basic exercises of the classical school, involving as they do movement in both longitudinal and lateral directions.

Longitudinal exercises "unite" the horse: they develop connection; as muscles strengthen in response to load, the frame stabilises. Secondary to this stability is an improvement in the ability to shift the centre of gravity.

Lateral exercises result in improved flexibility. The effect of the exercises is to target and so strengthen muscles with a normal function, i.e. in general, to work, not in an active, but in a static/stabilising, mode.

Following sufficient lateral work, horses are considered to have become supple, or to move easier, with increased range. This improved range is possible because their joints are ably supported due to the improved condition of the muscle groups targeted by lateral work, and known collectively as adductor and abductor muscles. Lateral exercises can also be used to influence one-sidedness, and/or build one side of the back.

Early rehabilitation

The horse should be worked in straight lines when active rehabilitation commences: work off a straight line gradually introduced, first by incorporating serpentines, then lateral work and finally circles. *Long reins* are preferable to the *lunge* due to the ability to control the hindquarters, in particular the outside hindleg, when work off a straight line is introduced. A horse does not, as a natural activity, perform circles. To execute a 10-m circle, in perfect balance and perfect cadence, is probably one of the most difficult coordinations demanded and circle work should be avoided in early rehabilitation. Indeed horses working in small circles often have areas of skeletal stress (Plate 39a).

There is an apparent lack of understanding about the direct effects of individual exercises. Those described in texts state "X exercise improves X movement", or that the activities described "improve performance". Unfortunately these statements do not identify the muscles affected by the particular exercise, explain the requirement for joint stability in order to improve general suppleness, or describe linkage between the influence of muscles on activity, stability and/or movement range. Understanding the effects of exercises, in particular *serpentines, lateral work* and *transitions down*, enables appropriate selection.

Why classical exercises?

The exercises of the classical school were designed to recruit differing muscle combinations, in order to stabilise the axial skeleton, so enabling a safe change of gravitational position; this was necessary, before the introduction of the difficult movements demanded by Haute Ecole (all human dancers start their training using the basics of classical ballet!).

The use of an arena, equipped with poles and cavalletti, enables the RT to vary the limb action of the horse, not only changing the work of active muscles, from outer to middle range, but also as a result of the change of head and neck position influencing the position of the centre of gravity.

Muscle loading

Added to an understanding of the effects of the basic classical exercises is the appreciation that increased resistance or loading is necessary for muscle recovery, and appropriate loading is the only way to address unilateral muscle atrophy. Weight, either by the use of a heavy shoe or boot, increases the load of the selected limb (Plates 39b and 40a), with a secondary requirement for the stabilising musculature to also work against an increased load.

In addition to the addition of weights directly to the limb, the introduction of water and slopes can be employed to provide variety of resistance. Increased loading is used for both muscle recovery and movement re-education because proprio-

ceptive stimulation is affected by unnatural weight. Proprioceptive stimulus can also be enhanced by varying both terrain and footing.

There is no programme formula appropriate for all cases, even when considering a single body area. Each case requires an individual, specific programme. This programme should be appropriate for:

- the type of injury
- the primary site of damage
- location of pain
- muscles involved
- eventual requirement.

The RT should remember that he or she is dealing with a recovery situation and that the speed of recovery will vary with each case, as will the ability to restore muscle competence.

Lateral work

The muscle masses of the hindquarters may be considered as two pistons, each of which should produce equal power; to achieve this, the hindlimb thrust must be even, and the horse moves forward as design intended, with the vertebral column straight. If one hindlimb produces less thrust, the vertebral column will be subjected to a torque-type stress and the horse, as it moves forward, will not move truly straight.

With the *left hindquarter* affected the gluteal tongue and the deep musculature of the *right loins* (the antagonistic stabilisers) *atrophy* (Plate 40b). If the problem in the hindquarter is not addressed or noticed, the horse rapidly becomes a "back pain" case, because, due to muscular imbalance, vertebral stress has occurred. The horse has become one sided, displaying back discomfort/pain, usually at the thoracolumbar junction, the range of vertebral movement is compromised and the horse's performance suffers. To counteract this situation, it is necessary to create an activity that loads the weaker hindquarter and works the back musculature unilaterally. To achieve this, the horse must be made to move off a straight line. By moving diagonally forward, one hindleg will need to exert a greater force in order to project the body mass, laterally, over the underloaded, contralateral limb. The requirement for the horse to move laterally has increased the workload of one leg, the leg of thrust, powered by the musculature of the appropriate hindquarter. The antagonistic, stabilising muscles of the vertebral column, sited on the opposite side to the muscles of thrust, are activated, because they work to retain the vertebral column in its functional position, straight.

Thrust supplied by the *left hindlimb* will load the *left hindquarter* muscles, and the movement will automatically influence the muscles down the *right side* of the back. Thus, by working to the right, employing the classic half-pass, the desired result, that of strengthening the musculature of the left hindquarter and right loins, is achieved.

Serpentines

The natural horse relies, for survival, on flight, necessitating a straight rather than a curved alignment of the vertebrae. When the horse performs a series of curves or loops a slight curve/rotation is created in the vertebral column, secondary in part to the movement of the weight of the abdominal mass.

The vertebral column is naturally designed to remain straight. If subjected to forces that create a curve, the subconscious reflex muscular response is to remove the curve and straighten the vertebral column. Thus work necessitating a series of loops or curves achieves increased activity within the muscle groups lying on the created convexity. Where the RT is aiming to treat a situation of bilateral muscle atrophy, even curves are employed, i.e. true serpentines. In cases with unilateral atrophy, the convexity is created on the same side as the muscle atrophy; the horse is then driven straight for a few strides, before executing another identical curve.

Transitions down (deceleration)

Movement at the lumbosacral junction recruits, among other muscles, iliopsoas and the gluteal tongue. A downward transition requires movement at the lumbosacral joint and these muscles, as they work to control the force generated by deceleration, are strengthened.

Early rehabilitation

This is best described as the period immediately following injury, surgery or during the acute phase of muscle disease. Movement will be affected as a result of inflammatory responses (i.e. pain, muscle spasm, oedema).

At this stage it is the physiotherapist who uses his or her skills to reduce pain, retain optimum mobility and prevent excessive muscle atrophy. Activity, in the acute phase, unless box rest has been ordered, should be curtailed to hand walking, and/or turn-out in a small paddock or cage, rather than an immediate gymnastic approach.

Why is a period of rest important in the rehabilitation programme?

Before initiating a carefully controlled exercise programme it is best to observe a period of rest. This is recommended because, although the horse is still painful (from surgery or injury), it may recruit muscles other than those normally used when asked to perform specific activities by the RT or rider. The adaptation of incorrect muscle recruitment leads to an incorrect, inefficient, movement pattern. The adaptation is subconscious and adopted to attempt to reduce the pain experienced during movement. *In the author's opinion, persuading a horse that has changed its way of going to readopt the appropriate economic biomechanical pattern is one of the most exacting and difficult tasks for the RT.*

Examples of inefficient patterns

Forelimb pain

The horse with pain in a forelimb, may shorten the length of normal forelimb protraction, and by so doing will reduce the weight-bearing period at each stride, but will create uneven vertebral stress in and just caudal to the withers. Standing base narrow and placing the forelimbs along a central line, rather than standing and moving four square, is another change observed; these horses often show as having a "cold back" when mounted.

Hindlimb pain

A horse with hindquarter discomfort may attempt to overcome a loss of hindquarter impulsion by recruiting forelimb musculature, e.g. the brachiocephalic muscle may be used to exert traction at the sternal origin and pull the thoracic cage forward. In such cases, over time, an upside-down neck develops creating incorrect neck positioning, compromising nuchal ligament function and leading to a hollow, painful back.

Incorrect patterns rapidly become established, in the cortex, as normal, *and will be retained*, even after the condition giving rise to the pain has subsided, and often after a rehabilitation programme has been initiated and delivered. This is not successful rehabilitation.

Introduction of active rehabilitation

It is important to ensure that the acute injury phase is subsiding before a programme of active rehabilitation, involving as it does specific movements to order, is initiated. The time involved in each stage of specific tissue healing must always be considered.

The aims at this stage are to design a programme of exercises incorporating, at the appropriate time, varied aids and activities to encompass the following:

- Prevent development of soft tissue contractures
- Prevent adhesions
- Minimise ongoing loss of muscle
- Restore muscle competence in all groups following atrophy
- Restore normal levels of mobility
- Re-educate to restore normal movement.

Throughout the programme, it is important that the RT liaise with the veterinary surgeon, owner, trainer and/or rider to ensure that the anticipated outcome, and the time required to achieve this, are understood and agreed by all concerned.

Failure

The prime reason for an unsuccessful outcome (Plate 41a) is that the RT has failed to:

- recognise incorrect movement patterns
- identify and re-build appropriate muscle groups

- re-educate movement
- re-establish normal biomechanics.

Another common mistake, if an incorrect movement pattern has been noticed, is to introduce 'training aids' when trying to re-educate a way of going, e.g. the Chambon, de Gogue or Abbot Davies. In a rehabilitation programme, horses rapidly learn to rely on these, using them as a balance aid, rather as a child uses stabilisers when learning to ride a bicycle. Remove the stabiliser and the programme falls apart *because static positioning does not build muscle.* In some cases:

- the pain of injury is still present, inhibiting movement
- the primary cause of the pain has not been elicited and addressed
- the condition causing the pain has been so long term that cortical adaptation may have become irreversible.

Diagnosis and prognosis should have indicated whether the condition will resolve or whether irreversible changes are present. In the latter case any rehabilitation programme should be tailored appropriately

Slopes as a rehabilitation aid

Walking a horse across a slope, either led or in long reins, can be used to exercise, strengthen and restore function in the long back muscles. The slope needs to be sufficiently steep to cause the positioning of a pair of limbs to be below, or downhill to, the contralateral pair; the body weight will then exert a "down-hill" pull, creating a mild lateral or convex curve in the thoracolumbar spine, with the convexity downhill. The cortical pattern automatically attempts to restore equilibrium, and re-establish the normal, straight configuration of the vertebral column. This attempt is achieved by the muscles on the "down-hill" side of the column working to reduce the convexity and pull the column straight. The muscle activity is similar to that achieved by the use of serpentines – restoration of a straight column – but demand is increased. Due to the use of a slope, the body weight is shifted laterally and the length of time for holding the position can be manipulated by the distance travelled across the slope; both these factors increase muscle loading.

The activity has been used not only for rehabilitation after atrophy of the back musculature, but also by a number of international riders to strengthen their horse's loins. The specificity of this activity is not fully known; however, rectal examination suggests that iliopsoas is the prime muscle targeted. In addition, in cases of iliac wing fracture, repeated rectal examination has suggested that this activity reverses the atrophy that occurs after fracture.

Treadmill

A treadmill can provide a very useful method of controlled exercise during rehabilitation (Plate 41b). In some cases, rehabilitation exercises in the arena using poles will restore a balanced cadence; however, some cases fail to respond and retain an unlevel gait sequence. One of the advantages of the treadmill is that the horse requires more balanced stride sequence, when on the treadmill, in order to remain upright, than it would on solid ground. A treadmill with an uphill slope, as found in most rehabilitation centres, necessitates a lift to advance each individual limb rather than the normal swing through, making the limb and its muscles work harder than on a flat surface.

Balance becomes established after three to five 5-minute sessions at walk, and is normally retained when the horse is worked over ground.

Hydrotherapy – water as a rehabilitation aid

As previously stated, to improve muscle efficiency work effort needs to be increased. The swimming pool, hydrospa, water treadmill and water walker all make use of the weight of water as an aid to recovery, i.e. to increase muscle efficiency. Before the invention/marketing of the above devices, rivers, lakes and the sea were incorporated by some RTs into their rehabilitation programmes. All rehabilitation programmes using water have been reported as being very effective, although unfortunately little or no scientific research has been published detailing their efficacy.

Cardiovascular and muscular effects of water therapy

Equine pools

The shape of equine pools vary: some are round, some straight with a ramp for entry and exit at each end, and some oval but with a straight section that can be used either as a straight section on its own or incorporated into the oval. The straight section is useful when teaching horses to swim and is the preferred option for rehabilitation. The ease with which horses adapt to swimming varies from individual to individual. However, even in horses that do learn to swim, unfortunately not all horses follow the required limb pattern in order to swim with a straight spine (Plate 42a); some swim using front legs only, others just kick from behind, trailing their front legs, or screw the hindquarters to one side, and then kick both hindlimbs simultaneously sideways.

Benefits of swimming

The resistance supplied by water is even, but, when swimming is incorporated as a rehabilitation aid, it is suitable only for horses that adopt a one-, two-, three- or four-limb pattern, or four-limb sequence, similar to the walk. The horses should also swim in a manner that keeps their back just out of the water, with head and neck comfortably positioned. Swimming benefits include the following:

- The muscles of the shoulders and hindquarters, and to a degree those of the loins and possibly the abdominal tunic.
- Joints: human studies suggest that movement of joints in a non-weight-bearing situation is of value in rehabilitation. Thus, the equine knee and hock, subjected to considerable stress in all competition animals, and often the primary cause of vertebral stress, may well benefit.
- Swimming does not benefit the tendons of the distal limbs. Movement in the distal limbs is

entirely reliant on tendon stretch and recoil, affected only by weight bearing and weight transference.

Cardiovascular stress

Ray Hutchinson, MRCVS was one of the first to build a hydrotherapy pool in the UK in the 1980s. As a veterinary surgeon he was interested in the response of the cardiovascular system to swimming and he observed that a straight pool was preferable, raising the heart rate to over 200 beats/min, and that a circular/oval pool might stress the horse excessively. Thus the hydrotherapy pool does cause a marked cardiovascular effort; however, swimming should not replace ground-based exercise but should be considered useful as a cardiorespiratory adjunct to rehabilitation.

Side effects of swimming

It is possible that stress to the cervicothoracic and lumbosacral junctions can occur, particularly in bad or poor swimmers. It is also postulated that possible damage to the back may result, secondary to the loss of proprioceptive input and when a horse is tired. A tired horse usually begins to drop its back and becomes noisy as it gasps for air. Experienced swimming personnel should never allow a horse to reach this stage of exhaustion. Excessive chilling is also a theoretical problem to the equine swimmer, although this is a rarity. In an ideal situation, in cold weather, a horse should be put on a walker or stood under heat lamps to be dried off.

The dense mineral water of the thermal spas of Europe is warm, so there is no danger of muscle damage due to chilling, in mid-winter.

Pools obviously have their place but it should be accepted that swimming does not activate all over ground muscles; the prime benefit of swimming must be considered to be a non-weight-bearing, cardiovascular activity.

Water walking

To improve muscular efficiency it is necessary to increase the workload of the muscle. This can be done in a number of ways, as described above. Water walking achieves this by using the resistance of water to increase the work required by the muscle to move the limb. Walking in a stream provides some resistance; walking in the sea is harder work due to the density of the water. The depth of the water that is being walked through does affect the work done. Water that is only fetlock deep does not change the action of the limb, but it has been noted that the splashing created appears to stimulate abdominal sensors and achieve abdominal muscle contraction. Work in deeper water, e.g. mid-cannon, does change the action. Mid-cannon work requires recruitment of the musculature of the loins to help lift the hindlimb and also activates the musculature at the base of the neck. In contrast, observation of horses wading shoulder deep suggests that they utilise normal limb activity, albeit with a shortened stride. For horses that, despite extensive rehabilitation from the ground, have failed to readopt a balanced cadence, water walking can be very helpful. They appear to rapidly recover and re-establish balance and normal limb sequence.

The sea walker

The sea walker (Plate 42b) brings the benefits of the sea to the rehabilitation yard. Rather than walking on rubber or matted surface, as on the normal walker, horses walk in a trough filled with a filtered, chilled, saline solution. Depth and speed can be adjusted in order to create varied recruitment of muscle, e.g. fetlock deep does not radically change normal limb action, but 19 inches (48 cm) of depth does, the limb movement adopted increasing activation of back and abdominal musculature; thus, if the point of the exercise is to strengthen the back, an increase in water depth will achieve this.

The water treadmill

The rehabilitation unit's water treadmill is a modified version of the standard treadmill originally designed for respiratory research. The addition of the water increases the amount of work that has to be done in order to ambulate at the required speed. The horse on a treadmill does not recruit its musculature exactly as it does when walking over the ground, because the moving belt repositions the weight-bearing limb/limbs to some extent: the front limb is taken back under the body and the hindlimb is carried behind the horse immediately the foot has been placed under the body mass. In the water treadmill, the tank is usually filled to mid-chest level, so, in order to move individual limbs, each is required to be lifted up rather than swung normally due to the resistance of the water. In the forelimb this is achieved by recruiting trapezius, normally acting in a pivotal rather than a lifting manner. The different usage eventually makes the horse appear thick through the withers, due to muscle overbuild; this has also demonstrated an apparent reduced stride length.

In the hindlimb (also required to be lifted) muscle recruitment occurs primarily in the loins, the horse reversing the normal function of a part of longissimus. When in deep water the horse must lift the hindquarter of the advancing hindlimb, then use the hip flexors, not required normally as a strong muscle group, to bring the leg forward under the body. Over ground, this positioning occurs just before the hindquarter musculature creates the tremendous backward thrust, delivered as the limb straightens, to push the body mass over the planted forelimb. On the treadmill there is no need for this thrust – the leg is taken backwards by the moving belt.

It is difficult to build the muscles of the back when the horse is being ridden, because, in order to carry rider weight, the back muscles need to achieve considerable tension, functioning in a holding or static, rather than active, manner; the static hold is necessary to resist a weight-induced downward curve. Static work does not build muscle, so, for a horse with a weak back, active recruitment of the back musculature in the water treadmill is very beneficial.

With the device and programme carefully chosen, the use of water to increase resistance can be of great benefit within a rehabilitation programme and may be utilised by the rider following an initial rehabilitation programme given by the RT.

Conclusion

A request for rehabilitation should follow accurate diagnosis by a veterinary surgeon. The diagnosis should result in the appropriate medical or surgical intervention, followed by treatment from an appropriate practitioner such as an osteopath, chiropractor, physiotherapist or masseur.

As previously stated rehabilitation is directed at restoration of pre-injury function and is effected by selecting appropriate active exercise regimes; these are designed, first, to target the muscle groups compromised as a result of accident, injury or disease, and then to restore normal biomechanics.

Following any disruption from normal, multifactorial dysfunction occurs; all skeletal components are affected to a greater or lesser degree: bone, joints, ligament, tendon, nerve, muscle, and circulatory and lymphatic systems.

The person undertaking rehabilitation requires an understanding of the muscular skeletal system, healing mechanisms and possible restrictions, precluding the restoration of full function in order to achieve the best possible outcome (Plate 42c).

References

1. Comas, A.J. *Skeletal Muscle: Form and Function.* Champaign, IL: Human Kinetics Publishers, 1996.
2. Back, W. Development of equine locomotion from foal to adult. PhD thesis, University of Utrecht, 1994.
3. Back, W. and Clayton, H.M. *Equine Locomotion.* Philadelphia: Saunders Co., 2000.
4. Becher, R. *Schooling by the Natural Method.* London: J.A. Allen, 1963.
5. Belasik, P. *Exploring Dressage Technique: Journeys into the art of classical riding.* London: J. A. Allen, 1994.
6. Budras, K-D., Rock, S. and Sack, W.O. *Anatomy of the Horse: An illustrated text*, 4th edn. Hannover: Schlütersche, 2003.
7. De Lahunta, A. *Veterinary Neuroanatomy and Clinical Neurology*, 3rd edn. Philadelphia: W.B. Saunders Co., 2008.
8. Delforge, G. *Musculoskeletal Trauma: Implications for sports injury management.* Champaign, IL: Human Kinetics Publishers, 2003.
9. Decarpentry, A.E. *Academic Equitation: A preparation for international dressage tests.* Tonbridge: J.A. Allen & Co., 1971.

10. Fonesca, B.P.A., Alves, A.L.G., Nicoletti, J.L.M. et al. Thermography and ultrasonography in back pain diagnosis of equine athletes. *Journal Equine Veterinary Science* 2006;**26**:507–516.

11. Goody, P.C. *Horse Anatomy: A pictorial approach to equine structure.* Tonbridge: J.A. Allen & Co Ltd, 1976.

12. Hinchcliff, K.W., Kaneps, A.J. and Geor, R.J. *Equine Sports Medicine and Surgery.* Philadelphia: W.B. Saunders, 2004.

13. Jones, W.E. *Equine Sports Medicine.* Philadelphia: Lea & Febiger, 1989.

14. Klimke, R. *Cavalletti.* Canaan, NY: Sydney R. Smith, 1995.

15. Olivera, N. *Classical Principles of the Art of Training Horses.* Tonbridge: J.A. Allen, 1983.

16. Oliviera, N. *Reflections on Equestrian Art.* Tonbridge: J.A. Allen & Co Ltd, 1976.

17. Rooney, J.R. *Mechanics of the Horse.* Malabar, FL: Krieger Publishing Co., 1980.

18. Schoen, A.M. and Wynn, S.G. *Complementary and Alternative Veterinary Medicine.* Philadelphia: Mosby, 1998.

19. Sissons, S. and Grossman, J.D. *The Anatomy of the Domestic Animals.* Philadelphia: W.B. Saunders Co., 1975.

20. Short, C.E. and Van Poznak, A. *Animal Pain.* New York: Churchill Livingstone, 1992.

21. Stanier, S. *The Art of Long Reining.* Tonbridge: J.A. Allen, 1975.

22. Harris, S.E. *Horse Gaits, Balance and Movement.* Toronto: John Wiley & Sons Ltd, 1993.

23. Stodulka, R. *Medizinische Reitlehre.* Stuttgart: Parey Bei Mvs, 2006.

24. Podhajsky, A. *The Complete Training of Horse and Rider.* Chatsworth, CA: Wilshire Book Co., 1965.

25. Edwards, E.H. *Training Aids in Theory and Practice.* Tonbridge: J.A. Allen, 1990.

Index

Note: bold page numbers refer to figures and plates.